TOOTH or IMPLANT?

The **recovery** or **replacement** of the severely compromised natural tooth

TOOTH or IMPLANT?

The **recovery** or **replacement**
of the severely compromised natural tooth

Pio **BERTANI**
Paolo **GENERALI**
Fabio **GORNI**
Tiziano **TESTORI**

With the collaboration of
Renato **COCCONI**

Editor
Massimo **GAGLIANI**

Foreword by
Clifford J. **RUDDLE**

edra
PUBLISHING

Original title
Dente o Impianto? Il recupero o la sostituzione del dente naturale gravemente compromesso

ISBN: 978-88-214-5432-5

Editor: **Paola Sammaritano**, Edra S.p.A.
Project Manager: **Sandra A. Calarota**, Edra S.p.A.
Paper, Printing and Binding Manager: **Paolo Ficicchia**, Edra S.p.A.
Graphic design: **Katja Lupinc**
Cover illustration: **Alessandro Meggio - 3DShift srl, Vicenza**

This edition first published 2024

ISBN: 978-1-957260-52-5
eISBN: 978-1-957260-70-9

edra
PUBLISHING

Edra Publishing US LLC
3309 Northlake Boulevard,
Suite 203, Palm Beach Gardens,
FL, 33403
EIN: 844113980
info@edrapublishing.com
www.edrapublishing.com

Printed in Italy in March 2024 by "Erregiemme printing" S.r.l.

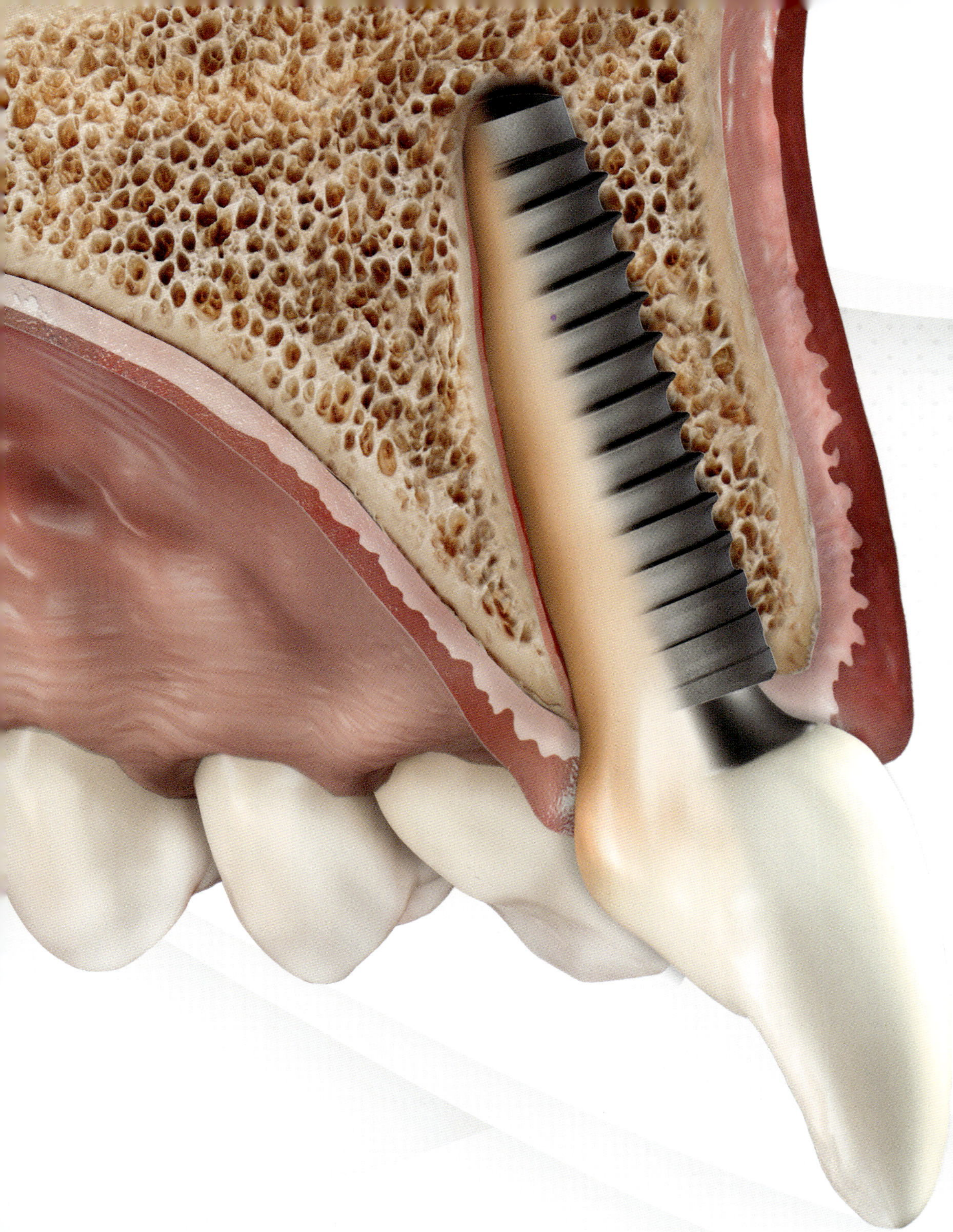

AUTHORS

Pio **Bertani**

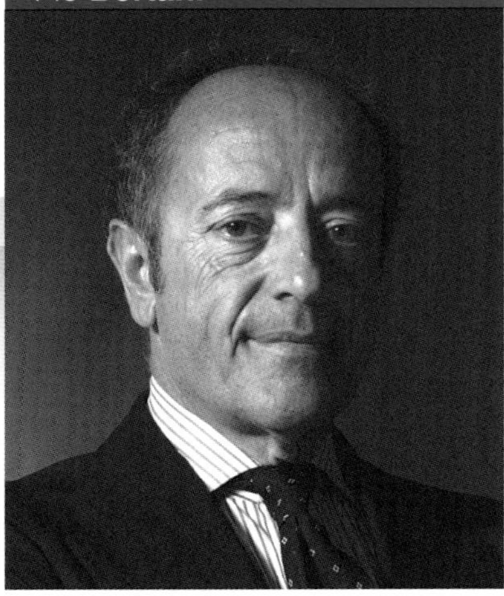

Medical Doctor, Specialist in Odontostomatology. Professor a.c. of Conservative Dentistry at the University of Modena and Reggio Emilia from 2003 to 2008. Professor of the Specialization Course in Conservative Dentistry in 2004-2005 at the University of Modena and Reggio Emilia. Professor of the Advanced Training Course in Prosthesis from 2009 to 2013 at the University of Bologna.
Professor a.c. of Endodontics at the University of Parma. Active member of the Italian Academy of Aesthetic Dentistry. Active member of the Italian Society of Endodontics (SIE), of which he is Past President. Active Member of the European Society of Endodontics. Co-author of the book "Illustrated Manual of Endodontics" (Masson, 2003) and of the "Manual of Endodontics" (Edra, 2013).

Paolo **Generali**

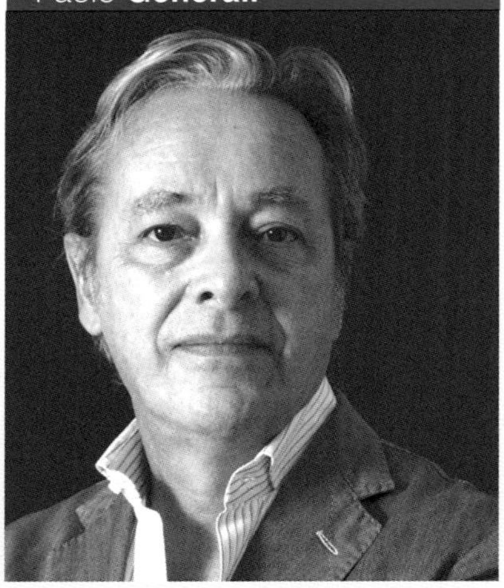

Graduated in Medicine and Surgery with honours and Specialist in Odontostomatology. Effective member of the Amici di Brugg and active member of the Italian Society of Endodontics (SIE).
ANDI member. Author of texts, articles and reports at Congresses in Italy and abroad. Professor of Conservative Dentistry at the CLSOPD, former professor of specialization courses and masters.
Lecturer at the II level Master in Endodontics and Restorative Dentistry at the University of Siena.

Fabio **Gorni**

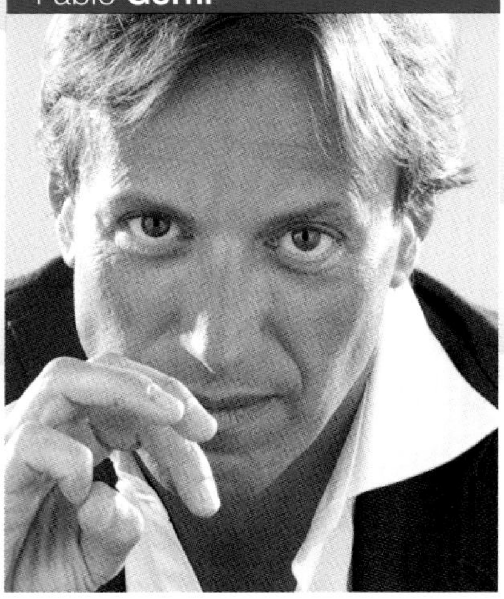

Head of the Micro Endodontic Surgery Course - Dental School - University Vita Salute San Raffaele, Milan. He is the founder of Style Italiano Endodontics. Private practice in Milan, Italy. He graduated from the University of Milan Dental School in 1984. He was visiting Professor for the Department of Endodontics of the S. Paolo Hospital, Milan. From 1994-1998, he was a member of the admission committee of the Italian Society of Endodontics (SIE). From 1998-2001, he was the cultural secretary of the SIE, and President from 2003 to 2005. International lecturer, author of scientific publications in national and international journals and scientific videos. Together with C.J. Ruddle, he has published a video series called "The Endodontic Game", which was distributed in Europe, USA, Canada, Australia, and Asia. He has written chapters for five different endodontics books, and this year author of a new international book on retreatment.

Tiziano **Testori**

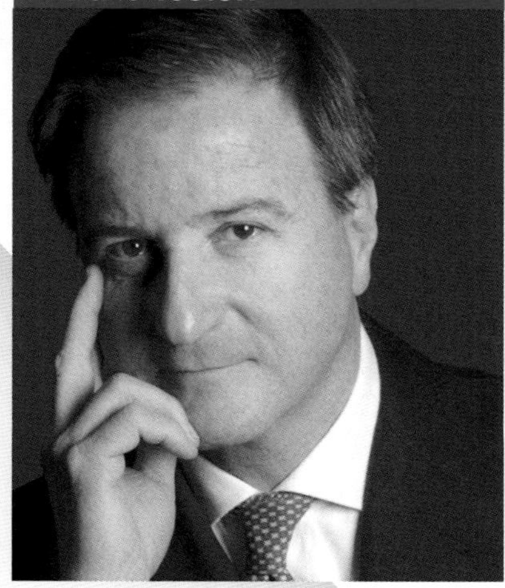

Graduated in Medicine and Surgery in 1981, specialized in Odontostomatology in 1984 and Orthodontics in 1986 at the University of Milan.
Head of the Department of Implantology and Oral Rehabilitation Dental Clinic (Director Prof. Francetti), IRCCS Galeazzi Orthopaedic Institute, University of Milan.
Adjunct Clinical Associate Professor, Department of Periodontics and Oral Medicine, University of Michigan, School of Dentistry. Author of 123 scientific articles indexed on PubMed.

EDITOR

Massimo **Gagliani**

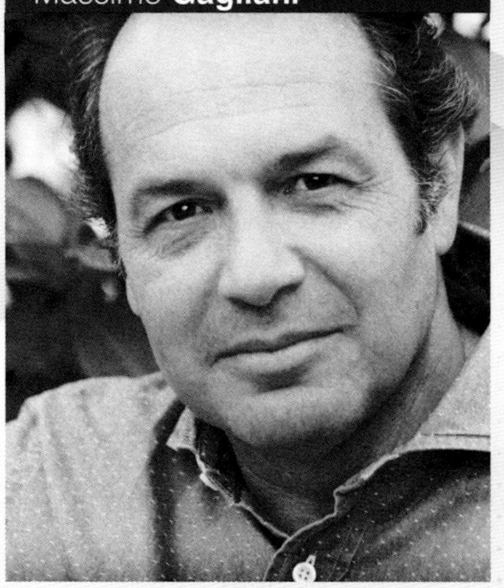

Graduated in Medicine and specialized in Dentistry, with particular focus on Conservative Dentistry and Endodontics, within the Degree Course in Dentistry and Dental Prosthesis of the University of Milan. As an Associate Professor of Odontostomatological Diseases since 2000 at the same University, he practices at the "Giorgio Vogel" Dental Clinic in Milan. He is the author of numerous scientific publications in national and international journals, including the International Endodontic Journal, the Journal of Endodontics and the Italian Journal of Endodontics. He is Editorial Coordinator of the EDRA group for Dentistry, former Editor-in-Chief of the Italian Journal of Endodontics and Founding member of the Digital Dental Academy (www.digitaldentalacademy.it).

CO-AUTHORS

Renato **Cocconi**

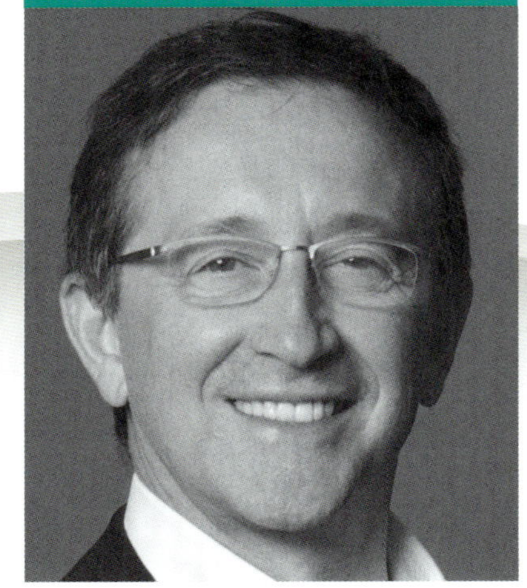

Specialized in Orthodontics at the University of Milan in 1992. During the university period, he underwent a 3-year internship in San Diego, USA, with Dr. L.F. Andrews (father of the Straight Wire technique). Collaborated with Dr. Terry Tanaka, at U.S.C. Centre for Craniomandibular Disorders in Los Angeles, and with Dr. Bill Arnett, at the Centre for Orthognathic Surgery in Santa Barbara (USA). Two-year post-specialization course dedicated to the Straight Wire technique, according to Dr. Roth's philosophy, at the Roth-Williams Centre in Burlingame, California. For over 20 years he has dedicated to orthodontics, with particular focus on innovations related to the treatment of malocclusions for enhancing facial aesthetics. He has an intense teaching activity at the national and international levels. In the last ten years he has been a keynote speaker of the major international orthodontic societies and is a frequent guest of the most prestigious American and European universities. Active member of the Angle Society of Europe and the European Academy of Aesthetic Dentistry (EAED). Founding member and Honorary President of the Face Association (FACExp - Experts in Orthodontics). Member of SIDO (Italian Society of Orthodontics).

Matteo Antonio **Deflorian**

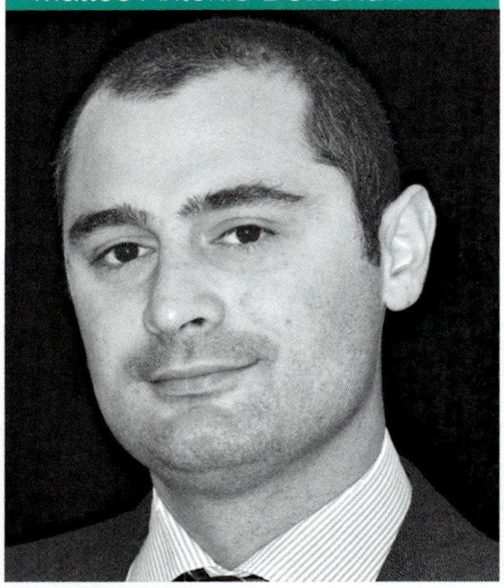

Graduated in Dentistry and Dental Prosthetics at the University of Milan in 2007. Tutor at the Department of Implantology and Oral Rehabilitation (Head Prof. T. Testori), University of Milan, Department of Biomedical Sciences , Surgical and Dental, IRCCS Galeazzi Orthopedic Institute, Odontostomatology Service (Director Prof. L. Francetti). Scientific co-director of "I&J". Active member of the Italian Academy of Osseointegration (IAO).

Fabio **Galli**

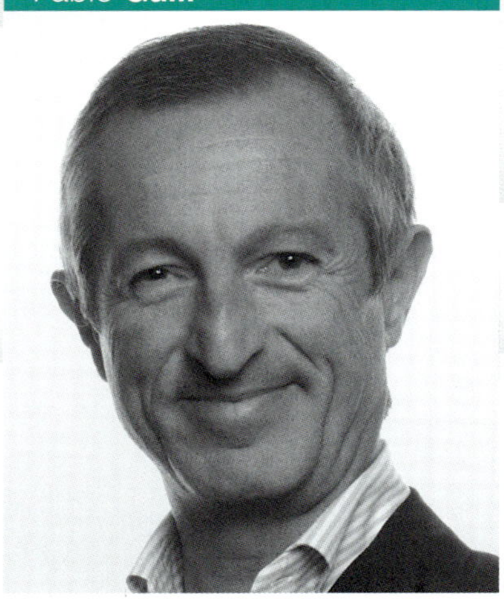

Medical Doctor, Odontostomatologist. Expert in Oral Surgery and Implant Prosthesis at IRCCS, Galeazzi Orthopedic Institute. Head of the Prosthesis Department in the Implantology and Oral Rehabilitation Department (Head Dr. T. Testori) at the University of Milan, Department of Biomedical, Surgical, Dental Sciences, Dental Clinic (Director Prof. L. Francetti). Lecturer in masters and courses in Implantology and Prosthetics at the Universities of Milan, Padua, Genoa, Trieste, and Bologna. Active member of SIO, SICOI, IPA, and IAO (Italian Academy of Osseointegration). Founding member of AISG, SISBO, and SIPRO. Member of the IAO Board of Directors (2017-2018), the IAO Board 2022, the Reading Committee of the Q.I., and the Scientific Committee of "I&J". Speaker at national courses and congresses of ANDI, CAO and scientific societies in the implant-prosthetic field. Author of over 160 publications in national and international journals. Author and co-author of six implant-prosthesis books. Freelancer in Monza.

Pierfrancesco **Zuffetti**

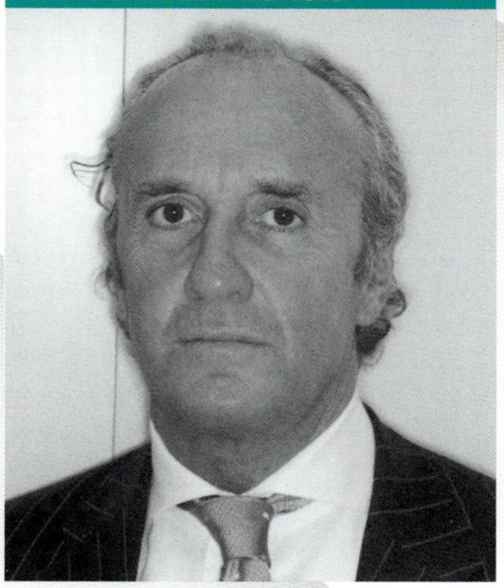

Surgeon, specialist in dentistry at the University of Milan. Lecturer in the Implantology Department of the San Paolo Hospital in Milan from 1995 to2001. Since 2002, Professor at the Department of Implantology and Oral Rehabilitation, University of Milan, Department of Health Technologies, IRCCS Galeazzi Orthopaedic Institute (Director Prof. Luca Francetti). Lecturer in the course in implantology at the University of Milan from 2006 to 2007. Member of Sidp (Italian Society of Periodontology) and SISBO (Italian Society for the Study of Bisphosphonates in Dentistry). Active member of SIE (Italian Society of Endodontics), IAO (Italian Academy of Osseointegration), AO (Academy of Osseointegration), EAO (European Association of Osseointegration), the European Board of Oral Surgery (EFOSS), BBA (Bone Beyond Academy), IPA (International Piezosurgery Academy). Winner of the William R. Laney Award in 2007 for best scientific article in the JOMI magazine. Speaker at national and international courses and conferences in the field of implantology and oral surgery. Author of more than 80 scientific works in national and international journals. He works as a freelancer in Crema and Milan.

Andrea **Pittaluga**

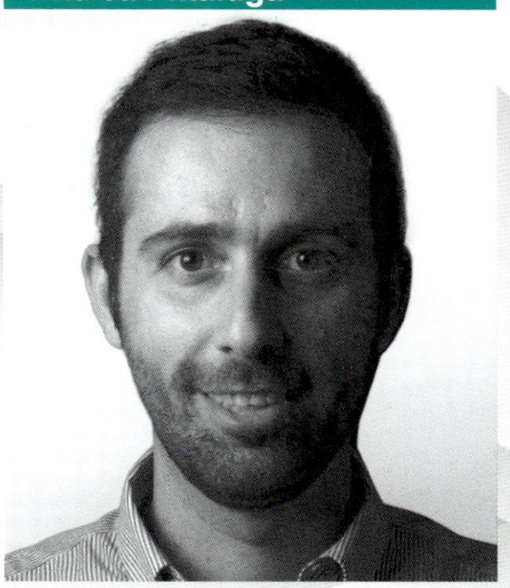

Graduated in 2015 from the Alfonso X El Sabio University of Villanueva de la Canada (Madrid) with the thesis "Anatomical and surgical revision of the maxillary sinus lift". In 2016 he began working in dental offices in Milan and its province and attending post-graduate courses with the best Italian professionals and speakers: Dr. Federico Ferraris, Dr. Stefano Gracis, Prof. Fabio Gorni. From 2017 to 2018, he attended the Oral Surgery Department of the San Raffaele Hospital in Milan directed by Prof. Raffaele Vinci (Rector Prof. E. Gherlone). From 2019, he tutored at the postgraduate courses of orthograde, microscopic and surgical Clinical Endodontics of Prof. Fabio Gorni. Representative of the Dentistry Department of the Auxological Institute of Milan. Speaker in Italy and abroad, as well as "Lecturer" at the Lake Como Institute. He currently privately practices as a microscopic endodontics specialist in the private practice of Dr. M. Imelio, a specialist in conservative, endodontic and prosthetic dentistry in the study of Dr. Prof. Tiziano Testori and in his private practice in Sesto San Giovanni.

Riccardo **Scaini**

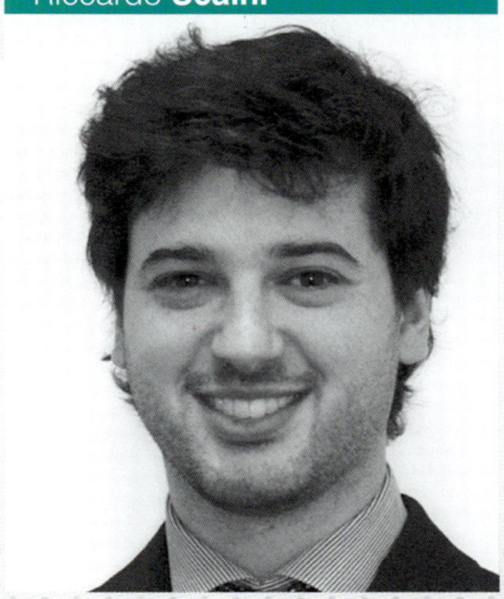

Degree in Dentistry and Dental Prosthetics at the University of Milan, where he obtained the Specialty in Odontostomatological Surgery. Tutor at the Department of Implantology and Oral Rehabilitation (Head Prof. T. Testori), University of Milan, Department of Biomedical, Surgical and Dental Sciences, IRCCS Galeazzi Orthopedic Institute, Odontostomatology Service (Director Prof. L. Francetti). Scientific co-director of "I&J". Active member of the Italian Academy of Osseointegration (IAO).

TABLE OF CONTENTS

FOREWORD

When properly performed, interdisciplinary treatment is the foundation for oral health, function, and esthetics. Predictably successful outcomes may be attributable to advancements in biological and material science, technological innovation, and better trained general dentists and specialists alike. Necessary for this unfolding story is the public's growing expectation that dental treatment can be painless, efficient, and predictably successful. This success story should be expected to massively grow in the years ahead given the fact that the best that dentistry has to offer will be disseminated on all platforms, including the utilization of the immense power of the internet and social media. An educational renaissance will result and serve to accelerate all phases of clinical treatment forward scientifically, clinically, and commercially.

To this end, it is a pleasure and honor for me to write the Foreword for this textbook, "**Tooth or Implant? The recovery or replacement** of the severely compromised natural tooth." The principal authors, Pio Bertani, Paolo Generali, Fabio Gorni, Tiziano Testori, Renato Cocconi and Massimo Gagliani, as well as many other impressive contributors are all recognized experts in this subject matter. This textbook contains seventeen (17) chapters that admirably cover endodontic and periodontal treatment, and implant, restorative, and reconstructive dentistry. Each chapter provides an intriguing glimpse into the imagination and critical thinking utilized by these authors to guide each case toward a successful conclusion. Chapters 1-4 emphasize the critically essential importance of the diagnostic process and how to decide between saving a tooth or placing an implant. Chapters 5-8 eloquently describe and illustrate endodontic treatment of the severely compromised tooth, with emphasis on how to manage various complications. Chapters 9-13 provide a step-by-step description, enhanced by beautifully documented images and high value illustrations, of how to replace a severely compromised tooth with immediate implant replacement. Finally, Chapters 14-17 provide intriguing concepts, useful information, and innovative techniques for replacing hopelessly compromised teeth.

In every instance, the contributors worked diligently despite many other heavy professional responsibilities. All are teachers and authors of considerable note, and many also devote substantial time to clinical practice. They have contributed with enthusiasm and their efforts will undoubtedly inspire generations of dentists as to the value of interdisciplinary treatment. This textbook is well-organized and balances intelligent scholarly text with outstanding clinical visual material. **Tooth or Implant?** is not just another textbook; rather, a call to action to reach the summit of your dental potential ... "Whatever you can do or dream you can, begin it. Boldness has genius, power, and magic in it!" - The Scottish Himalayan Expedition, W. H. Murray.

Clifford J. Ruddle, DDS
Santa Barbara, California USA

INTRODUCTION

Even in advanced cultures, a tooth is often considered a marginal "organ". Its abundance probably makes it less "interesting" than vital organs. Interestingly, we will find out the opposite.

Paradoxically, avoiding the loss of the first tooth can prevent toothlessness (edentulism)!

Furthermore, every single tooth is a biological organ. Although they are part of the oral system, each tooth can individually perceive and participate in its function. This is because each tooth has a direct "connection" to the central nervous system that helps transmit sensations like pain, temperature, pressure, and more,[1] which are then sent to their corresponding representative areas of the brain.[2] However, tooth loss can cause these regions to atrophy.[3] Moreover, the pulp is considered a sensory organ due to its advanced neurosensory structure. Odontoblasts share genetic similarities with sensory cells, including the presence of glial cells that maintain the homeostasis of sensory organs. The capillaries in the central sensory organs resemble those in the blood-brain (haemato-encephalic) barrier. This has even led to the hypothesis that teeth evolved from craniofacial sensory organs that originally served to locate and distinguish food in an ancestral aquatic environment. This hypothesis suggests that these organs then adapted to synthesise the dentinal matrix.[4] Teeth are sensory organs, perhaps best exemplified by the narwhal tusk's thermal, chemical, physical and proprioceptive sensitivity. The trophic and non-trophic functions of teeth are still being explored. The profound biological fascination with the extraordinary environmental, physiological and evolutionary characteristics of teeth has led to a recent congress being named "Biology at the Cusp: Teeth as a Model Phenotype for Integrating Developmental Genomics, Biomechanics, and Ecology".[5] This focused on the studying the dental organ in various animal species. Furthermore, teeth are a permanent biological record of metabolic stresses that may alter mineralisation from birth to adulthood. Therefore, they are considered to play a central role in the theory of the foetal origin of adult diseases[6] (DOHaD, Developmental Origins of Health and Diseases). Burgio defines this as "a potentially unifying pathogenetic model for all emerging chronic disease epidemics like obesity, type 2 diabetes, neurodevelopmental disorders and neurodegenerative pathologies, which necessitate immediate primary prevention strategies to reduce maternal-foetal exposure to the ever-increasing risk factors".[7] Dysmetabolic conditions, like Vitamin D deficiency, can affect developing teeth by forming partially mineralised interglobular dentin. Detecting this dentin in deciduous or permanent teeth helps to determine the time of deficit onset with reasonable accuracy. This information can be useful in bioarchaeology to gain insights into the health status of ancient communities.[8]

In human dentistry, even minor cerebral atrophy can have significant consequences. Extensive or complete tooth loss can have significant consequences, i.e., possibly significant cognitive deficiencies.[9] If these happen in older individuals already suffering from cognitive deficits of other pathological origins, it can cause significant problems. Edentulism is a global phenomenon, with an estimated 500,000 people in 2013[10] not using prosthetic tooth replacements! Scientific studies have confirmed that edentulism is associated with negative neurophysiological conditions, like reduced mental abilities, increased frailty, poor nutritional status and mortality.[11-17] In 2021, Qi et al. conducted a systematic review with meta-analysis and found a dose-dependent association between tooth loss and dementia.[18] This could be reduced by using a prosthetic replacement.

Therefore, it is evident that this has significant implications for the economy, socio-sanitary conditions and community management, with age, pathologies and edentulism all contributing to the issue.

The question arises: how can we solve these problems? The answer is simple - avoid losing the first tooth!

But how can we avoid losing any teeth in the first place? Clearly, prevention in all its aspects should be the starting point.

However, this book explores the different possible therapeutic solutions instead.

Let us divide our efforts into three different phases.

The first phase involves all strategies devised for complex retreatments resulting from previous endodontic failures, like complex anatomy, technical errors, instrument fractures, false pathways and perforations. While an orthograde approach may suffice for some of these problems, surgery is necessary for others. Endodontic surgery *is crucial in extreme cases where preserving natural teeth is still feasible.*

In the second phase, a natural tooth is taken from a different area (transposition) and auto-transplanted into an area of high aesthetic and functional value. This tooth has been "sacrificed" for various reasons, including contra-lateral agenesis, orthodontic extractions, wisdom teeth lacking an antagonist and teeth in osseous inclusion.

The third phase entails using natural teeth portions to support the periodontium and the bone volume, which in turn holds the supporting structures in tooth substitution strategies with implants.

This volume will cover tooth replacement with implants after carefully considering all the previously mentioned solutions in a multidisciplinary approach.

We are often tempted to prioritize our preferences above the patient's expectations. Therefore, it is necessary to be well-balanced and consider all the possibilities, first and foremost, the biological factors, along with patient expectations, their aptitudes and wishes, the practitioner's skills and economic evaluations.

Our goal is to provide readers with a complete evaluation of all options for saving a natural tooth and identifying the best alternatives.

Bibliography

1. Trulsson M, Francis ST, Bowtell R, McGlone F. Brain activations in response to vibrotactile tooth stimulation: a psychophysical and fMRI study. *J Neurophysiol.* 2010;104(4):2257-2265.
2. Chen H, Iinuma M, Onozuka M, Kubo KY. Chewing Maintains Hippocampus-Dependent Cognitive Function. *Int J Med Sci.* 2015;12(6):502-509.
3. Goto T, Kuramoto E, Dhar A, et al. Neurodegeneration of Trigeminal Mesencephalic Neurons by the Tooth Loss Triggers the Progression of Alzheimer's Disease in 3×Tg-AD Model Mice. *J Alzheimers Dis.* 2020;76(4):1443-1459.
4. Farahani RM, Simonian M, Hunter N. Blueprint of an ancestral neurosensory organ revealed in glial networks in human dental pulp. *J Comp Neurol.* 2011;519(16):3306-3326.
5. Fraser GJ, Hulsey CD. Biology at the Cusp: Teeth as a Model Phenotype for Integrating Developmental Genomics, Biomechanics, and Ecology. *Integr Comp Biol.* 2020;60(3):559-562.
6. Barker DJ. The origins of the developmental origins theory. *J Intern Med.* 2007;261(5):412-417.
7. Burgio E. 2015, 2 ottobre. Sanità 24-Sole24ore https://www.sanita24.ilsole24ore.com/art/medicina-e-ricerca/2015-10-02/l-impatto-determinanti-ambientali-cronicita-e-malattie-neurodegenerative-impone-pediatra-salto-qualita-130715.php?uuid=ACM2Kt8, consultato il 12 dicembre 2021.
8. Brickley MB, Kahlon B, D'Ortenzio L. Using teeth as tools: Investigating the mother-infant dyad and developmental origins of health and disease hypothesis using vitamin D deficiency. *Am J Phys Anthropol.* 2020;171(2):342-353.
9. Kato H, Takahashi Y, Iseki C, et al. Tooth Loss-associated Cognitive Impairment in the Elderly: A Community-based Study in Japan. *Intern Med.* 2019;58(10):1411-1416.
10. Ricorso alle cure odontoiatriche e la salute dei denti in Italia. ISTAT 2015. https://www.istat.it/it/files//2015/07/salute_dei_denti_DEFINITIVA.pdf consultato il 12 dicembre 2021.
11. Qi X, Zhu Z, Plassman BL, Wu B. Dose-Response Meta-Analysis on Tooth Loss With the Risk of Cognitive Impairment and Dementia. *J Am Med Dir Assoc.* 2021;22(10):2039-2045.
12. Appollonio I, Carabellese C, Frattola A, Trabucchi M. Influence of dental status on dietary intake and survival in community-dwelling elderly subjects. *Age Ageing.* 1997;26(6):445-456.
13. Appollonio I, Carabellese C, Frattola A, Trabucchi M. Dental status, quality of life, and mortality in an older community population: a multivariate approach. *J Am Geriatr Soc.* 1997;45(11):1315-1323.
14. De Andrade FB, Lebrão ML, Santos JL, da Cruz Teixeira DS, de Oliveira Duarte YA. Relationship between oral health-related quality of life, oral health, socioeconomic, and general health factors in elderly Brazilians. *J Am Geriatr Soc.* 2012;60(9):1755-1760.
15. De Andrade FB, Lebrão ML, Santos JL, Duarte YA. Relationship between oral health and frailty in community-dwelling elderly individuals in Brazil. *J Am Geriatr Soc.* 2013;61(5):809-814.
16. Velázquez-Olmedo LB, Borges-Yáñez SA, Andrade Palos P, García-Peña C, Gutiérrez-Robledo LM, Sánchez-García S. Oral health condition and development of frailty over a 12-month period in community-dwelling older adults. *BMC Oral Health.* 2021;21(1):355.
17. Albani V, Nishio K, Ito T, et al. Associations of poor oral health with frailty and physical functioning in the oldest old: results from two studies in England and Japan. *BMC Geriatr.* 2021;21(1):187.
18. Lopez-Jornet P, Zamora Lavella C, Pons-Fuster Lopez E, Tvarijonaviciute A. Oral Health Status in Older People with Dementia: A Case-Control Study. *J Clin Med.* 2021;10(3):477.

PART I

The diagnostic process of deciding between a tooth and an implant

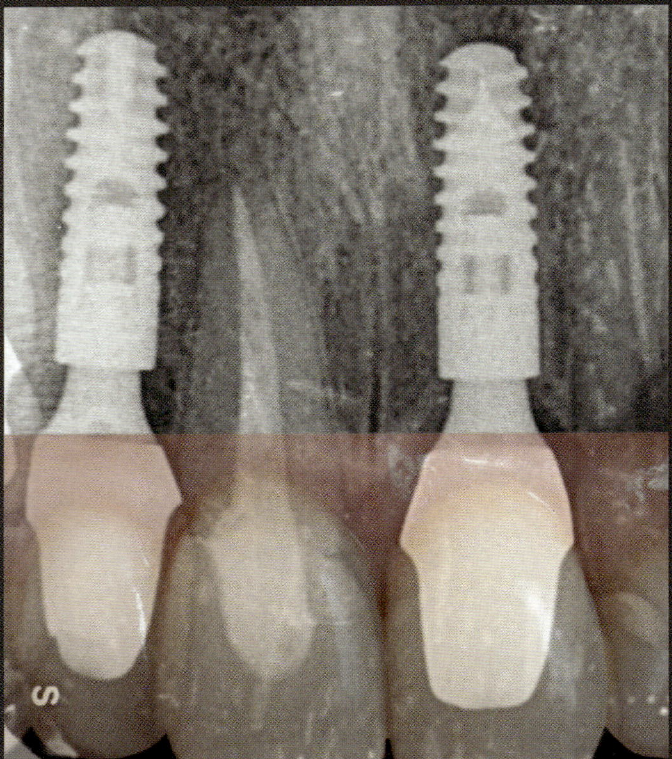

Pio **Bertani**

Paolo **Generali**

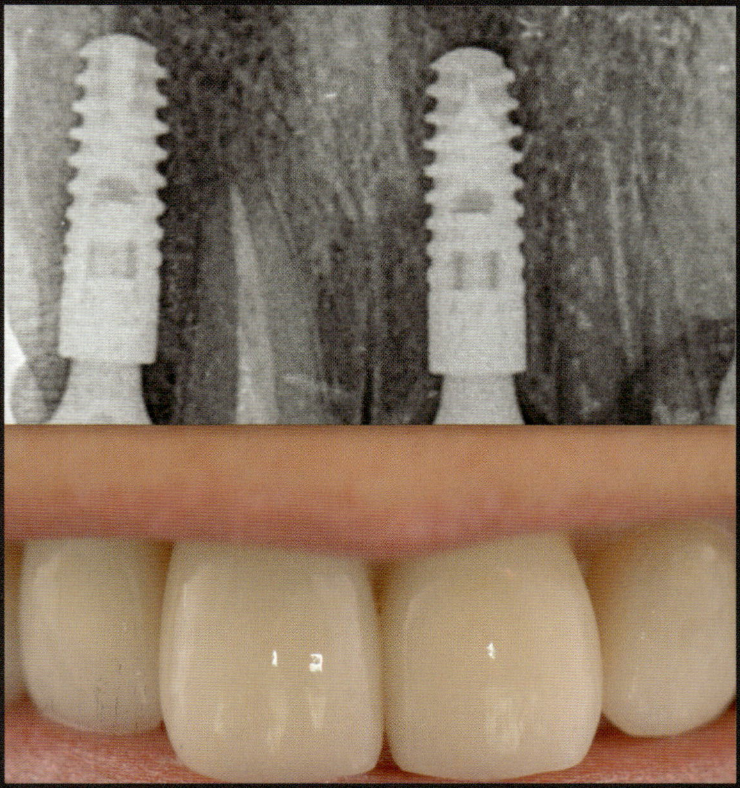

Introduction

The first part of this text covers the decisional process for clinically evaluating a severely compromised single tooth to determine whether it can be saved or extracted and replaced with an implant, which involves multiple phases.
Developing the treatment plan involves multiple phases, which will be elaborated on the subsequent chapters. The proposed therapy must consider three levels of evaluation during development.
Firstly, the patient's general health status, lifestyle, and modifiable risk factors (that may or may not be eliminated) are evaluated. Secondly, the overall oral health condition was evaluated, which included the current bacterial load, the associated damage, the possibility of plaque control, the elimination of factors promoting its accumulation, an examination of the occlusal situation, and a general aesthetic and functional evaluation. Finally, the third level involves diagnosing and examining the possibility of correcting or eliminating each tooth's endodontic, restorative, or periodontal pathology. Therefore, a prognosis is made concerning the survival and possible early or late onset of complications for each tooth, along with evaluating the effect of a successful strategy on these complications and the need for additional treatment to cope with them.
This evaluation process is quite complex and warrants careful consideration, including understanding the patient's motive for seeking dental consultation and a solution.
Once the emergency is resolved, a treatment plan will be established in a sequence that prioritises the elimination of causal factors and address minor emergencies, such as reconstructing a fractured tooth that causes aesthetic problems, or has cutting edges or sharp points (even if it is not painful). Furthermore, extractions of root remnants or unsalvageable teeth should be carried out in this first phase.
In the early stages of treatment planning, instrumental examinations are necessary to finalise the treatment plan. Here, 3D radiology and intraoral scanners are recent innovations that can greatly simplify and speed up the planning process while also providing a realistic pre-visualisation of the achievable results and improving communication with the patient.
When devising a treatment plan, it is important to consider all factors that can impact the outcome. Healthcare providers must offer alternative treatment options and thoroughly discuss all relevant aspects with the patient based on ethical and economic considerations. While it is unnecessary to delve into every technical detail, it is essential to specify timeframes, costs, potential side-effects, and inconveniences associated with each phase, along with the expected outcome.
An evidence-based approach incorporates the literature, clinical experience, and patient-related factors. However, the "patient-centred approach" only focuses on the patient and eventually aims for a shared decision-making process called Shared Decision Making (SDM).
Ultimately, this approach leads to a better clinical decision that prioritises the patient's interest and preferences and benefits the dentist, thus establishing a "therapeutic alliance" that serves as a mutually satisfactory solution for both the patient and the dentist.

1

Treatment planning for severely compromised teeth

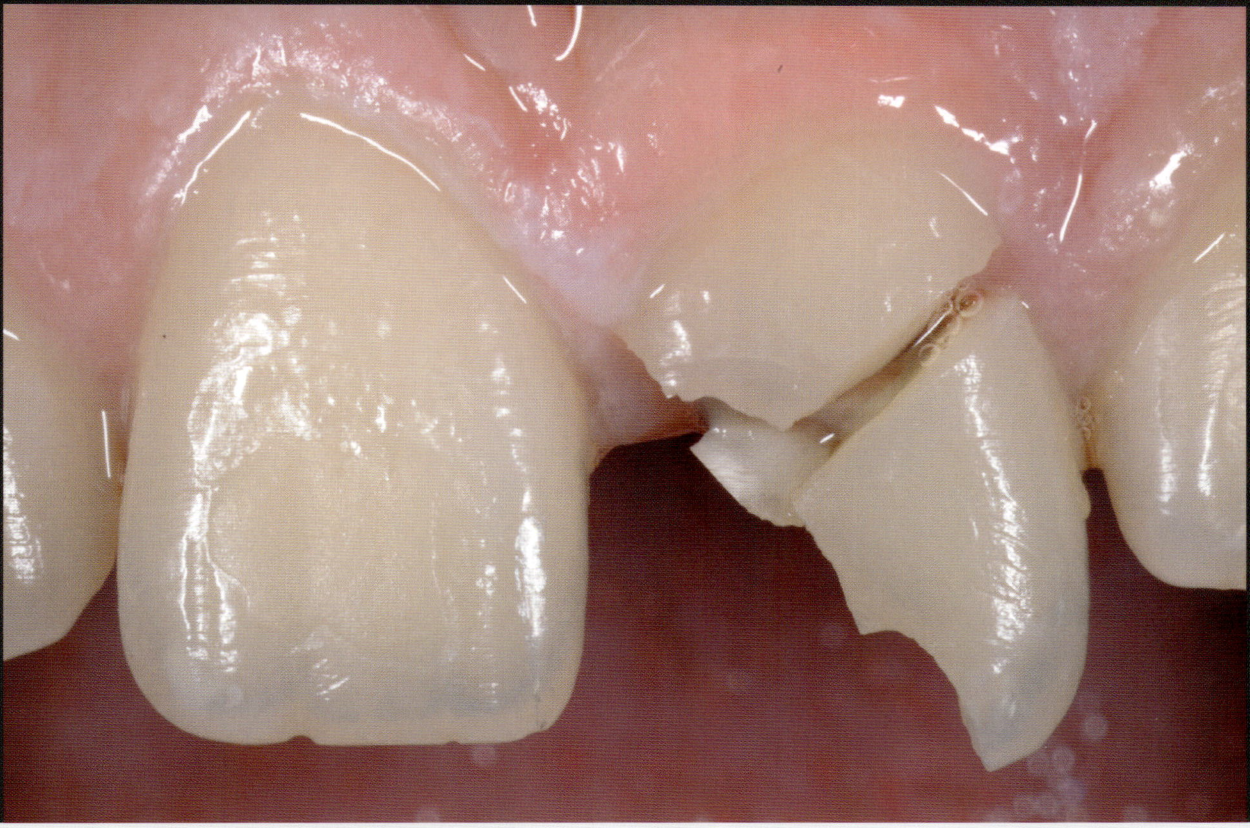

Developing a dental treatment plan is a complex process that begins with identifying the patient's primary concern (which prompted them to seek our dental advice) and following a diagnostic protocol to explain the treatment sequence to resolve their oral health problems, regardless of their awareness. The diagnostic protocol involves a thorough assessment of the patient's overall health status, bad habits, caries susceptibility, oral hygiene standard and bacterial plaque control, periodontal health, orthodontic and occlusal condition, presence of parafunction, non-carious and other lesions affecting the patient's oral cavity Besides these factors, an important aspect of the assessment pertains to the evaluation of the single tooth, including its prognosis, possibility of treatment, and expected outcome.

Anticipating the fate of a single tooth may not be as easy as it seems[1,2] as there are numerous uncontrollable factors to consider, particularly relating to the patient's future and their general oral health and effective regular maintenance therapy. A Norwegian study on over 500 patients[3] found that the ability of healthy teeth surrounded by healthy inflammation-free tissues has a high survival rate. This was evident from the fact that 99.5% of such teeth were still present after 51 years. Conversely, 93.3% of teeth with occasional gingival inflammation survived after 50 years, while only 63.4% of teeth with constant inflammation survived after 47 years.

Therefore, gingival inflammation is a major factor that increases the risk of tooth loss by 46 times. However, various factors, especially domiciliary and professional oral hygiene procedures, can change unpredictably during the patient's life, thus highlighting the importance of managing gingival inflammation for tooth survival. Unfortunately, the current literature lacks clear data regarding restored teeth. Most scientific studies tend to focus on the effectiveness of a particular restoration technique rather than analysing the fate of the tooth itself.[4,5]

Preparation of the treatment plan

When creating a treatment plan for each tooth, it is necessary to classify them as certain, doubtful, and not worth treating,[6] based on endodontic, periodontal, and prosthetic criteria.

A 1978 retrospective study by Hirschfeld and Wasserman[7] on 600 periodontal patients with a 22-year follow-up generated two patient groups: 1) certain prognosis and 2) doubtful prognosis. However, Samet and Jotkowiz[8] proposed a more complex and articulate evaluation in 2009 that categorises teeth into five groups based on prognosis: good (Class A), reasonable (Class B), guarded (Class C), compromised (Class D), and hopeless (Class X). This classification was based on four criteria, namely, periodontal evaluation, restorability, endodontic status, the occlusal relationship and position of the teeth. Furthermore, two extra factors can be added - anatomical anomalies and aggravating iatrogenic factors.

In the past, severely compromised teeth were often extracted and replaced with prosthetics instead of being treated, especially for disadvantaged socio-economic groups. Although this resulted in partial and total edentulism being common among the adult and geriatric populations,[9] the improved living standards, prevention efforts, increased access to treatment, and other factors are reducing its prevalence.[10,11] Therefore, nowadays, the decision to treat a tooth compromised by caries, endodontic, and periodontal problems is not solely based on the location and extent of the issues or their severity. Additionally, the value placed by the dentist and patient on maintaining the affected tooth, the required financial commitment, and various behavioural and socio-economic factors are also crucial in shaping the final clinical decision.[12]

Prognosis of the severely compromised tooth

Tooth damage can result from diverse factors, such as genetic or infective diseases, iatrogenic and traumatic problems, as well as prosthetic failure. However, dental caries, affecting 90% of the world's population,[13] is the most common cause of tooth structural damage, thereby making it the second most prevalent disease after the common cold. Although poor oral hygiene is the primary cause, other possible contributing causes include radiotherapy, chemotherapy, and certain medications that reduce salivary flow. The caries-causing bacteria create an acidic environment that degrades hydroxyapatite, thereby undermining the tooth structure. If left untreated, the disease then adversely affects the pulpal tissue. Despite the dental pulp (a highly differentiated tissue) producing primary, secondary, and tertiary dentine in response to harmful stimuli, which transmit mechanical and thermal stimuli, their ability to regenerate lost dentine is limited. If there is irreversible inflammation or necrosis, endodontic treatment then becomes necessary. This comprises removing the infected or necrotic pulp tissue, shaping and cleaning the endodontic space, and subsequent tooth restoration. Unfortunately, a tooth treated this way loses its vitality, sensitivity, and, consequently, its ability to react to future infections. A carious infiltration could, therefore, spread undetected into the surrounding tissues, thereby causing chronic periradicular lesions. Moreover, the caries-induced primary or recurrent structural damage of the tooth and restorative interface, or a fracture, combined with the necessity of preparing an endodontic access cavity, could further weaken the tooth.

Despite these negative aspects, endodontic treatment has a very good prognosis. This was supported by a study with a 20-27-year follow-up, which reported a long-term success rate of 86.4%.[14] Moreover, after 20-27 years of retreatment, 95.5%[15] roots were found to have a normal radiographic appearance. Studies done on an insurance database have confirmed very high medium to long-term survival[16,17] rates above 90% at ten years for molars treated by endodontic specialists.[18]

Restoration of the severely compromised tooth

A severely compromised tooth is traditionally restored with a full crown. However, endodontically-treated teeth often require direct or indirect crown reconstruction with prefabricated or non-prefabricated metal intracanal retention. Despite the substantial loss of tooth structure and the eventual endodontic treatment due to caries, teeth treated with full crowns have a very good long-term prognosis. A longitudinal study found that crown success rates were high at 5, 10, 20, and 25 years, with 97%, 80%, 70%, and 65%, respectively. However, repair or re-veneering due to decay was required in 12% of the crowns, while 10% of vital teeth needed endodontic treatment.[19] Moreover, a 17-year study[20] has shown a good clinical prognosis for metallic posts. Recent research and interest have shifted towards the possibilities offered by partial coverage indirect restorations luted with adhesive, thus reducing the need for mechanical intracanal retention. Furthermore, fibre-reinforced composite[21] posts are now commonly used, which are less rigid than traditional posts.

Partial adhesive restorations are favourable as they preserve more dental tissue, require less mechanical retention, and eliminate the need for hiding metallic margins. Fibre posts also present advantages, as they are less damaging to the root integrity, and even if they fracture, one can often still save the root, unlike metal posts.[22] However, few *in vivo* studies in the literature examined the long-term performance of posts with a low modulus of elasticity. Ferrari et al.[23] found a good 6-year survival rate, while another study found that after 10 years, failure rates were high, especially for anterior teeth[24]. Although traditional restoration with a cast post and full crown is currently still widely used in clinical practice[25], a recent systematic review recommends metal posts in specific cases.[26] Despite this, a tooth needing endodontic treatment or even retreatment can still be crucial for achieving a complete dentition from both functional and aesthetic perspectives.[27] Finally, precise restoration coupled with effective endodontic treatment has shown a remarkable 97.3% survival rate at 18 years, as per a recent study.[28]

Conclusions

As mentioned earlier, the diagnostic phase is crucial and, therefore, must be carefully performed. It involves evaluating the condition of each tooth and also the risk factors associated with the patient's overall health and lifestyle habits.

To illustrate this, **Figs. 1.1** and **1.2** demonstrate a diagnostic-treatment path that outlines a possible treatment plan and involves the patient in the decision-making process. Therefore, this approach ensures that patients are fully informed about treatment options, allowing them to make informed decisions about their dental care.

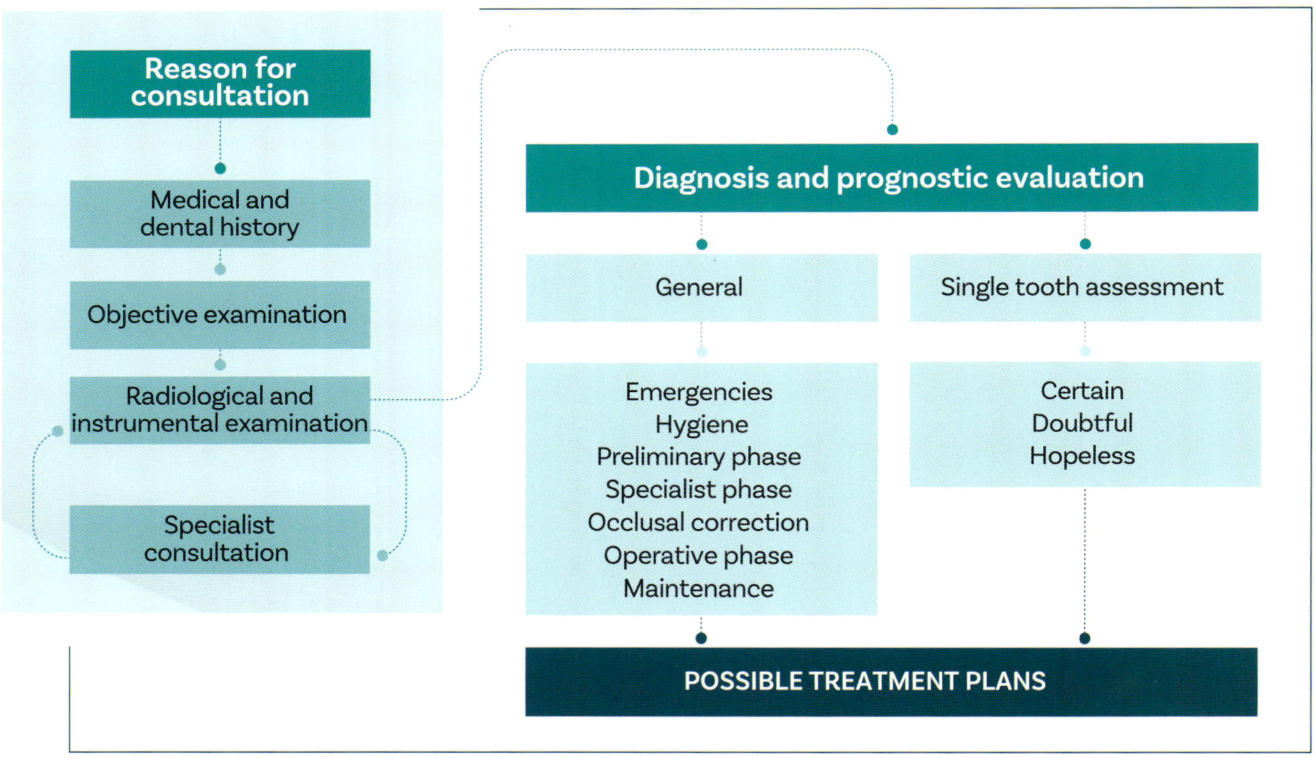

Fig. 1.1 ■ The formulation of a treatment plan involves passing through the various medical and dental diagnostic phases using instrumental and radiological examinations and eventual specialist consultations. This helps in reaching a diagnosis and a prognostic evaluation that will be both general at the level of the organ, and precise at the level of the single tooth which should be classified as certain, doubtful and hopeless. From this evaluation, possible treatment plans are formulated.

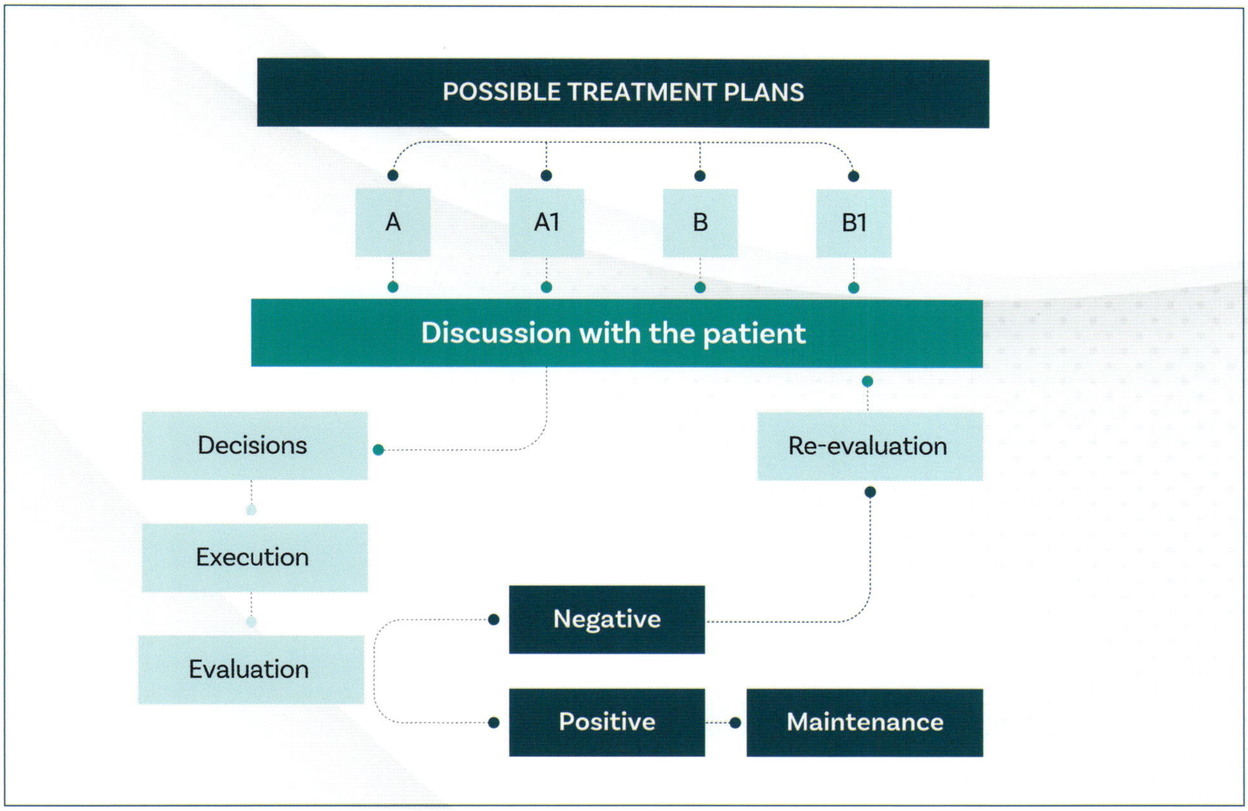

Fig. 1.2 ■ There is almost always more than one possible treatment plan, and each one of these can have different variations. From discussions with the patient, the choice of plan that at that moment best suits the patient will arise. The plan will then be carried out, and the results thereof will be evaluated. If unsatisfactory, a re-evaluation will lead to further phases, after which, following completion, maintenance will start.

Bibliography

1. Mordohai N, Reshad M, Jivraj S, Chee W. Factors that affect individual tooth prognosis and choices in contemporary treatment planning. *Br Dent J.* 2007;202(2):63-72.
2. McGuire MK. Prognosis vs outcome: Predicting tooth survival. *Compend Contin Educ Dent.* 2000;21(3):217-220, 222, 224 passim; quiz 230.
3. Schätzle M, Löe H, Lang NP, Bürgin W, Ånerud Å, Boysen H. The clinical course of chronic periodontitis: IV. Gingival inflammation as a risk factor for tooth mortality. *J Clin Periodontol.* 2004;31(12):1122-1127.
4. Pjetursson BE, Sailer I, Zwahlen M, Hämmerle CH. A systematic review of the survival and complication rates of all-ceramic and metal-ceramic reconstructions after an observation period of at least 3 years. Part I: Single crowns. *Clin Oral Implants Res.* 2007;18(Suppl 3):73-85.
5. Sailer I, Pjetursson BE, Zwahlen M, Hammerle CH. A systematic review of the survival and complication rates of all-ceramic and metal-ceramic reconstructions after an observation period of at least 3 years. Part II: Fixed dental prostheses. *Clin Oral Implants Res.* 2007;18(Suppl 3):86-96.
6. Zitzmann NU, Krastl G, Hecker H, Walter C, Waltimo T, Weiger R. Strategic considerations in treatment planning: deciding when to treat, extract, or replace a questionable tooth. *J Prosthet Dent.* 2010;104(2):80-91.
7. Hirschfeld L, Wasserman B. A long-term survey of tooth loss in 600 treated periodontal patients. *J Periodontol.* 1978;49(5):225-237.
8. Samet N, Jotkowitz A. Classification and prognosis evaluation of individual teeth. A comprehensive approach. *Quintessence Int.* 2009;40(5):377-387.
9. Holm-Pedersen P, Lang NP, Müller F. What are the longevities of teeth and oral implants? *Clin Oral Implants Res.* 2007;18(Suppl 3):15-19.
10. Petersen PE, Yamamoto T. Improving the oral health of older people: the approach of the WHO Global Oral Health Programme. *Community Dent Oral Epidemiol.* 2005;33(2):81-92.
11. Vilstrup L, Holm-Pedersen P, Mortensen EL, Avlund K. Dental status and dental caries in 85-year-old Danes. *Gerodontology.* 2007;24(1):3-13.
12. Joshipura KJ, Ritchie C. Can the relation between tooth loss and chronic disease be explained by socio-economic status? *Eur J Epidemiol.* 2005;20(3):203-204.
13. Islam B, Khan SN, Khan AU. Dental caries: from infection to prevention. *Med Sci Monit.* 2007;13(11):RA196-RA203.
14. Molven O, Halse A, Fristad I, MacDonald-Jankowski D. Periapical changes following root-canal treatment observed 20-27 years postoperatively. *Int Endod J.* 2002;35(9):784-790.
15. Fristad I, Molven O, Halse A. Nonsurgically retreated root filled teeth - radiographic findings after 20-27 years. *Int Endod J.* 2004;37(1):12-18.
16. Salehrabi R, Rotstein I. Endodontic treatment outcomes in a large patient population in the USA: an epidemiological study. *J Endod.* 2004;30(12):846-850.
17. Lazarski MP, Walker WA 3rd, Flores CM, Schindler WG, Hargreaves KM. Epidemiological evaluation of the outcomes of nonsurgical root canal treatment in a large cohort of insured dental patients. *J Endod.* 2001;27(12):791-796.
18. Burry JC, Stover S, Eichmiller F, Bhagavatula P. Outcomes of Primary Endodontic Therapy Provided by Endodontic Specialists Compared with Other Providers. *J Endod.* 2016;42(5):702-705.
19. Valderhaug J, Jokstad A, Ambjrnsen E, Norheim PW. Assessment of the periapical and clinical status of crowned teeth over 25 years. *J Dent.* 1997;25(2):97-105.
20. Fokkinga WA, Kreulen CM, Bronkhorst EM, Creugers NH. Up to 17-year controlled clinical study on post-and-cores and covering crowns. *J Dent.* 2007;35(10):778-786.
21. Dietschi D, Duc O, Krejci I, Sadan A. Biomechanical considerations for the restoration of endodontically treated teeth: a systematic review of the literature, Part II (Evaluation of fatigue behavior, interfaces, and in vivo studies). *Quintessence Int.* 2008;39(2):117-129.
22. Fokkinga WA, Kreulen CM, Vallittu PK, Creugers NH. A structured analysis of in vitro failure loads and failure modes of fiber, metal, and ceramic post-and-core systems. *Int J Prosthodont.* 2004;17(4):476-482.
23. Ferrari M, Vichi A, Fadda GM, et al. A randomized controlled trial of endodontically treated and restored premolars. *J Dent Res.* 2012;91(Suppl 7):72S-78S.
24. Naumann M, Koelpin M, Beuer F, Meyer-Lueckel H. 10-year survival evaluation for glass-fiber-supported post-endodontic restoration: a prospective observational clinical study. *J Endod.* 2012;38(4):432-435.
25. Agrafioti A, Giannakoulas DG, Kournetas N, Grigoriou S, Kontakiotis EG. Different Patterns of Restoration Provision Between Initial Endodontic Treatment and Retreatment: A Retrospective Clinical Study. *Int J Prosthodont.* 2017;30(4):354-356.
26. Sarkis-Onofre R, Fergusson D, Cenci MS, Moher D, Pereira-Cenci T. Performance of Post-retained Single Crowns: A Systematic Review of Related Risk Factors. *J Endod.* 2017;43(2):175-183.
27. Gulabivala K, Ng YL. Value of root-filled teeth in maintaining a functional dentition for life. *Br Dent J.* 2019;226(10):769-784.
28. Pontoriero DIK, Grandini S, Spagnuolo G, et al. Clinical Outcomes of Endodontic Treatments and Restorations with and without Posts Up to 18 Years. *J Clin Med.* 2021;10(5):908.

2

Periodontal, endodontic and reconstructive evaluations

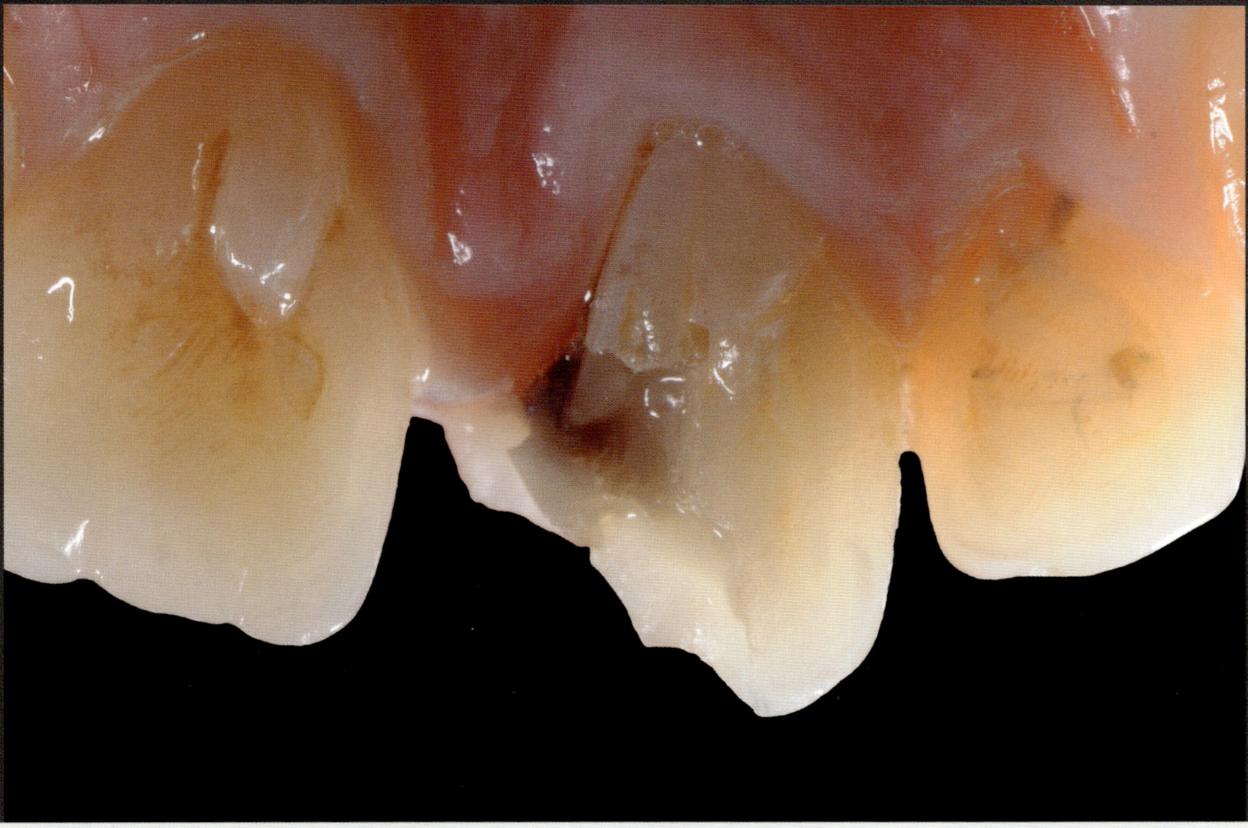

A tooth may be severely compromised due to various reasons, such as loss of periodontal support, persistent periradicular infection (with or without pain), or structural loss from wear, caries or fracture.[1,2] However, before technically addressing these factors, it is necessary to identify and rectify the underlying cause of the severe tooth damage, which may be due to poor plaque control, occlusal parafunction, systemic pathologies or other causes.[3,4]

Periodontal evaluations

From a periodontal point of view, many studies have focused solely on the survival of a treated compromised tooth without considering its role in a treatment plan and its impact on dental function and aesthetics.[5,6] However, in 2018, Martinez-Canut and Llobell found that the prognostic indexes for predicting tooth loss from periodontal disease had relatively low accuracy. The false positive rates ranged from 19.6% to 38% for the "hopeless" prognosis, and for teeth with a "doubtful" prognosis, the possibility of error varied from 37% to 74%. In contrast, the prognosis was more precise for teeth with a good prognosis, with a maximum error of only 2%.[7] This poor accuracy is attributed to insufficient consideration of patient-related factors, although a systemic literature review identified only smoking and old age as risk factors.[8] Recently, new algorithms have been developed to quantitatively define periodontal prognosis, with a systemic literature review[9] identifying five different models for evaluating periodontal risk:

- DEPPA, DenPlan Excel/Previsor® Patient Assessment[10]
- HIDEP, Health Improvement in Dental Practice[11]
- RABIT, Risk Assessment Based Individualised Treatment[12]
- DRS, Dentition Risk System[13]
- PRA, Periodontal Risk Assessment[14]

Among these, the Periodontal Risk Assessment and its varying modifications have been validated globally and can determine the best frequency for maintenance sessions in various patient groups. However, these algorithms do not help us evaluate the prognosis of a single tooth.

To address this, the recent classification of periodontal pathologies[15] aims to link diagnosis, prevention, and treatment by introducing five diagnostic categories. The possible diagnoses include 1) periodontal health, 2) gingivitis, 3) effectively treated periodontitis (reduced but healthy periodontium), 4) gingivitis in a periodontal patient (persistent inflammation after periodontal treatment), 5) periodontitis, 6) periodontitis as a manifestation of systemic disease, 7) necrotizing periodontitis. Once a diagnosis is made, the staging and grading phases follow, which determine the disease's severity and its risk of progression, respectively.

The staging phase can be divided into four levels:

- I: Initial stage of attachment loss: <15% bone loss, 1-2 mm attachment loss.
- II: Periodontitis with bone loss of 15–33% and 3-4 mm attachment loss.
- III: Significant periodontal damage with bone loss up to the middle third of the root or beyond, attachment loss of 5 mm or more, up to 4 teeth lost due to periodontitis and at least 10 pairs of teeth in occlusion without occlusal collapse, migration, flaring or severe crestal defects.
- IV: Loss of masticatory function due to periodontitis, with over 4 teeth lost, less than 10 pairs of teeth in occlusion having occlusal collapse, migration, flaring or severe crestal defects.

The grading phase is divided into three levels:

- Slow disease progression
- Normal disease progression
- High risk of disease progression.

This recent classification emphasizes the need for new decisional algorithms, like Sanz and Tonetti's proposed algorithm in 2019.[16] However, the evaluation focuses on the patient and the disease as a whole without addressing the single tooth affected by periodontal disease.

To overcome this limitation, Martinez-Canut and Llobell[7] proposed a predictive model in 2018 to improve periodontal prognosis by analysing the survival probability of the single tooth based on 11 criteria. Among them, five were patient-related factors (disease severity, smoking, bruxism, low tooth count, and age), and six were tooth-related (type of tooth, probing depth, bone loss, and presence of furcation lesions that can be probed, mobility and crown-root ratio). The model is available at http://www.perio-project.com. It has been retrospectively tested and shows a strong correlation between its predictions and actual tooth loss of periodontally compromised teeth. Paradoxically, the study found that tooth loss cases were less common when large amounts of plaque and calculus were removed as compared to those with fewer risks at the time of diagnosis. To date, the model proposed by the aforementioned website seems to be the most efficient in predicting the survival of a periodontally involved tooth by quantifying it in the number of years of survival before its probable loss.

Endodontic evaluations

Numerous scientific studies have analysed factors that impact prognostic evaluation of endodontically treated teeth, including pre-, intra-, and post-operative factors that can affect the endodontic treatment outcome by preventing or favouring the resolution of a periradicular lesion.[17] From a general point of view, Gulabivala and Ng[18] have argued that an endodontically treated or retreated tooth can be a valid long-term component of the masticatory apparatus due to its extremely high success and survival rates. Although the survival and success rates are high, it is challenging to predict which tooth is at risk of extraction or has the safest prognosis. The factors affecting successful endodontic treatment outcomes at the single tooth level are diverse, ranging from biological situations that influence the relation between host and pathogen to the appropriate treatment variables.

The development and the healing probability of an endodontic lesion[19,20] may be influenced by the patient's systemic pathologies, particularly diabetes mellitus and hypertension, which negatively impact the survival of endodontically-treated teeth.[21] Periapical lesion presence and size are among the most commonly cited prognostic factors, as confirmed by 50 years of endodontic literature.[22,23] Moreover, a large lesion suggests a prolonged infection in the endodontic space, where a well-organized biofilm may establish itself and become difficult to eradicate.[24] Additionally, the biofilm may spread beyond the canals lumen, causing an infection that is untreatable by an orthograde endodontic treatment.[25] However, this does not mean that large lesions cannot be healed with adequate endodontic therapy.

The technical feasibility of an efficient endodontic treatment is another vital prognostic factor. Efficiently shaping and irrigating the endodontic space depends on the instruments' ability to approach the apical constriction. In teeth with periapical pathology, every unshaped millimetre of the canal reduces the possibility of healing by 12–14%.[26] Incomplete canal shaping may be tied to technical errors committed during the initial phases of the treatment or unsurmountable obstacles like perforations in the apical third, instrument fragments, ledges or more. Prognostic endodontic criteria evaluation, as shown in **Table 2.1**, allows us to classify the tooth into different categories. The presence of one or more findings, as in columns C or D, suggests that we should favour retreatment or extraction, while columns A or B suggest treatment with an adequate follow-up plan.

Table 2.1 ■ Endodontic evaluations.

	A	B	C	D
Pain	Absent	Absent	Occasional	Persistent
Function	Optimal	Optimal	Not perfect	Not possible
Aesthetics	Satisfactory	Not satisfactory	Not satisfactory	Irreparable
Tissue loss	Minimal	Moderate	Severe	Severe or very severe
Periapical radio-translucency	Absent or reduced	< than twice the periodontal space	< than twice the periodontal space	> than twice the periodontal space
Canal obturation: extension	Coinciding with the apex	Within 2 mm	Within 2 mm	Over 2 mm from apex
Canal obturation: extrusion	None	None	Present	
Canal obturation: density	Uniform and high	Uniform and high	Scarce	Scarce
Respect for morphology	Yes	Slightly altered	Severely altered	Severely altered
Necessity for intracanal retention	No	Yes	Yes	Yes
Coronal seal	Yes	Yes	Doubtful	Doubtful

Reconstructive evaluations

Evaluating a severely compromised tooth presents some challenges in terms of its structural or reconstructive evaluation. The first problem is represented by the intrinsic imperfection of evaluating a previously restored and possibly root-canaled tooth. The presence of caries, fractures and infiltrations is often difficult to define during the diagnostic phase and treatment planning. Despite using modern inspection methods such as visual inspection, probing and radiographic examinations, the presence of a restoration can hinder their efficiency. Radiopaque restorations can obstruct visualization of neighbouring dental structures, which may lead to underestimating possible lesions. Even digital radiography is not free from overestimation errors, which may be due to the frequent artefacts. The dental radiography software integrates image processing systems to "enhance" the image quality by removing empty pixels and highlighting or hiding specific parts of the image. During this, the digital enhancement can occur without the operator's prior knowledge, who must then activate less intuitively accessible options to view the original image. The various software producers for visualizing and archiving dental radiology integrate their own algorithms to enhance definition, reduce background "noise", enlarge, colour, measure angles and lengths, and evaluate density. Furthermore, these filters may sometimes create images that simulate the presence of caries or marginal leakage at the interface between tooth structures and restoration. Therefore, it is crucial to critically evaluate digital radiological images and ntegrate them with the irreplaceable objective examination to avoid diagnostic errors.[27] Thus, retrieving the unfiltered original radiographic image could greatly help[28] here.

When evaluating a severely compromised tooth, the instrumental, radiographic and objective examinations may be subject to misinterpretation in the presence of extended restorations. In 2004, Abbott compared evaluations performed during the diagnostic phase to those after removal of restorations in 245 endodontically treated and then successively restored teeth. Initially, 19.2% of teeth had carious lesions, which increased to 86.1% post-restoration removal. Similarly, fractures increased from 23.3% to 60%, while marginal leakage rose from 39.2% to 99.6%.[29] Therefore, during the initial phase of treatment planning, it is crucial for the clinician to revaluate and revise the prognosis after removing the previous restorations. Any objective diagnostic difficulties should be shared with the patient while discussing the treatment plan and collecting their informed consent, along with providing alternative solutions.

Despite these difficulties, it is necessary to evaluate the quantity, quality and location of any residual dentine and enamel to determine if sufficient structural integrity is present for the expected restoration. This evaluation is crucial for guaranteeing stability and peripheral seal, which determine the necessary conditions to resist occlusal loading, which echoes back to our previously covered aspects. Additionally, the quality of the restoration and the coronal seal, like the biological width's effect on periodontal health, influence the prognosis of an endodontic treatment.

In a reconstructive evaluation, the amount of healthy residual dental tissue is a crucial factor in determining the prognosis of endodontically treated teeth.[30] According to a recent systematic literature review on the reconstruction of endodontically treated teeth, a residual dental volume of < 30% of the original tooth increases the risk of failure. Moreover, other unfavourable prognostic factors include having only one residual wall, lacking a contact point, and being in the terminal position in the dentition.[31]

Besides the quantity, the location of the residual dental tissue also affects the prognosis. In a near-ideal occlusal situation, the posterior and anterior teeth experience axial and transversal forces, respectively. Furthermore, a healthy palatal dentine is essential for providing the tooth-restoration complex with adequate occlusal loading resistance.[32] In 2005, The presence and the number of dentinal walls were studied in 2005 by McDonald and Setchell, who proposed a Tooth Restorability Index (TRI) to measure tooth restorability based on the presence and number of dentinal walls. This index assesses six parts of the tooth (two interproximal, two buccal and two lingual or palatal parts) on a scale from 0 to 3, with 0, 1, 2, and 3 corresponding to an absent wall, inadequate amount, doubtful amount and an adequate amount. A TRI score of 12 indicates a reliable tooth, scores between 9 and 12 indicate a doubtful tooth, while a score below 9 indicates that the tooth is inadequate for restoration, even with a fibre post.[33]

In 2017, Dawood and Patel[34] proposed "The Dental Practicality Index" to evaluate all the restorative aspects of dentition in its local and general context. A matrix assigns scores to the structural, periodontal, endodontic and general evaluations, with 0 for unnecessary treatment cases, 1 for simple treatment cases, 2 for complex treatment cases, and 6 for severe cases with "impractical" or contraindicated treatment. Several studies have validated the Dental Practicality Index's effectiveness in predicting the outcome of endodontically involved teeth[35] and from the point of view of the residual dentine quantity.[36]

An aspect that has been widely discussed in scientific literature is the need for an adequate amount of healthy dentine at the cervical level to generate the ferrule effect. From Sorensen and Engelman's studies in 1990[37] to the most recent data,[38] *in vitro* research has established a unanimous consensus that the ferrule effect is associated with a higher resistance of the tooth-restoration complex. The ferrule effect is defined as a "360° metal crown collar surrounding parallel dentine walls and extending coronally to the shoulder of the preparation". On the other hand, *in vivo* studies have produced more controversial results, which can be attributed to various confounding factors, with the presence or absence of a post being predominant. A meta-analysis of the *in vitro* and *in vivo* studies on the ferrule effect concludes that it is clinically noticeable only in premolars *in vivo* and not at all in molars.[39] A randomized controlled study on 360 teeth demonstrated that endodontically treated and successively restored premolars had a significantly better prognosis when at least one healthy dentine wall was present, while the presence or absence of the ferrule effect did not seem to affect the restoration's survival probability.[40] However, recently revised literature concludes that the ferrule effect is extremely important for the good prognosis of restored teeth.[41]

Conclusions

Many attempts have been made to objectively quantify a tooth's prognosis based on its compromised structural, endodontic, and periodontal states, as well as its functional requisites. In this regard, the authors of this book intend to present their own method of evaluating the tooth's prognosis (**Tables 2.2a,b**), which involves assigning numerical scores to the different degrees of compromise and finally classifying the tooth as certain, doubtful or untreatable (**Fig. 2.1**).

Tables 2.2a,b ■ Evaluation system proposed by the authors of this text. The periodontal, restorative, endodontic and functional aspects are evaluated separately for their most significant features.

a	PERIODONTAL	RESTORATIVE	ENDODONTIC	FUNCTIONAL
A	No bleeding on probing Probing <3 mm	2 marginal crests 4 valid walls	Tooth untreated endodontically	Normal, 2 adjacent teeth
B	Occasional bleeding on probing Probing <3 mm	1 marginal crest 2 valid walls	Retreatment with intact roots	1 adjacent tooth
C	Occasional bleeding on probing Probing <5 mm Grade II furcation	No marginal crests 1-2 valid walls	Retreatment with root alterations	No adjacent teeth
D	Bleeding on probing Probing >5 mm Grade III furcation	<2 mm of supragingival dental structure	Long-term endodontic lesion	Parafunction
E	Conditions mentioned above + abscess	Absence of supragingival dental structure	Untreatable endodontic abscess	Severe parafunction

b	PERIODONTAL	RESTORATIVE	ENDODONTIC	FUNCTIONAL
A	1	1	1	1
B	2	2	2	2
C	4	4	4	4
D	8	8	8	8
E	16	16	16	16

4-8	8-32	32-64
CERTAIN	DOUBTFUL	UNTREATABLE

Fig. 2.1 ■ The sum of all points allows us to classify the tooth as certain, doubtful and untreatable.

Treatment of a corono-radicular fracture complicated by pulp exposure

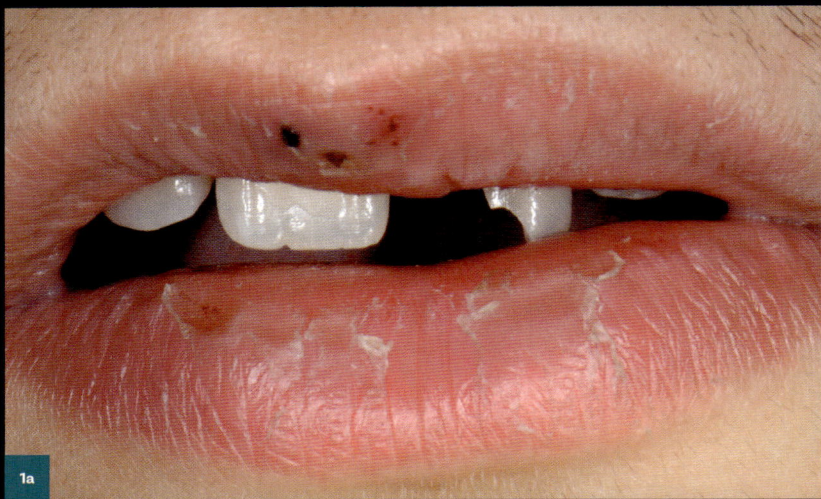

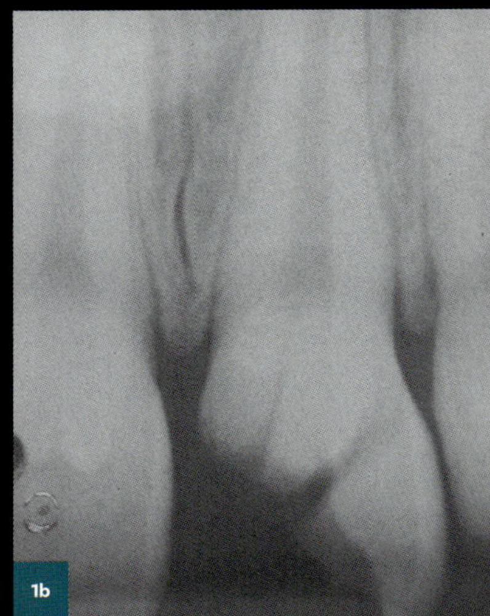

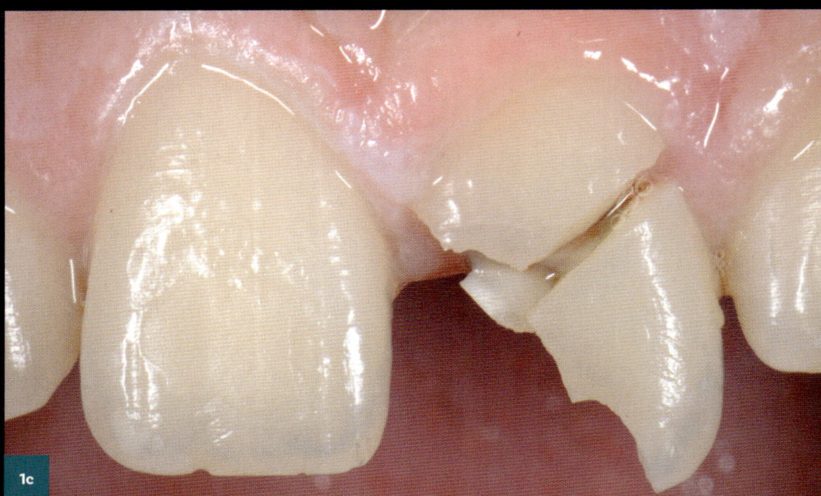

Fig. 1a ■ Following a motorcycle accident, patient C.L. (14 years of age) presents a deep and complex corono-radicular fracture of the upper left central incisor.

Fig. 1b ■ Rx that shows the root integrity.

Fig. 1c ■ Deep fracture line that involves a portion of the root.

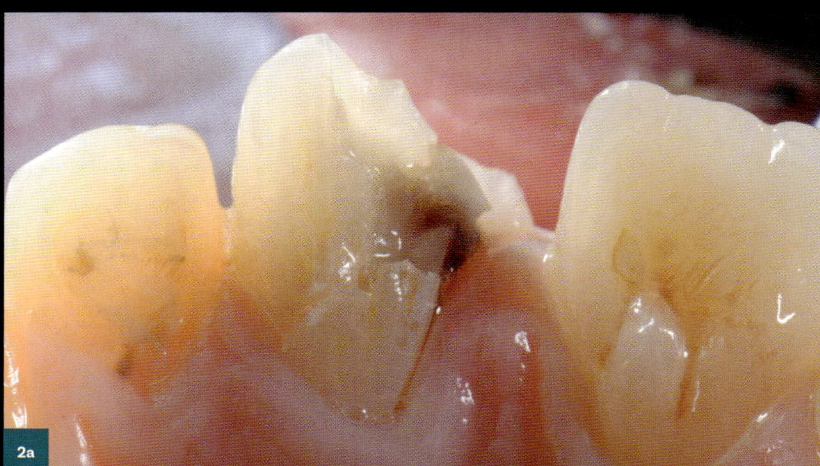

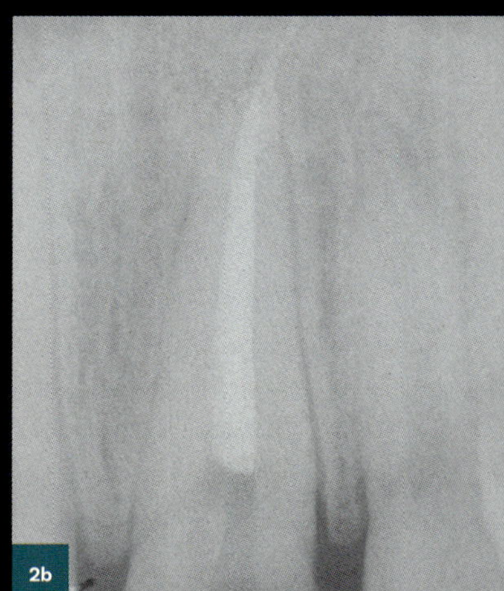

Fig. 2a ■ Palatal view that shows the fracture depth and pulp involvement.

Fig. 2b ■ The Rx shows the essential endodontic treatment.

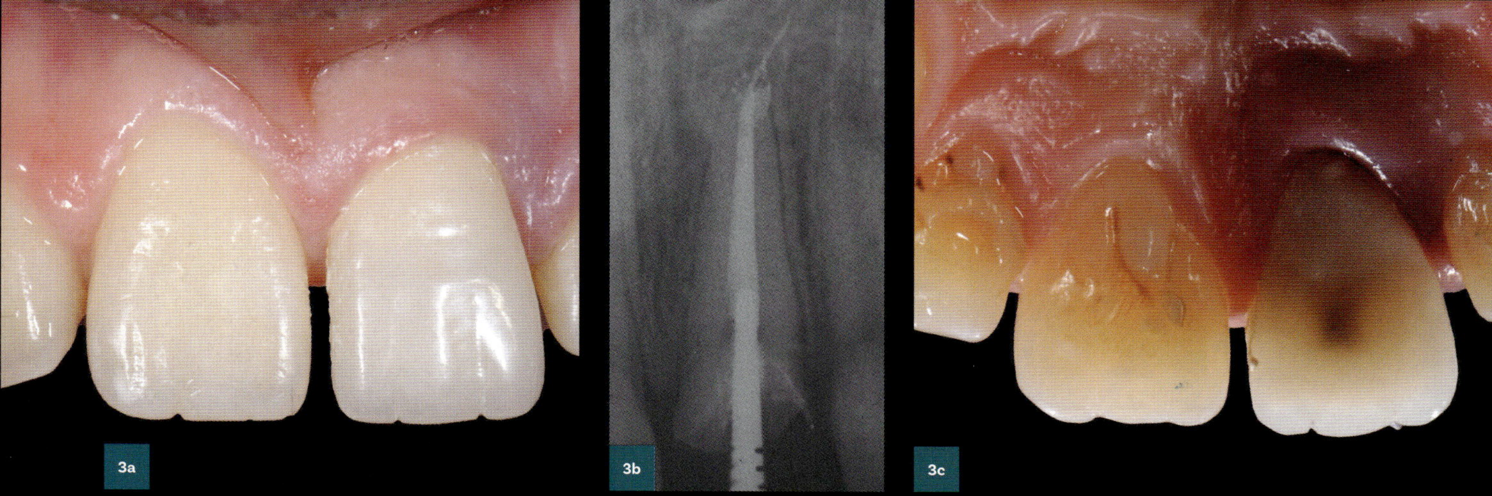

Fig. 3a ■ A temporary crown is placed to quickly resolve any aesthetic issues.

Fig. 3b ■ Rx with post in place for the temporary crown.

Fig. 3c ■ Palatal view which highlights the gingival inflammation caused by the deep fracture line.

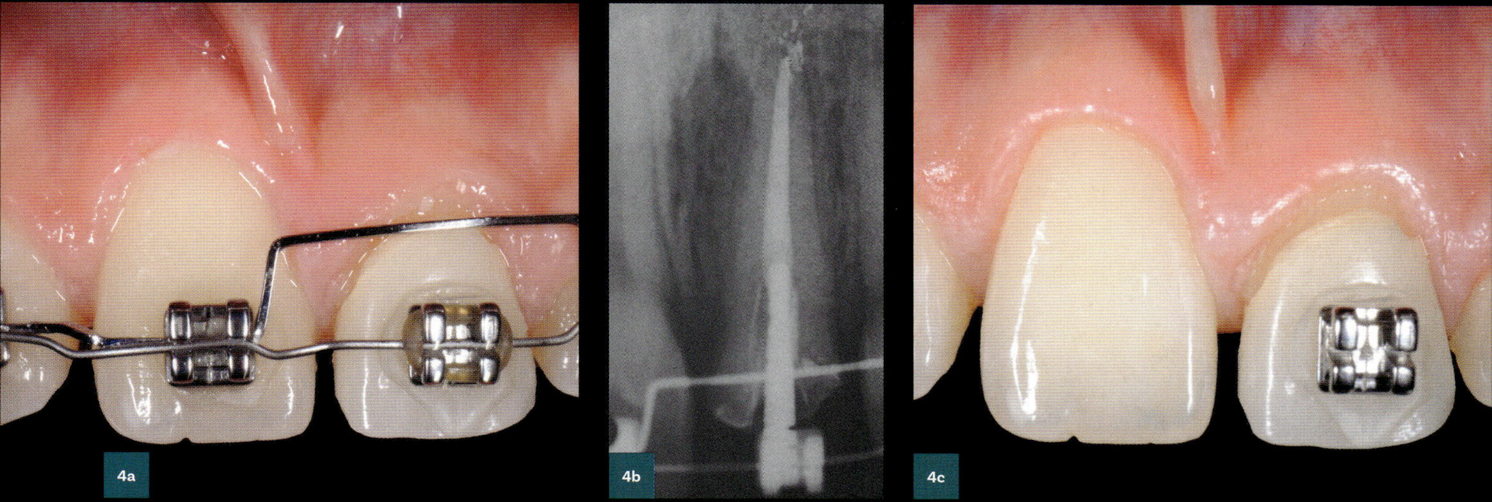

Fig. 4a ■ Considering the patient's young age it is decided to orthodontically extrude the root to have the correct biological width and restore it correctly. **4a**: orthodontic device.

> *CONT'D*

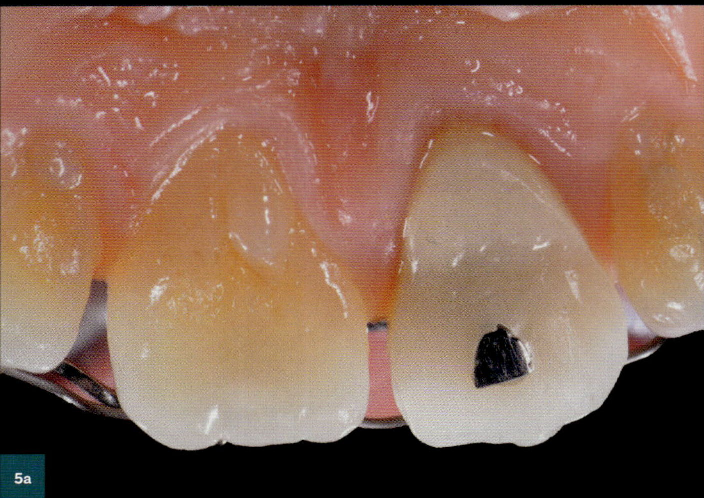

5a

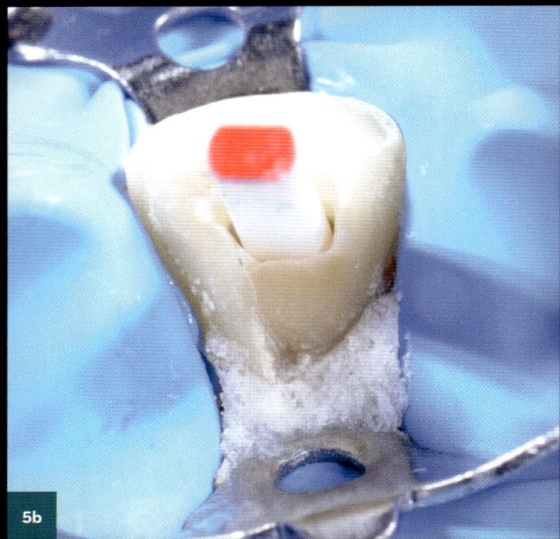

5b

Fig. 5a ■ Post-exposure after the temporary crown's progressive occlusal reduction demonstrates how much the root has been extruded and the ensuing resolution of the periodontal inflammation.

Fig. 5b ■ Since a good amount of dentine is now present, a direct restoration is decided.

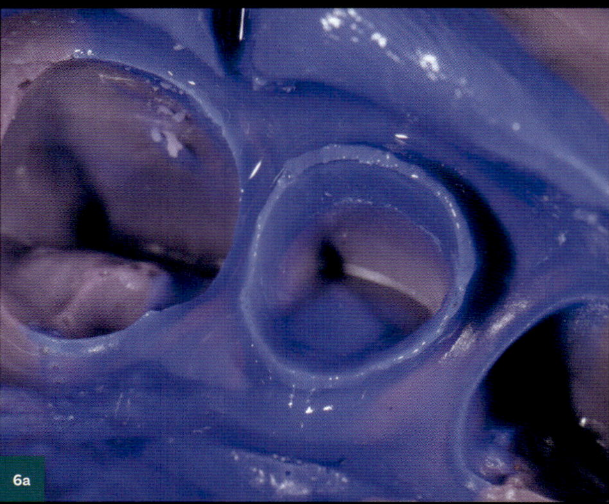

6a

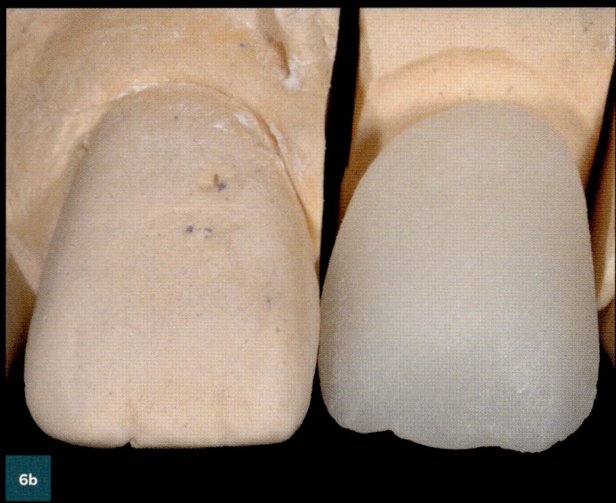

6b

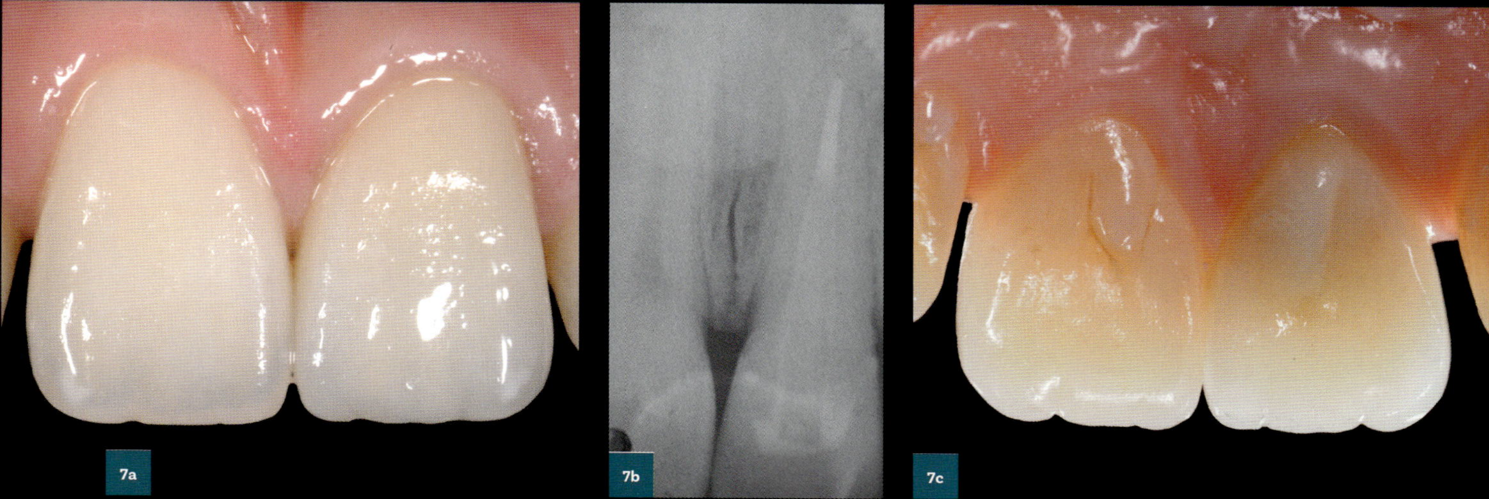

Fig. 7a ■ Buccal view of the final restoration. Aesthetics and periodontal health are restored.

Fig. 7b ■ Final radiographic check-up.

Fig. 7c ■ Palatal view of the naturalness of the restoration.

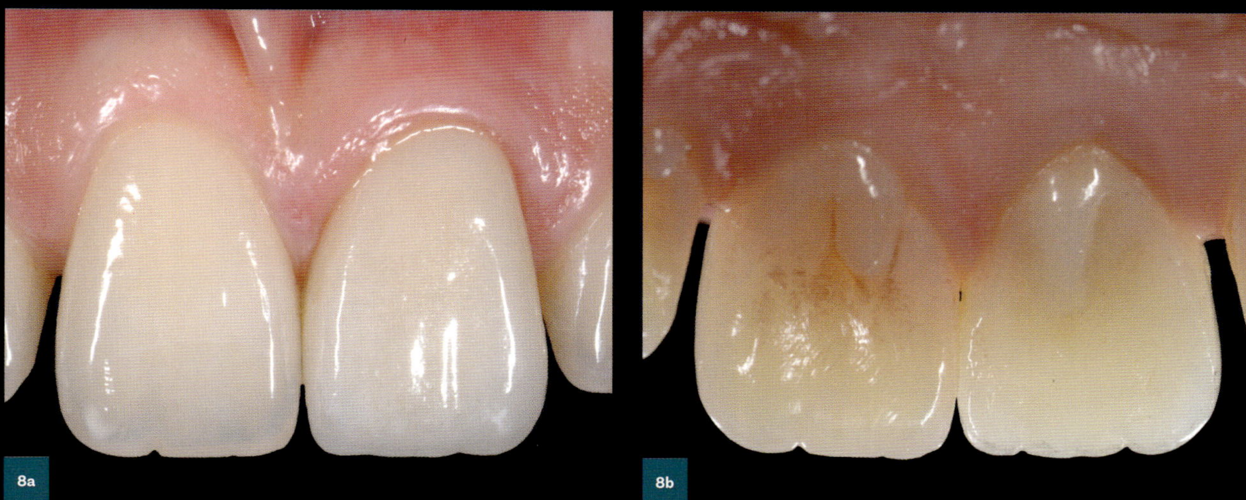

Figs. 8a,b ■ Buccal and palatal check-up at 9 years.

Bibliography

1. Caplan DJ, Weintraub JA. Factors related to loss of root canal filled teeth. *J Public Health Dent.* 1997;57(1):31-39.
2. Olcay K, Ataoglu H, Belli S. Evaluation of Related Factors in the Failure of Endodontically Treated Teeth: A Cross-sectional Study. *J Endod.* 2018;44(1):38-45.
3. Aquilino SA, Caplan DJ. Relationship between crown placement and the survival of endodontically treated teeth. *J Prosthet Dent.* 2002;87(3):256-263.
4. Skupien JA, Opdam N, Winnen R, et al. A practice-based study on the survival of restored endodontically treated teeth. *J Endod.* 2013;39(11):1335-1340.
5. Kwok V, Caton JG. Commentary: Prognosis revisited: A system for assigning periodontal prognosis. *J Periodontol.* 2007;78(11):2063-2071.
6. Tonetti MS, Steffen P, Müeller-Campanile V, Suvan J, Lang NP. Initial extractions and tooth loss during supportive care in a periodontal population seeking comprehensive care. *J Clin Periodontol.* 2000;27(11):824-831.
7. Martinez Canut P, Llobell A. A comprehensive approach to assigning periodontal prognosis. *J Clin Periodontol.* 2018;45(4):431-439.
8. Chambrone L, Chambrone D, Lima LA, Chambrone LA. Predictors of tooth loss during long-term periodontal maintenance: a systematic review of observational studies. *J Clin Periodontol.* 2010;37(7):675-684.
9. Lang NP, Suvan JE, Tonetti MS. Risk factors assessment tools for the prevention of periodontitis progression a systematic review. *J Clin Periodontol.* 2015;42(Suppl 16):S59-S70.
10. Page RC, Krall EA, Martin J, Mancl L, Garcia RI. Validity and accuracy of a risk calculator in predicting periodontal disease. *J Am Dent Assoc.* 2002;133(5):569-576.
11. Fors UG, Sandberg HC. Computer-aided risk management - a software tool for the Hidep model. *Quintessence Int.* 2001;32(4):309-320.
12. Teich ST. Risk Assessment-Based Individualized Treatment (RABIT): a comprehensive approach to dental patient recall. *J Dent Educ.* 2013;77(4):448-457.
13. Lindskog S, Blomlöf J, Persson, et al. Validation of an algorithm for chronic periodontitis risk assessment and prognostication: risk predictors, explanatory values, measures of quality, and clinical use. *J Periodontol.* 2010;81(4):584-593.
14. Lang NP, Tonetti MS. Periodontal risk assessment (PRA) for patients in supportive periodontal therapy (SPT). *Oral Health Prev Dent.* 2003;1(1):7-16.
15. Caton JG, Armitage G, Berglundh T, et al. A new classification scheme for periodontal and peri-implant diseases and conditions. Introduction and key changes from the 1999 classification. *J Periodontol.* 2018;89(Suppl 1):S1-S8.
16. Tonetti MS, Sanz M. Implementation of the new classification of periodontal diseases: decision-making algorithms for clinical practice and education. *J Clin Periodontol.* 2019;46(4):398-405.
17. Joe Editorial Board. Success and failure in endodontics: an online study guide. *J Endod.* 2008;34(5 Suppl):e1-e6.
18. Gulabivala K, Ng YL. Value of root-filled teeth in maintaining a functional dentition for life. *Br Dent J.* 2019;226(10):769-784.
19. Segura-Egea JJ, Martin-Gonzalez J, Castellanos-Cosano L. Endodontic medicine: connections between apical periodontitis and systemic diseases. *Int Endod J.* 2015;48(10):933-951.
20. Svetlozarova S. Association between systemic diseases and endodontic treatment outcome- review of literature. *Adv Dent & Oral Health.* 2019;11(5):148-152.
21. Mindiola MJ, Mickel AK, Sami C, Jones JJ, Lalumandier JA, Nelson SS. Endodontic treatment in an American Indian population: A 10-year retrospective study. *J Endod.* 2006;32(9):828-832.
22. Strindberg LZ. The dependence of the results of pulp therapy on certain factors: an analytic study based on radiographic and clinical follow-up examinations. *Acta Odontol Scand.* 1956;14(21):1-175.
23. Ng YL, Mann V, Gulabivala K. A prospective study of the factors affecting outcomes of nonsurgical root canal treatment: part 1: periapical health. *Int Endod J.* 2011;44(7):583-609.
24. Ricucci D, Siqueira JF Jr. Biofilms and apical periodontitis: study of prevalence and association with clinical and histopathologic findings. *J Endod.* 2010;36(8):1277-1288.
25. Tronstad L, Barnett F, Riso K, Slots J. Extraradicular endodontic infections. *Endod Dent Traumatol.* 1987;3(2):86-90.
26. Chugal NM, Clive JM, Spångberg LS. Endodontic infection: some biologic and treatment factors associated with outcome. *Oral Surg Oral Med Oral Pathol Oral Radiol Endod.* 2003;96(1):81-90.
27. Clark JL, Wadhwani CP, Abramovitch K, Rice DD, Kattadiyil MT. Effect of image sharpening on radiographic image quality. *J Prosthet Dent.* 2018;120(6):927-933.
28. Brettle D, Carmichael F. The impact of digital image processing artefacts mimicking pathological features associated with restorations. *Br Dent J.* 2011;211(4);167-170.
29. Abbott P. Assessing restored teeth with pulp and periapical diseases for the presence of cracks, caries and marginal breakdown. *Austr Dent J.* 2004;49(1):33-45.
30. Dietschi D, Duc O, Krejci I, Sadan A. Biomechanical considerations for the restoration of endodontically treated teeth: A systematic review of the literature - Part 1. Composition and micro- and macrostructure alterations. *Quintessence Int.* 2007;38(9):733-743.
31. Bhuva B, Giovarruscio M, Rahim M, Bitter K, Mannocci F. The restoration of root filled teeth: a review of the clinical literature. *Int Endod J.* 2021;54(4):509-535.
32. Ng CC, Dumbrigue HB, Al-Bayat MI, Griggs JA, Wakefield CW. Influence of remaining coronal tooth structure location on the fracture resistance of restored endodontically treated anterior teeth. *J Prosthet Dent.* 2006;95(4):290-296.
33. McDonald A, Setchell D. Developing a tooth restorability index. *Dent Update.* 2005;32(6):343-344, 346-348.
34. Dawood A, Patel S. The Dental Practicality Index - assessing the restorability of teeth. *Br Dent J.* 2017;222(10):755-758.
35. Tifooni A, Al-Nuaimi N, Dawood A, Mannocci F, Patel S. Validation of the effectiveness of the Dental Practicality Index in predicting the outcome of root canal retreatments. *Int Endod J.* 2019;52(10):1403-1409.
36. Al-Nuaimi N, Ciapryna S, Chia M, Patel S, Mannocci F. A prospective study on the effect of coronal tooth structure loss on the 4-year clinical survival of root canal retreated teeth, and retrospective validation of the Dental Practicality Index. *Int Endod J.* 2020;53(8):1040-1049.
37. Sorensen JA, Engelman MJ. Ferrule design and fracture resistance of endodontically treated teeth. *J Prosthet Dent.* 1990;63(5):529-536.
38. Tribst JPM, Dal Piva AMO, de Jager N, Borges ALS, Bottino MA. Full-Crown Versus Endocrown Approach: A 3D-Analysis of Both Restorations and the Effect of Ferrule and Restoration Material. *J Prosthodont.* 2021;30(4):335-344.
39. Skupien JA, Luz MS, Pereira-Cenci T. Ferrule Effect: A Meta-analysis. *JDR Clin Trans Res.* 2016;1(1):31-39.
40. Ferrari M, Vichi A, Fadda GM, Cagidiaco MC, Tay FR, Breschi L. A randomized controlled trial of endodontically treated and restored premolars. *J Dent Res.* 2012;91(7 Suppl):72S-78S.
41. Juloski J, Radovic I, Goracci C, Vulicevic ZR, Ferrari M. Ferrule effect: a literature review. *J Endod.* 2012;38(1):11-19.

3

Patient and operator dependent variables

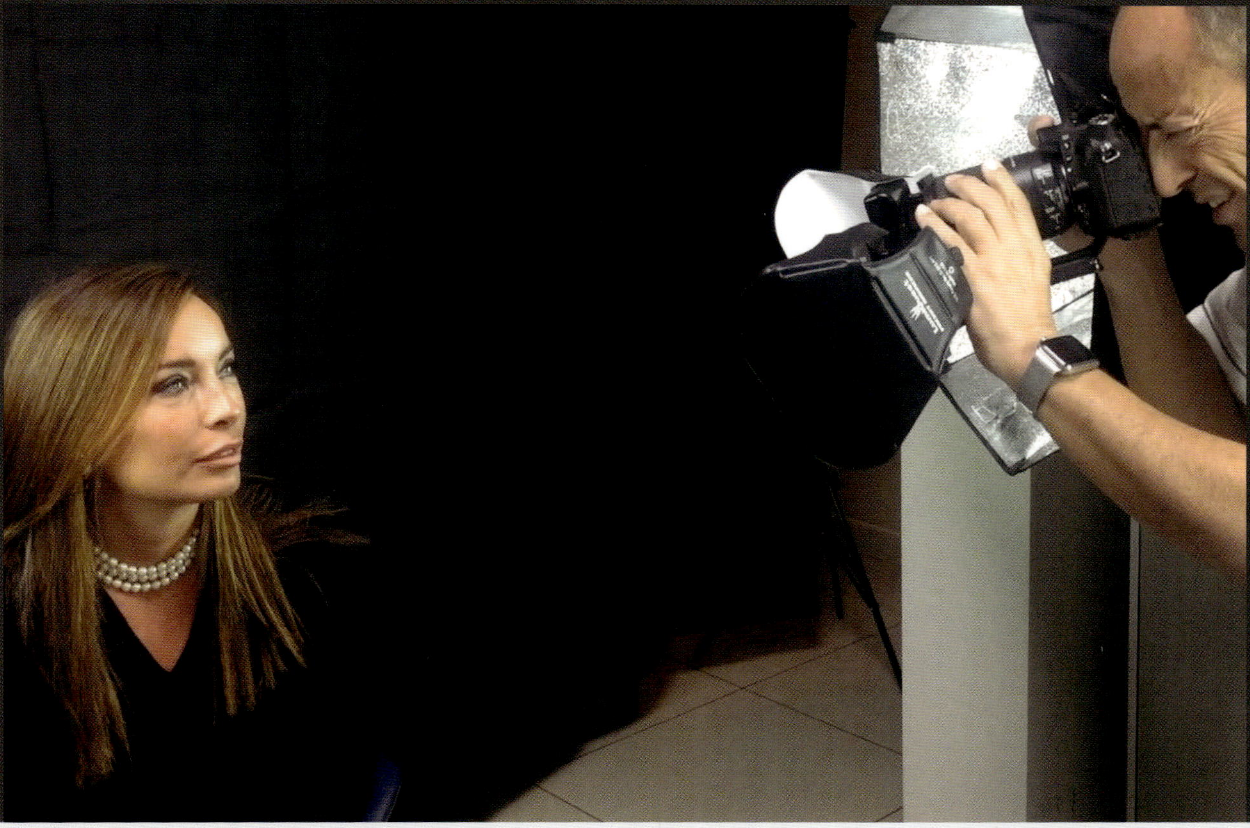

The choice of decision between treating or extracting a severely compromised tooth depends on more than just its condition. It is obvious that one's general health condition and lifestyle can influence the decision. For instance, systemic disease, smoking or previous therapy could contraindicate surgical intervention, thereby necessitating a more conservative treatment. Additionally, it is important to adequately consider the patient's attitude towards dental treatment, including past experiences (positive or negative) with conservative or implantology treatment, as it could considerably impact the final decision. Previous experience may not directly consider the patient but rather a discussion with related people, with the increasing cultural and ethnic diversity of patients possibly creating difficulties in communication and mutual understanding. Therefore, the common objective of the dentist and patient should be to choose the most appropriate treatment, re-establish the oral health condition, and establish a maintenance programme that can help avoid new treatment. Thus, to ensure successful treatment and maintenance, it is necessary to understand and respect the patient's attitude towards dental care to avoid being too forceful in the short term, which could lead to patient distancing in the long-term successive phases.

Compared to the past, patients nowadays have more access to vast amounts of potentially misleading information than ever before, which has caused them to question themselves and us, thereby leading to increased autonomy in their decision-making ability. As a result, the dentist must provide precise and current information about available therapies to help patients choose the most effective solution for their specific case and long-term prognosis. We are dealing with the evolution of dentistry from a standardized, one-size-fits-all approach to a more personalized, tailor-made approach.

One should not dismiss the possibility of adopting an ultraconservative approach, as it canreduce oral and extraoral pathogens through an adequate domiciliary and professional oral hygiene regime, the application of a reversible occlusal device or silver diamine fluoride, or even the implementation of an anti-smoking programme. Dentistry's remarkable and rapid progress has led to the development of innovative techniques for achieving previously unimaginable results. Adopting this attitude over time enables one to overcome distrust and scepticism that may disrupt the dentist-patient relationship over time.

Fear and anxiety associated with dental treatment can significantly impact the patient's perception and, consequently, their decisions. Negative experiences, whether personal or transmitted, could contribute to an apparently persistent negative attitude towards dental care,[1] which could lead to a vicious circle where the patient, frightened of treatment, avoids and delays it, thereby aggravating the clinical situation and ends with them needing a more complex and bothersome dental treatment.[2] Therefore, the medical history taken should include an evaluation of their anxiety and fear level. For some particularly sensitive patients, even the time in the waiting room, with the noise of the rotary instruments, typical dental surgery odours,[3] or the sight of instruments, in particular needles, can be traumatic.[4]

When it comes to treatment alternatives, patient attitudes play a significant role. In 2020, Wigsten et al.[5] compared the impact of endodontic treatment and extraction on the patient and found that endodontics made a better impact. Usually, extraction is considered a sign of functional senescence,[6] implying negative general health consequences,[7] which causes negative psychological[8] implications that have been associated with an increased risk of dementia.[9] Therefore, patients generally prefer conservative treatments, such as endodontic treatment, for teeth affected by apical periodontitis.[10] This tendency is confirmed in the experimental studies. In 2017, Re et al.[11] used a questionnaire that focused on the volition of patients to undergo treatment to restore a compromised tooth when compared to having an extraction and an implant. They found that 76% of patients preferred restorative treatment involving endodontic treatment or re-treatment, pre-prosthetic reconstruction, clinical crown lengthening and crown placement,[11] over having a compromised tooth extracted and replaced with an implant.

Similarly, even dentists tend to favour root canal treatment over-extraction for teeth affected with apical periodontitis. Furthermore, this tendency is more prevalent among young dentists and specialist endodontists, while those with 25 years of experience and general dentists prefer extraction more.

When considering evidence-based literature, Torabinejad et al.[13] published a systematic literature review in 2007 comparing treatment options for a severely compromised single tooth, including endodontics and restoration to a single implant and crown, to a fixed prosthesis and to extraction without replacement. The study showed higher longevity for the endodontic reconstructive treatment or implant compared to a fixed prosthesis, with not replacing a lost tooth possibly leading to a negative psycho-social outcome. In 2015, Walton[14] compared a 15-year outcome of single crowns on implants and fixed bridges of three units and found crowns on implants performing better, with statistically results for the anterior dentition. However, the decision to extract or treat periodontally compromised teeth is even more problematic. Although randomized clinical studies showed that regenerative treatment is effective even in severe periodontal impairment.[15] However, in reality, it seems that teeth with a 50-70% attachment loss are commonly extracted.[16] This is likely due to the fact that the patient's adherence to a precise domiciliary and professional oral hygiene protocol is crucial for a good long-term periodontal treatment outcome. In the absence of compliance and adequate maintenance, the treatment will fail,[17] and therefore, the currently available effective regenerative techniques would not be recommended. Conversely, with maintenance care following active periodontal treatment, the long-term survival of the teeth, even teeth affected by advanced periodontal disease, can have a very satisfactory long-term survival.[18] It is worth noting that the level of the operator's periodontal competence would seem to influence the final decision over the treatment plan, with lower-trained dentists[19,20] more likely to opt for extraction.

In conclusion, the patient plays a vital role in the development of the treatment plan for the severely compromised tooth, and their involvement is necessary for identifying the best solution for them by cooperating with the professional (**Fig. 3.1**).

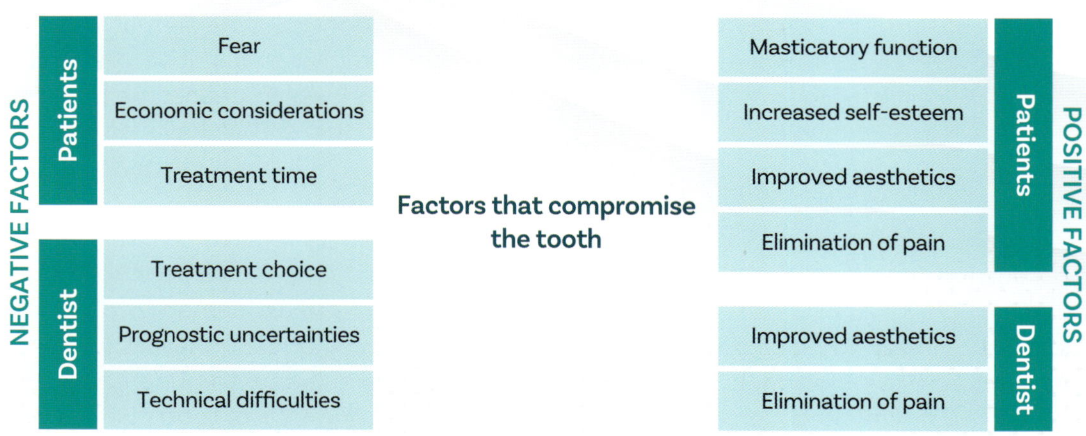

Fig. 3.1 ■ Negative factors (*left*) and positive factors (*right*) that condition the choices made by the dentist and patient.

In this process, the dentist's role is to instruct and advise patients, considering the various factors that influence the choices, including age, gender, socio-economic status, lifestyle, oral hygiene standard, attitude towards dental treatment and maintenance care, motivation, expectations and responsibility for their own health.[21] Therefore, to achieve the best outcome, it's important to prioritize the patient's lifestyle improvement and discontinuation of bad habits[21] before or alongside dental treatment.

Bibliography

1. de Jongh A, Muris P, Horst G, Duyx MP. Acquisition and maintenance of dental anxiety: the role of conditioning experiences and cognitive factors. *Behav Res Ther.* 1995;33(2):205-210.
2. Armfield JM, Stewart JF, Spencer AJ. The vicious cycle of dental fear: exploring the interplay between oral health, service utilization, and dental fear. *BMC Oral Health.* 2007;7:1.
3. Robin O, Alaoui-Ismaili O, Dittmar A, Vernet-Maury E. Basic emotions evoked by eugenol odor differ according to the dental experience. A neurovegetative analysis. *Chem Senses.* 1999;24(3):327-335.
4. Johnson B, Mayberry WE, McGlynn FD. Exploratory factor analysis of a sixty-item questionnaire concerned with fear of dental treatment. *J Behav Ther Exp Psychiatry.* 1990;21(3):199-203.
5. Wigsten E, Kvist T, Jonasson P, et al. Comparing quality of life of patients undergoing root canal treatment or tooth extraction. *J Endod.* 2020;46(1):19-28.
6. Osterberg T, Carlsson GE, Sundh V, Steen B. Number of teeth - a predictor of mortality in the elderly? A population study in three Nordic localities. *Acta Odontol Scand.* 2007;65(6):335-340.
7. Sheiham A, Steele JG, Marcenes W, et al. The relationship among dental status, nutrient intake, and nutritional status in older people. *J Dent Res.* 2001;80(2):408-413.
8. Eckerbom M, Magnusson T, Martinsson T. Reasons for and incidence of tooth mortality in a Swedish population. *Dent Traumatol.* 1992;8(6):230-234.
9. Stein PS, Desrosiers M, Donegan SJ, Yepes JF, Kryscio RJ. Tooth loss, dementia and neuropathology in the Nun study. *J Am Dent Assoc.* 2007;138(10):1314-1322.
10. Azarpazhooh A, Dao T, Figueiredo R, Krahn M, Friedman S. A survey of patients' preferences for the treatment of teeth with apical periodontitis. *J Endod.* 2013;39(12):1534-1541.
11. Re D, Ceci C, Cerutti F, Fabbro MD, Corbella S, Taschieri S. Natural tooth preservation versus extraction and implant placement: patient preferences and analysis of the willingness to pay. *Br Dent J.* 2017;222(6):467-471.
12. Lee J, Kang S, Jung HI, Kim S, Karabucak B, Kim E. Dentists' clinical decision-making about teeth with apical periodontitis using a variable-controlled survey model in South Korea. *BMC Oral Health.* 2020;20(1):23.
13. Torabinejad M, Anderson P, Bader J, et al. Outcomes of root canal treatment and restoration, implant-supported single crowns, fixed partial dentures, and extraction without replacement: a systematic review. *J Prosthet Dent.* 2007;98(4):285-311.
14. Walton TR. An up-to-15-year comparison of the survival and complication burden of three-Unit tooth-supported fixed dental prostheses and implant-supported single crowns. *Int J Oral Maxillofac Implants.* 2015;30(4):851-861.
15. Cortellini P, Stalpers G, Mollo A, Tonetti MS. Periodontal regeneration versus extraction and prosthetic replacement of teeth severely compromised by attachment loss to the apex: 5-year results of an ongoing randomized clinical trial. *J Clin Periodontol.* 2011;38(10):915-924.
16. Splieth C, Giesenberg J, Fanghanel J, et al. Periodontal attachment level of extractions presumably performed for periodontal reasons. *J Clin Periodontol.* 2002;29(6):514-518.
17. Becker W, Becker BE, Berg LE. Periodontal treatment without maintenance. A retrospective study in 44 patients. *J Clin Periodontol.* 1984;55(9):505-509.
18. Lindhe J, Nyman S. Long-term maintenance of patients treated for advanced periodontal disease. *J Clin Periodontol.* 1984;11(8):504-514.
19. Lang-Hua BH, McGrath CPJ, Lo ECM, Lang NP. Factors influencing treatment decision-making for maintaining or extracting compromised teeth. *Clin Oral Implants Res.* 2014;25(1):59-66.
20. Cairo F, Landi L, Gatti C, Rasperini G, Aimetti M; SIdP, the Italian Society of Periodontology and Implantology. Tooth loss and dental implant outcomes - Where is dentistry going? A survey by SIdP, the Italian Society of Periodontology and Implantology. *Oral Dis.* 2018;24(7):1379-1381.
21. Tachalov VV, Orekhova LY, Kudryavtseva TV, et al. Making a complex dental care tailored to the person: population health in focus of predictive, preventive and personalised (3P) medical approach. *EPMA J.* 2021;12(1):129-140.

4

From "Evidence-Based Medicine" to "Patient-Centred Care"

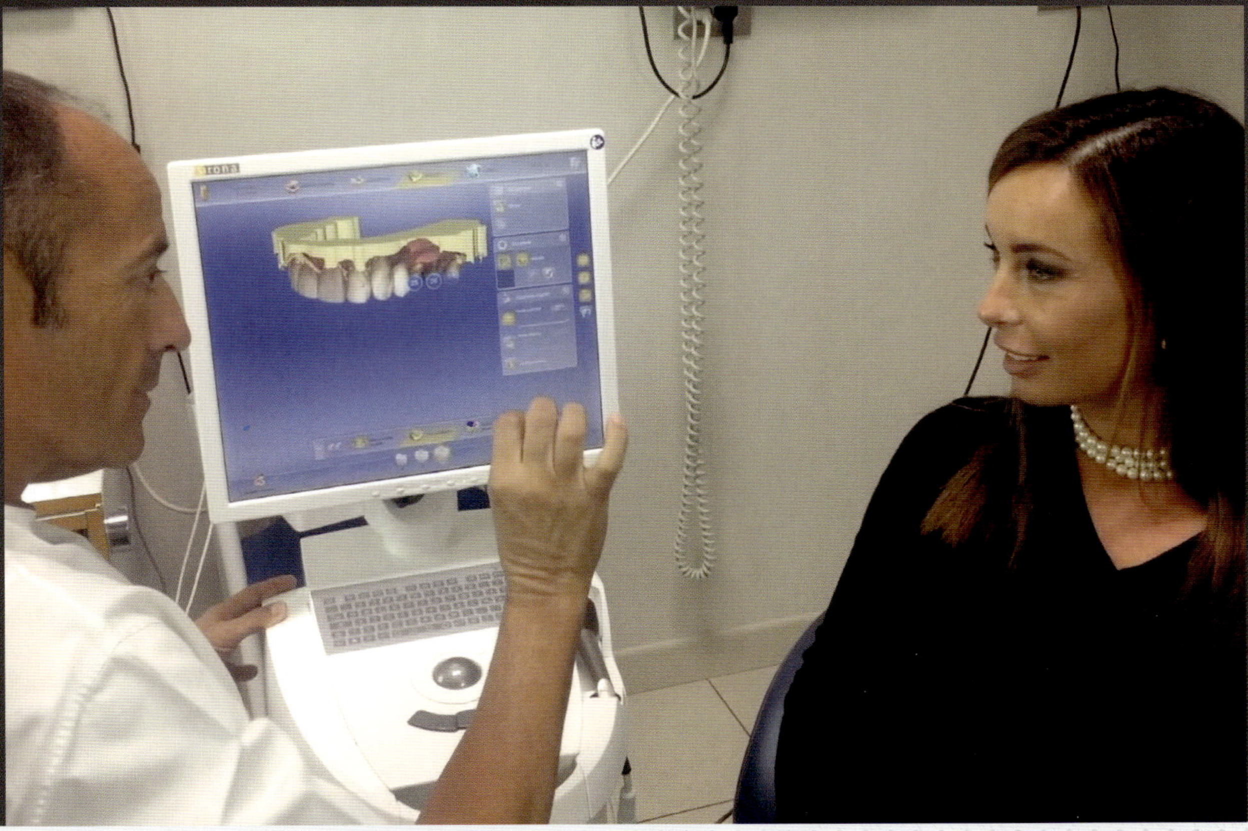

Evidence-Based Medicine

Evidence-Based Medicine (EBM) (**Fig. 4.1**) was conceptualised at the McMaster Canadian University in Hamilton, Ontario.[1] It was described via two sets of studies. The first set of studies was published from 1981 to 1984 in the Canadian Medical Association Journal (CMAJ), while the second collection was in the Annals of Internal Medicine.[2] Then, Guyatt coined the term EBM in 1990,[3] to define a university program at McMaster's University. This program was then introduced to a wider audience via a 1992 JAMA article by one of the University's Working Groups, where EBM is defined as an "emerging new paradigm" for medical practice.[4]

EBM has two areas of application: 1) Evidence-Based Health Care for macro-decisions concerning public health or groups of people homogeneous in terms of diseases or risk factors and 2) Evidence-Based Clinical Practice,[5] for single patient medical care (EBM proper), which interests us the most since it "starts and finishes with the patient" according to EBM.

EBM had an extraordinary impact in its first decade, with over 11,000 citations in MEDLINE, and gave rise to two genres of publications. The first genre focuses on the methodological criteria for researching, evaluating, and applying the "evidence." Specifically, this genre includes the 25 Users' Guides to the Medical Literature compiled and updated in their 3rd edition.[6] On the other hand, the second genre comprises "secondary" publications that summarise clinically relevant and methodologically validated RCTs (randomized clinical trials) and systematic reviews, including Clinical Evidence, ACP Journal Club and Evidence-Based Medicine, and Cochrane Library's meta-analysis summaries. In subsequent years, the concept of EBM became more cautious in its definition. It referred to "the conscientious, explicit and judicious use of current best [literary] evidence in making decisions about the care of individual patients,"

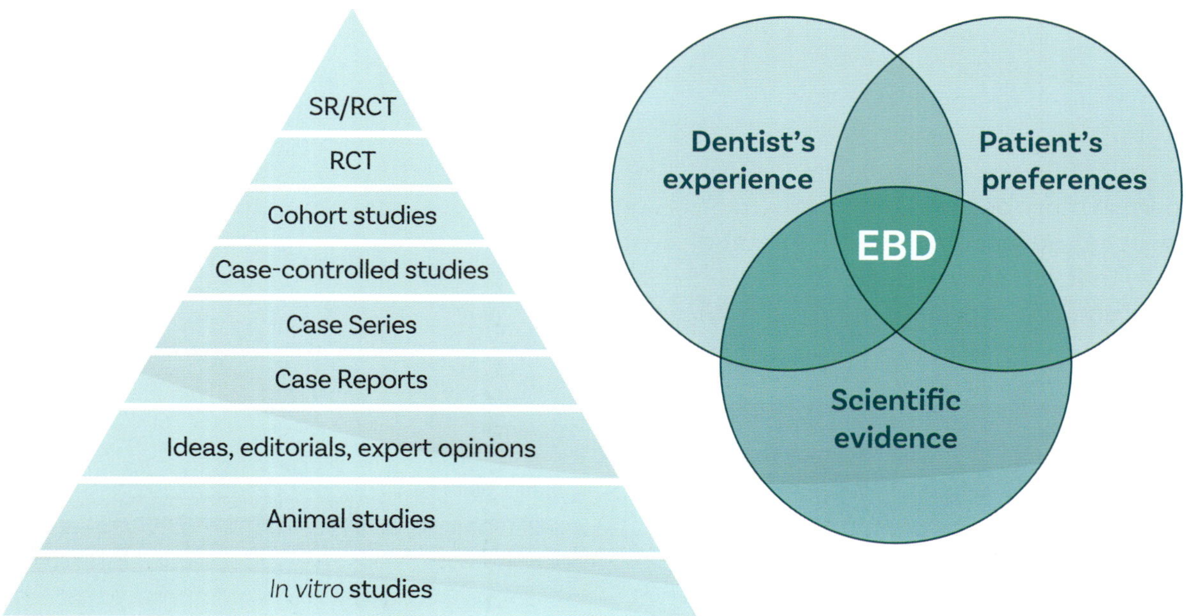

Fig. 4.1 ■ Evidence-based dentistry.

while acknowledging the need to combine the "evidence" with individual clinical expertise. Recently, the EBM Working Group now prioritises clinical expertise and patient preference as crucial clinical decision-making factors. This shift in importance is evident in various editorials[7] and more organically in a dedicated volume expanding upon the original 25 Users' Guides published in JAMA. This volume softens the philosophy behind EBM,[6] which expresses the concept that evidence alone is not enough in clinical decision-making through the book's title for the first chapter: "Clinical Decision Making: Evidence is never enough".

Initially, the EBM ideology prioritized the literature "evidence," especially clinical experiments, over the clinician's "expertise" and the patient's values. However, it has evolved over time, with the balance completely shifting. Currently, the "evidence" is viewed only as a component of clinical decisions: "Evidence does not make decisions, people do",[7] which is a more modern realistic take on EBM.

Despite the considerable literature on the concepts and practice of EBM, there is no evidence that following its precepts improves the quality of clinical practice,[8] thus creating a paradox[9] for "evidence"-based ideology. However, to evaluate the global effects of EBM, wider adoption could improve clinical practice compared to its current state.

For this to happen, EBM's integration into clinical expertise must become the norm, which is contingent on advancements in information technology that will allow us easier access to the "evidence" should the experimental methodology be available for evaluation before and after obtaining a degree. Furthermore, EBM should be integrated into a clinicians' expertise rather than being presented as an improbable "new paradigm".

Furthermore, as evident from multiple publications, EBM reportedly had a decisively important role in disseminating the methodology of evaluating the treatment studies and the "evidence" obtained exclusively from reliable studies like RCTs and systematic reviews.

However, when RCTs are either absent or inapplicable to the patient's individual characteristics, the evidence must be extrapolated from fields like pathophysiology and pharmacology. Nevertheless, these fields are often ignored in EBM literature, as they are ranked sixth out of seven in Guyatt's[10] classification of evidence validity.

Randomized trials are typically conducted in ideal conditions for evaluating treatments, with carefully selected patients based on "pure" pathologies (not presenting important comorbidities and their associated treatments), clinicians experts in the relevant field, closer and more complete supervision (compared to a routine environment), and high patient compliance.

However, the treatment that proves effective under these conditions may not translate to daily practice, with comorbidities possibly altering the risk/reward profile of a proven efficacious treatment. Although EBM-correlated literature can offer evidence-based information on choosing and interpreting indices and diagnostic hypothesis-verifying tests, it does not address the interpretation of signs and symptoms and the generation of a diagnostic hypothesis. This is because it overlooks descriptive observational studies and the diagnostic reasoning case reports, particularly those that present a Clinical Problem Solving structure, which explains both the development and the logical flow step-by-step.

For these reasons, despite extensive EBM-specific literature, its effect on clinical practice was not proportionate. This was due to multiple contributory hurdles identified by clinicians themselves, who are the theoretical recipients of EBM's message. Furthermore, this was accompanied by the important fact that therapeutic decisions are multidimensional in nature and cannot solely rely on literature-based "evidence."[11,12]

EBM can provide evidence-based information for choosing and interpreting indices and diagnostic hypothesis-verifying tests. Unfortunately, it does not address the interpretation of signs and symptoms and the generation of diagnostic hypotheses as it overlooks descriptive observational studies and diagnostic reasoning found in case reports.

Therefore, since EBM is an incomplete approach to medicine, it should be integrated with clinical competence, patient-specific biological characteristics and circumstances.[13] Furthermore, therapy selection should consider scientific evidence, experience, medical opinion, case specifics and patient preferences equally.

Patient-Centred Care

In recent years, patient subjectivity has been gaining importance, leading to a progressive rise in personalised therapies. Healthcare providers now recognise how pathologies and treatments impact the patient's psychological, social and socio-economic spheres, ultimately impacting their "quality of life". This gave rise to the concept of "Patient-Centred Care" (**Fig. 4.2**), which is now a fundamental aspect of healthcare quality.

The Picker Institute and the Harvard Medical School[14] researchers explained the concept of "Patient-Centred Care" through "eight principles of care". It involves listening, informing, and involving patients in their treatment. Additionally, the Harvard Medical School researchers, on behalf of the Picker Institute and the Commonwealth Fund, established "Picker's seven principles" to define Patient-Centred Care and promote a positive patient experience. The eighth principle, i.e., access to healthcare, was added later ("The Eight Principles of Patient-Centred Care," 2015).

Integrating experiential learning with humanistic content and promoting a "holistic vision of

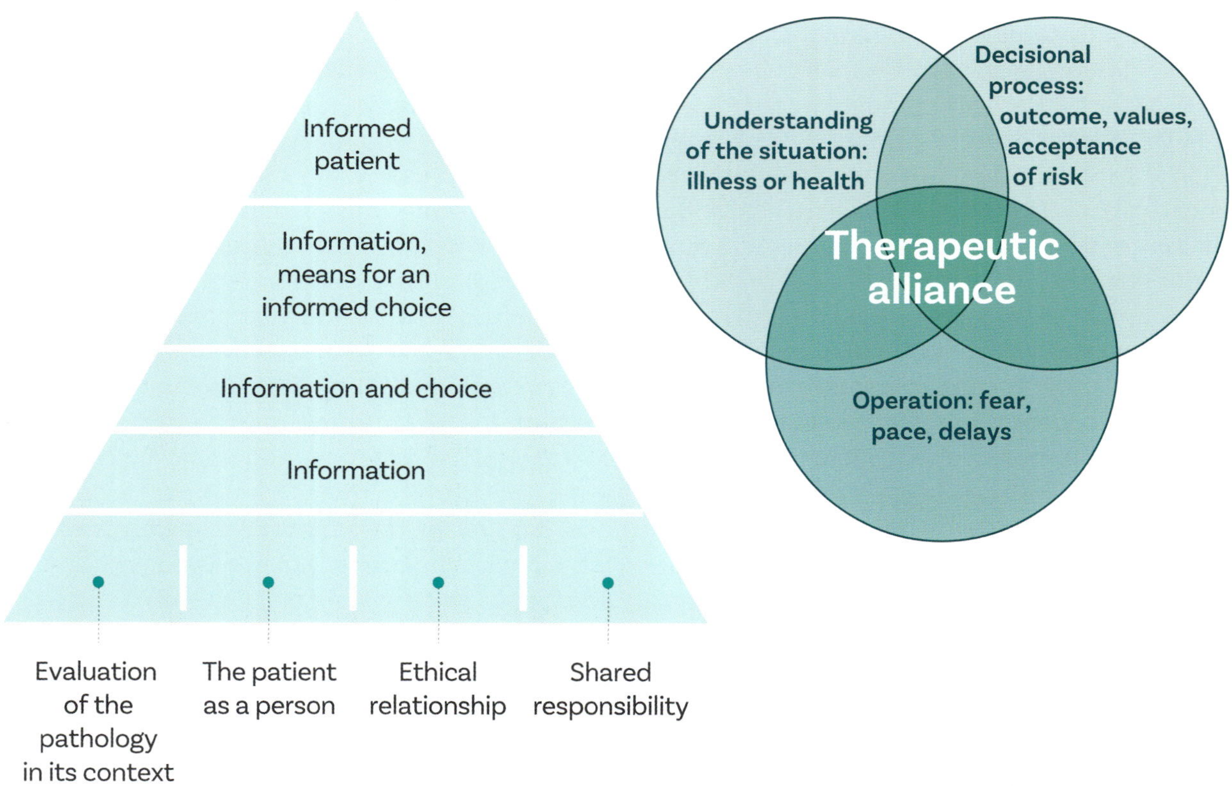

Fig. 4.2 ■ Patient-centred treatment.

patient experience"[15] can enhance skills such as communication, listening, cooperation, respect for diversity, and empathy in tomorrow's doctors and dentists.

A 2019 study showed that dental students who prioritized "Patient-Centred Care" during their studies gained empathy, sensitivity, improved communication skills, and learnt that providing mental and emotional care to patients is as important as their technical skills.[16]

The critical evaluation of EBM can be applied to its branch, Evidence-Based Dentistry (EBD). When analysing the argument of treating or replacing a severely compromised tooth, we may notice the differences between EBD and Patient-Centred Care in the literature. A search for the keywords "dental implant" produces 48,299 results, whereas "surgical endodontics" produces 9,221 results. Furthermore, the keyword searches for "endodontic retreatment" and "tooth autotransplantation" produced only 1597 and 1358 results, respectively. Since commercial interests evidently favour the most profitable solutions available to the dental industry, we are no strangers to such a wealth of literature on dental implants. An exclusively Evidence-Based approach would always guide the dentist to choose the "best" solution with the most support from medical literature. For instance, a severely compromised tooth can only be treated by replacing it with an implant. However, in reality, restorative and prosthetic options and lesser-known techniques like autotransplantation should be equally considered since each clinical case requires a specialist's evaluation to determine the most appropriate therapy. Furthermore, patient subjectivity is rarely studied in the literature, leading to a perception of it being a less scientific evaluation when compared to other more "academic" ones.

Precision tailored dentistry

There is no doubt that the future of dentistry will be shaped by new technologies, regenerative therapies, digitalization, and artificial intelligence.[17] However, a paradigm shift towards precision dentistry is necessary, which must go beyond either "the marginal seal around a crown" or "the working lengths in endodontics". Precision dentistry should be a science that precisely matches patient expectancies and characteristics, while predicting therapy outcomes, maintenance, and prevention of recurrence. Clinical decisions must be tailored to each patient, and standardized treatments should consider the unique characteristics of each patient and their impact on treatment outcomes. This approach can help avoid unsatisfactory final results, both clinically and financially.

Like the emerging direction in the medical field,[18] personalized dentistry, or precision dentistry, must prioritise the question, "What is the risk of disease progression, tooth loss, and poor treatment outcomes for this particular patient?",[19] before anything else. Schwendicke[20] asserts that tailored dentistry is not only advantageous but also necessary for the future of dentistry since many old concepts in dentistry are no longer valid. Caries, once concentrated mainly among the younger generations, has now polarized, with disadvantaged social groups presenting with caries instead of today's youth. Furthermore, elderly individuals who previously did not have caries due to extensive edentulism now often have widespread root caries due to poor plaque control from reduced manual ability, pharmaceutically-induced hyposalivation, and incorrect eating habits. Traditional restorative dentistry principles that focus on restoring carious lesions affecting the crowns of young individuals do not apply to preventing and treating radicular lesions in the elderly.[21]

Another growing concern is the prevention and treatment of occlusal surface wear, with uncertainties around the choice of technique and necessary materials selection.

In conclusion, "Patient-Centred Care" in dentistry needs further research based on tested and proven systems to become a well-defined concept that can be shared to truly put the patient at the centre of the treatment plan.[22]

An emblematic case of the integration between the concept of Evidence-Based Medicine and the criteria of Patient-Centred Care

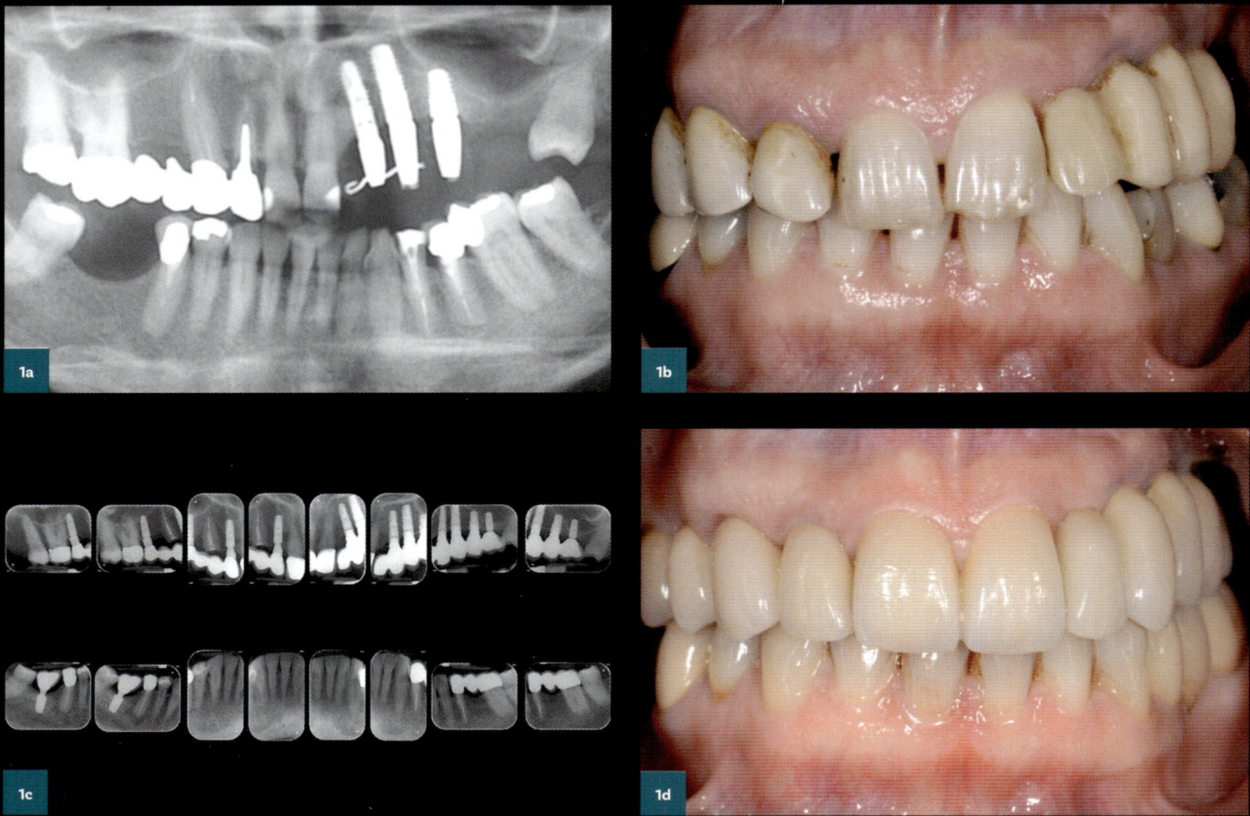

Figs. 1a-d ■ The coexistence of occlusal, aesthetic and functional problems, along with missing teeth and suboptimal implant positioning, influences the decisions made by both the operator and the patient. Consequently, extensive discussions are necessary to

Bibliography

1. Sackett D. How to read clinical journals: I. why to read them and how to start reading them critically. *Can Med Assoc J.* 1981; 124(5):555-558.
2. Canadian Task Force on the Periodic Health Examination. The periodic health examination. *Can Med Assoc J.* 1979; 121(9):1193-1254.
3. Guyatt G. Evidence-based medicine. *Ann Intern Med.* 1991;114(Suppl 2):A-16.
4. Guyatt G, Cairns J, Churchill D, et al. Evidence-Based Medicine: A New Approach to Teaching the Practice of Medicine. *JAMA.* 1992;268(17):2420-2425.
5. Sackett DL, Straus SE, Richardson WS, et al. Evidence-Based Medicine: How to Practice and Teach EBM. 2nd ed. Churchill Livingstone; 2000.
6. Guyatt G, Rennie D, Meade MO, Cook DJ. Users' Guides to the Medical Literature: A Manual for Evidence-Based Clinical Practice. 3rd ed. McGraw-Hill; 2015.
7. Haynes RB, Devereaux PJ, Guyatt GH. Physicians' and patients' choices in evidence-based practice. BMJ. 2002;324(7350):1350.
8. Norman GR. Examining the assumptions of evidence-based medicine. *J Eval Clin Pract.* 1999;5(2):139-147.
9. Norman GR. The paradox of evidence-based medicine. *J Eval Clin Prac.* 2003;9(2):129-132.
10. Guyatt G, Rennie D. Therapy and validity: surprising results of randomized controlled trials. In: Guyatt G, Rennie D, eds. Users' Guides to the Medical Literature: A Manual for Evidence-Based Clinical Practice. Chicago, AMA Press; 2002.
11. Djulbegovic B, Morris L, Lyman GH. Evidentiary challenges to evidence-based medicine. *J Eval Clin Pract.* 2000;6(2):99-109.
12. Gupta M. A critical appraisal of evidence-based medicine: Some ethical considerations. *J Eval Clin Pract.* 2003; 9(2):111-121.
13. GIMBE. https://www.gimbe.org/pagine/268/it/knowhow# (Published October 8, 2023. Accessed October 20, 2023).
14. Principles of Person Centered Care. Picker Institute. https://www.picker.org/about-us/picker-principles-of-person-centred-care/. Accessed October 5, 2021.
15. Irby DM, Cooke M, O'Brien BC. Calls for Reform of Medical Education by the Carnegie Foundation for the Advancement of Teaching: 1910 and 2010. *Acad Med.* 2010;85(2):220-227.
16. Michael K, Dror MG, Karnieli-Miller O. Students' patient-centered-care attitudes: The contribution of self-efficacy, communication, and empathy. *Patient Educ Couns.* 2019;102(11):2031-2037.
17. Khanagar SB, Al-Ehaideb A, Maganur PC, et al. Developments, application, and performance of artificial intelligence in dentistry. A systematic review. *J Dent Sci.* 2021;16(1):508-522.
18. Bartold PM. Personalized/precision dentistry – the future of dentistry? *Aust Dent J.* 2017;62(3):257-264.
19. Beck JD, Philips K, Moss K, et al. Advances in precision oral health. *Periodontol 2000.* 2020;82(1):268-285.
20. Schwendicke F. Tailored dentistry: from "one size fits all" to precision dental medicine? *Oper Dent.* 2018;43(5):451-459.
21. Lopez R, Smith PC, Gostemeyer G, Schwendicke F. Ageing, dental caries and periodontal diseases. *J Clin Periodontol.* 2017;44 (Suppl 18):S145-S152.
22. Scambler S, Delgado M, Asimakopoulou K. Defining patient-centred care in dentistry? A systematic review of the dental literature. *Br Dent J.* 2016;221:477-484.

PART II

Endodontic treatment of the severely compromised tooth

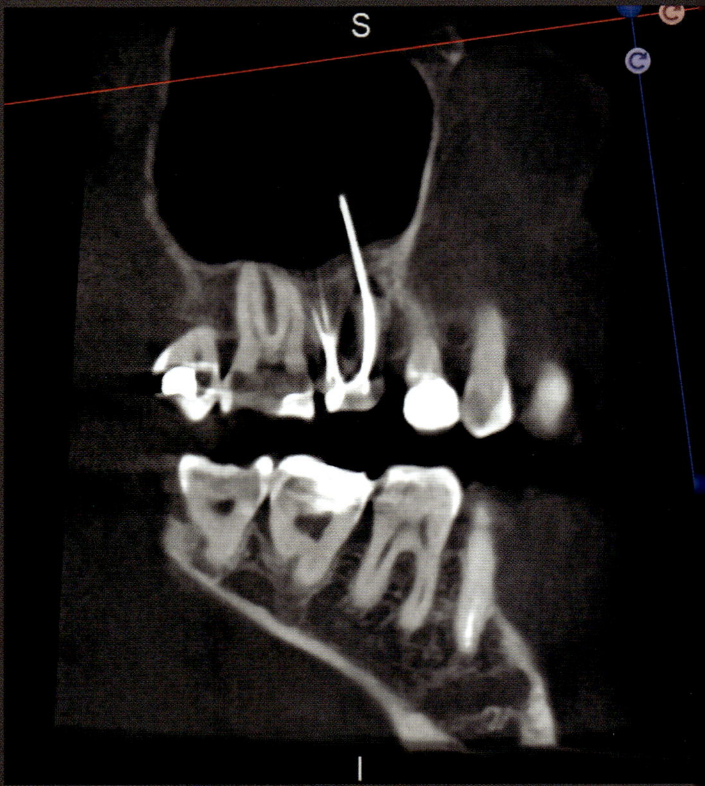

Massimo **Gagliani**

Paolo **Generali**

Fabio **Gorni**

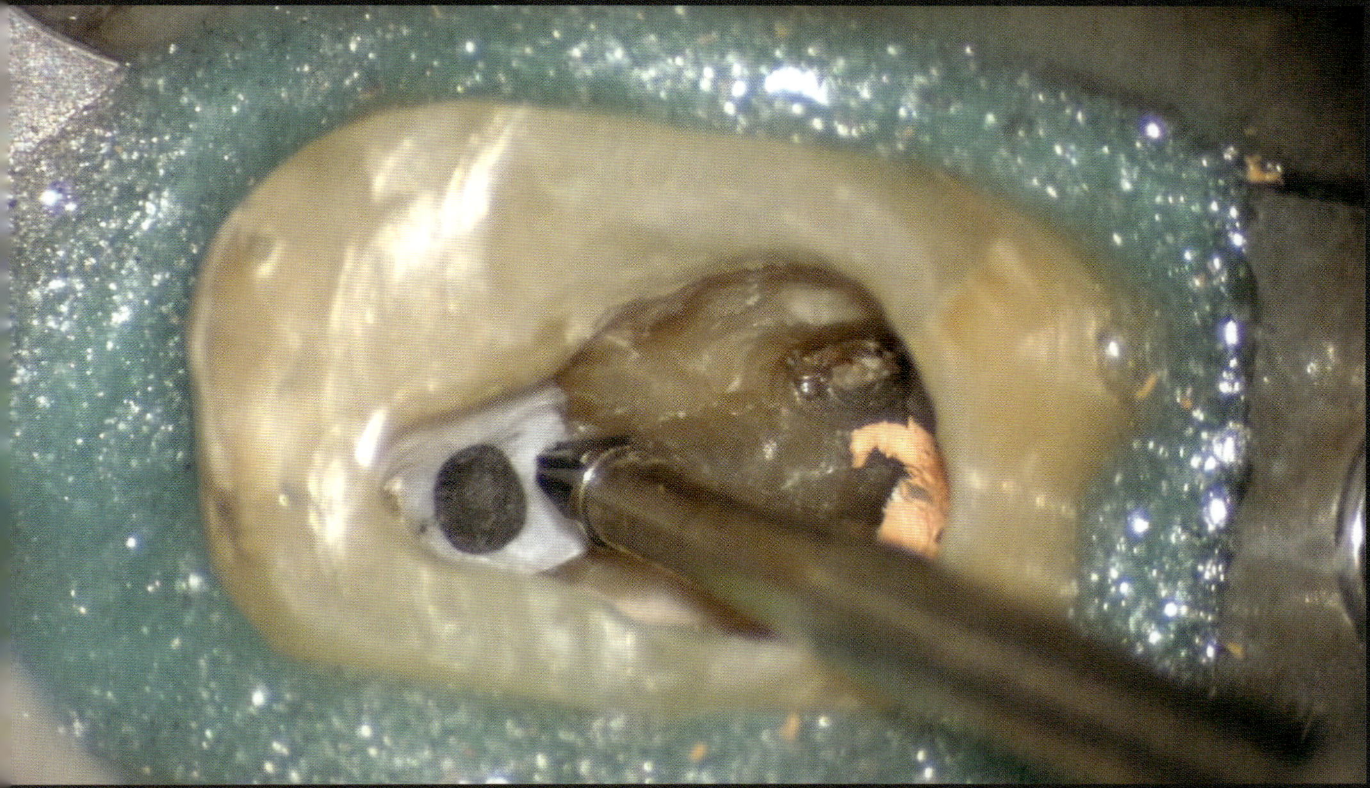

Introduction

When discussing a seriously compromised tooth, the first question to address is its definition. Although describing this clinical stage is challenging, certain factors help establish the classification criteria, and they fall into the dental and periodontal categories.
Dental factors include the shape and morphology of the dental crown. As highlighted in Chapter 1, the extent of hard tissue loss determines the severity of a compromised tooth. Additionally, its root length and periodontal support also impact its survival within the dental arch after endodontic treatment or retreatment.
Besides previously examined functional considerations, evaluating the impact of periodontal factors like the chronic periapical lesion commonly associated with highly compromised teeth is crucial. Although there are no definitive scales for measuring the lesion's size, large periapical inflammatory areas indicate a more severe impairment caused by difficult-to-eradicate, widespread and varied bacterial contamination.
In this context, it becomes crucial to highlight the unique characteristics of dental element damage and comprehensively explore suitable solutions to avoid lengthy, laborious and sometimes difficult treatments for the dentist and patient. Such treatments may not generate prognostically reproducible or favourable outcomes, often jeopardising successive implant procedures. This is partly described in this chapter and the next one.
Special emphasis will be placed on the selection criteria for proceeding with orthograde retreatment or surgical endodontics, better known as endodontic surgery. An operating microscope and appropriate retrograde obturation material are crucial for achieving satisfactory outcomes.
A dedicated section will address mechanical and anatomical problems, including broken instruments. Although once considered daunting, competent individuals can remove them using specialised tools like ultrasonic devices. Despite the successful resolution of iatrogenic perforations being anatomically relevant, their long-term prognosis may not be highly favourable. Nevertheless, these procedures should be considered part of a maintenance plan that can eventually extend the tooth's longevity until replacement, typically after eight to twelve years.
Teeth affected by internal or external resorption can cause complications of unknown origin, damaging dental hard tissue that often results in tooth loss, even in very young patients.
In summary, this section comprehensively covers all problems that can cause tooth impairment, which, if addressed promptly, can often save the affected tooth.

5

Complex endodontic cases

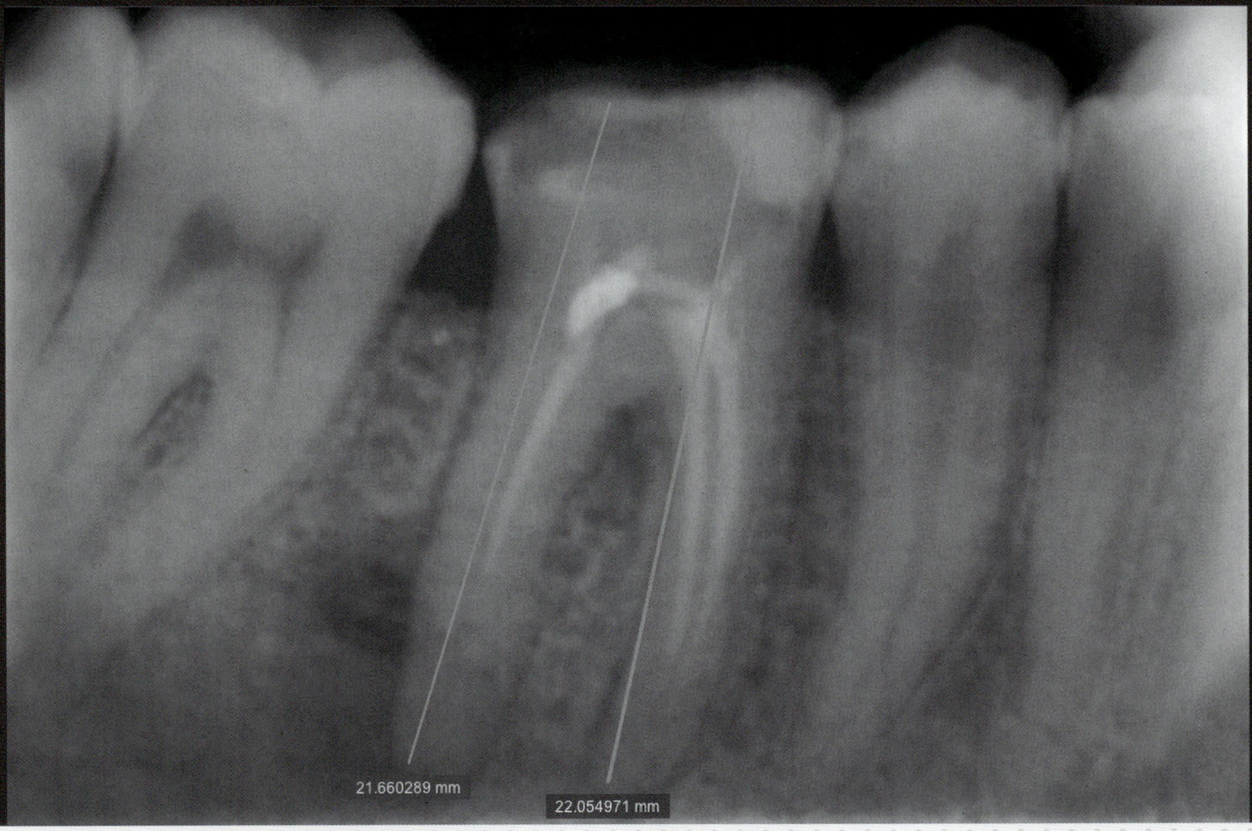

Clinical cases involving periapical pathologies of endodontic relevance can arise from diverse factors, with multiple cases apparently being associated with untreated teeth. However, recent epidemiological data indicates that the periapical lesions of endodontic origin are actually attributed to a higher percentage of teeth with inadequate prior treatment or unfortunate evolutionary outcomes.[1,2]
We will focus on the latter category with comprehensive documentation later on. In the introductory phase, the former category presents certain distinctions that often influence the preferred treatment choice in most cases. This is particularly true where the clinician favours extraction (avulsion) rather than heroically preserving the tooth, especially for posterior teeth like second molars (**Fig. 5.1**).
In daily clinical practice, extraction is not uncommon when facilitating the relocation of the wisdom teeth, either spontaneously or orthodontically, into the site of the second molar. Although this approach is strongly recommended in the upper jaw, it becomes more complex in the lower jaw, where the mesial migration is often more intricate and may require orthodontic appliances. However, this option remains the preferable choice. Preserving severely compromised teeth in the coronal aspect would require multiple interventions over a lifetime, potentially including the possible placement of osseointegrated implants, which can be avoided if healthy teeth are used as replacements.
In summary, as highlighted in the recent systematic review by Tiburcio-Machado,[1] the percentage of teeth affected by periapical lesions does not exceed 5%. However, these findings prompt us to reflect on the fact that over 50% of the described patients are significantly impacted by such issues, thus underscoring their relevance.
It is important to note that the success rates of these treatments vary based on the operators and the initial clinical conditions at the beginning of the treatment. Furthermore, teeth with extensive radiographically significant lesions have been found to have a proportionally significant success rate reduction in their treatments.
Therefore, it is crucial to address the difficulty in finding the variables involved in the decision-making process. This will be extensively explored in the following chapters.

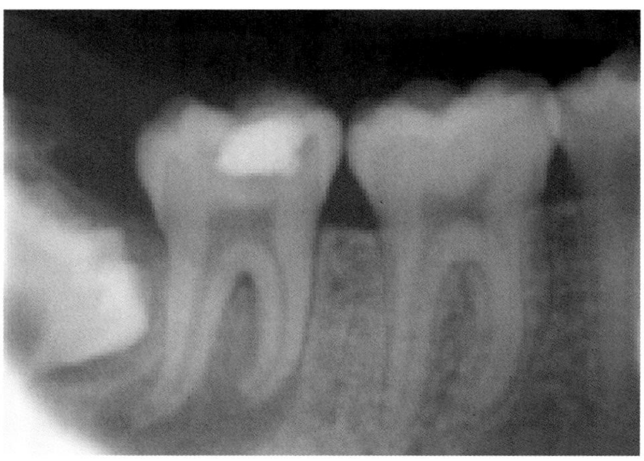

Fig. 5.1 ■ A case where a lower seven tooth had a significant periapical lesion, leading the clinician to extract it to allow the wisdom tooth to erupt.

Complex retreatment cases

From an endodontic perspective, defining the complexity of retreatment cases is challenging, and the choice becomes arbitrary regardless of the criteria used. In fact, despite the numerous analytic models examined, no definitive conclusions have been drawn.[3,4]

Nonetheless, establishing general criteria is vital to assist clinicians in determining whether the case can be resolved. Therefore, the final decision revolves around keeping the tooth, preparing it for endodontic surgery, or removing it to eliminate the associated pathology. These factors, as demonstrated by many, are influenced by colleagues' cultural backgrounds, training courses, and dental treatment planning during the decision-making process.[5,6]

We can identify different complexity levels in the preliminary phase, each contributing to the final judgment.

The first level involves the clinical severity of the pathology the patient presents. For example, a tooth with recurrent pain, significantly evident periapical radio-transparency, and pharmacologically managed acute abscesses will be considered more challenging than a clinically similar tooth but asymptomatic with modest radiological evidence. Similarly, a tooth with a history of previous retreatments or endodontic surgery requires careful evaluation before attempting another endodontic procedure.

Hence, microbiology should also be considered in the evaluation process, followed by anatomical considerations divided into macroscopic and microscopic categories. Since macroscopic anatomical ones are strongly related to the reconstructive phase, they will be examined separately. Although smaller anatomical details must be assessed through a two-dimensional radiographic examination, three-dimensional evaluation using Cone Beam Computed Tomography (CBCT) becomes essential for complex cases.

The Authors[7] dated study, supported by recent literature findings, undeniably confirms the importance of anatomical peculiarities (**Tables 5.1**, **5.2**). Understanding the condition of root canals and the outcomes of previous treatments through radiological analysis becomes decisive in choosing between tooth preservation and extraction. However, orthograde retreatment, surgical treatment, or a combination of both may be attempted to obtain the desired outcome.

During the preliminary evaluation phase, it is possible to summarize some of the salient prognostic data (**Table 5.3**).

Here is a list of potential outcomes related to periapical conditions in retreated teeth:

- Presence of new periapical radiolucency.
- Periapical radiolucency that can either be reduced or resolved/remain constant/increase in size.
- Healthy periapical state or no signs before and after therapy.

When considering "endodontic treatment," it is important to account for the anatomical reconstruction of the previously treated tooth. This includes factors such as the type of post-endodontic restoration, the possible presence of intracanal retention and its characteristics,[8] the type of endodontic cement inserted into the canal and the obturation methods used.[9-11]

Table 5.1 ■ Two-year results of retreatment cases: influence of root canal anatomy.

		N° teeth	Healed	Healing	Failed	% success	% failed
Teeth with preserved root canal morphology	Without periapical lesion	83	76	0	7	91.6	8.4
	With periapical lesion	167	136	4	27	83.8	16.2
Teeth with non-preserved root canal morphology	Without periapical lesion	32	27	0	5	84.4	15.6
	With periapical lesion	170	56	12	102	40	60

NOTE: 425 patients; 211 males; 214 females; mean age: 40.5 years; 452 teeth; control duration: 24 months.

Table 5.2 ■ Types of root canals in retreatments.

Classification of root canals	Type
Teeth with non-preserved root canal morphology	External or internal apical transport
	Root resorptions
	Perforations/stripping
Teeth with preserved root canal morphology	Missed canals
	Broken instruments with no obturation
	Intracanal calcifications with previous obturation

Table 5.3 ■ Prognostic elements of a retreatment.

Factors in FAVOUR of retreatment	Factors CONTRARY to retreatment
The lesion can flare up	No symptoms
The lesion could enlarge	Time and cost of treatment (retreatment)
The inflammatory lesion is in any case a risk	Post-treatment sequelae (symptoms)

Retreatment of lower molar with a large periapical lesion

The retreatment of a mandibular molar with consistent periapical pathology of endodontic origin requires careful evaluation. This treatment falls into the category where the tooth's anatomical structure remains largely intact, resulting in a favourable prognosis

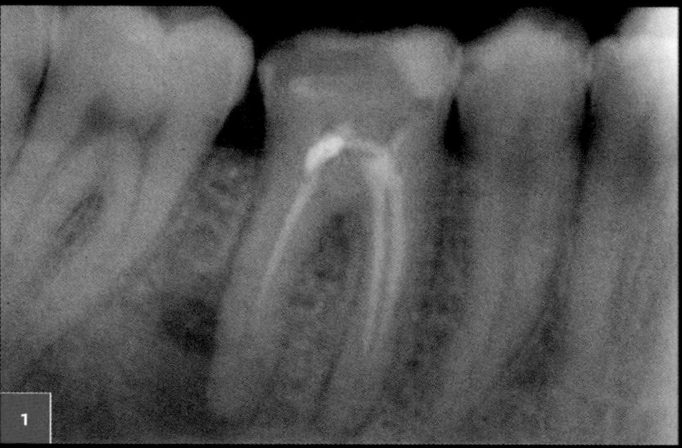

Fig. 1 ■ The radiographic findings indicate the widespread septic process involvement of the distal root, while the mesial root shows two canals that merge approximately 3-4 mm from the apex.

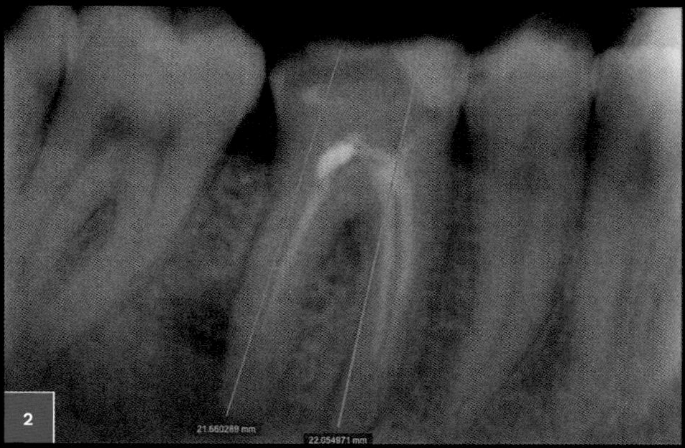

Fig. 2 ■ Radiographic analysis can be further supported by estimated "working lengths", which provide initial indications for the level of preliminary instrumentation. Confirmation will be obtained using the apex-locator.

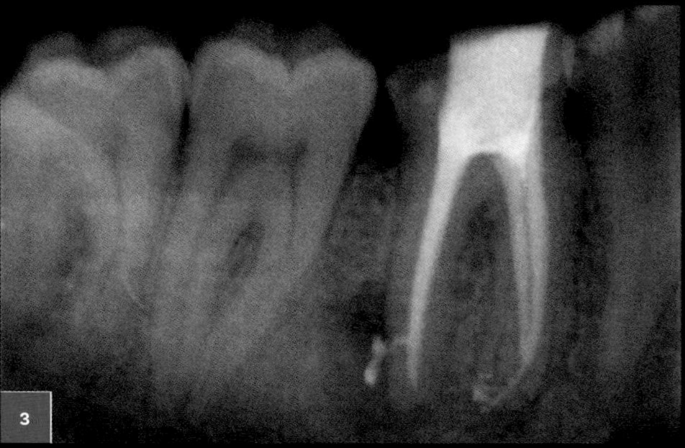

Fig. 3 ■ In the completed case, a prominent high posterior opening is clearly visible in the distal root where it is sealed with endodontic cement, whereas negotiating the confluent zone in the anterior area was challenging but still allowed for successful sealing of the endodontic space.

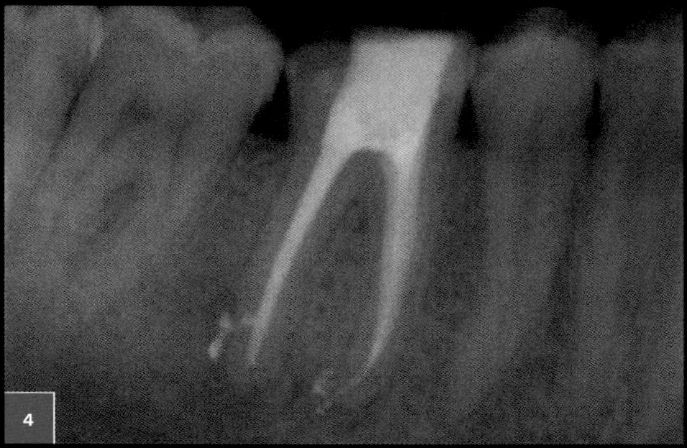

Fig. 4 ■ The resolution of the periapical inflammatory situation enables the completion of definitive restoration.

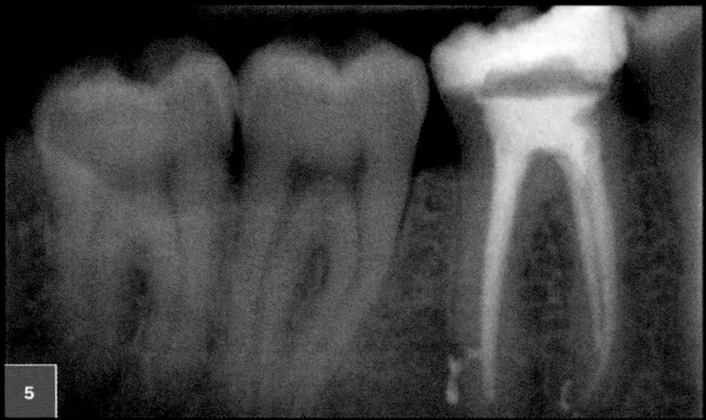

Fig. 5 ■ The follow-up examination after a few years confirms the long-term stability of the treatment performed.

The occurrence of broken instruments[12,13] does not always have a significant negative impact on assessing the difficulty level. This is because satisfactory results have been achieved in numerous cases after instrument removal.[14] In fact, instrument breakage often prompts the clinician to temporarily suspend the treatment, where if the maximum intracanal dentinal tissue is being preserved, it greatly favours the success of the retreatment.

Broken instrument – mesial root of a lower molar

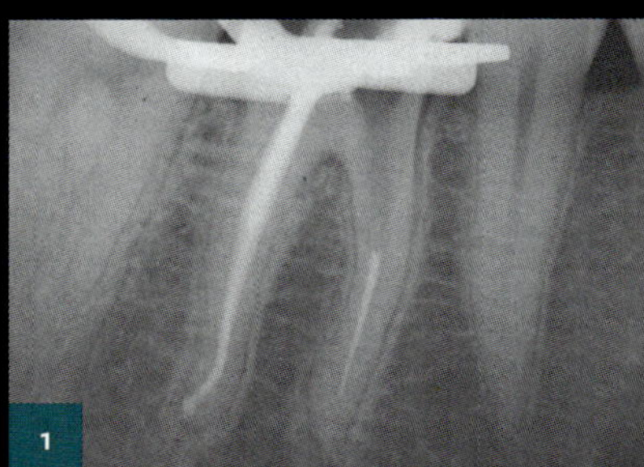

Fig. 1 ■ Large fragment of a rotary instrument broken in the mesio-buccal canal of a lower molar.

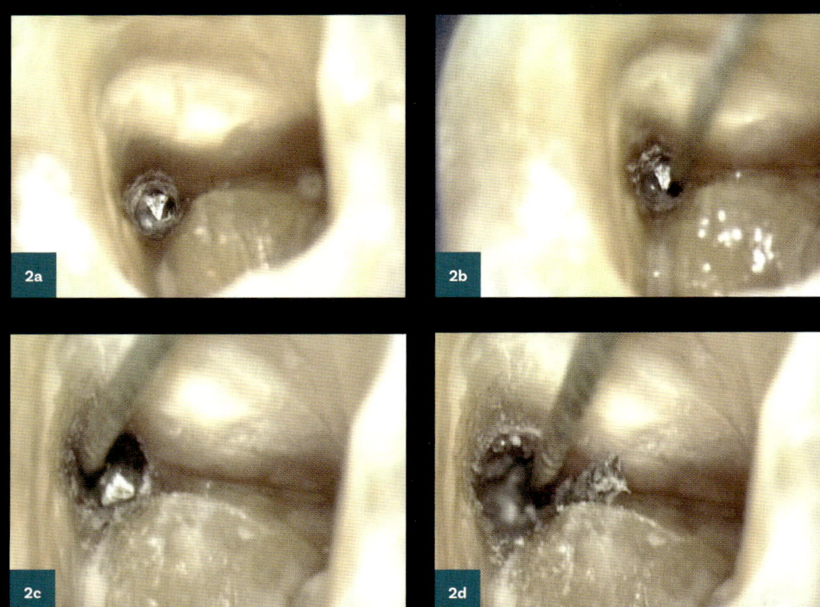

Figs. 2a-d ■ The images demonstrate the precise control achievable with the operating microscope in removing broken instruments. The combination of the microscope and ultrasonic tip enables the predictable extraction of instrument fragments, thereby preserving important teeth.

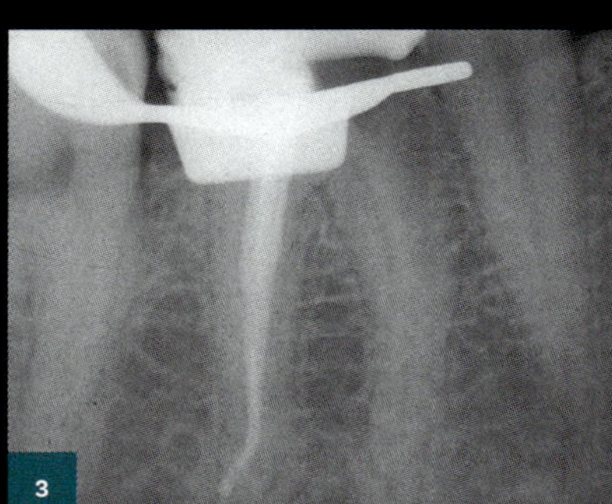

Fig. 3 ■ The radiograph shows the removal of the instrument.

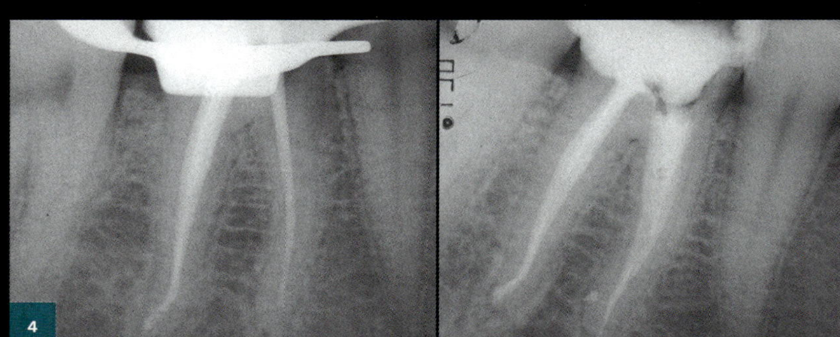

Fig. 4 ■ Cone fit and completion of treatment.

The third crucial consideration is the periapical health condition,[15-17] which is linked to the previous two points and reflects the microbiological status. Therefore, the more extensive the periapical radiolucent lesion, the more unfavourable the outcome. Furthermore, lesions affecting the dental structure, such as periapical resorption, add to the severity and complicate retreatment due to challenges encountered during the obturation phase.

A fourth point revolves around the future of the tooth. The complexity lies not only in the tooth itself but also in the reconstructive plan that depends on the tooth and its strategic involvement in the overall rehabilitation process of the patient.[18-20]

A premolar with a double radiolucent fibre post needs to be retreated for a large lateral inflammatory lesion

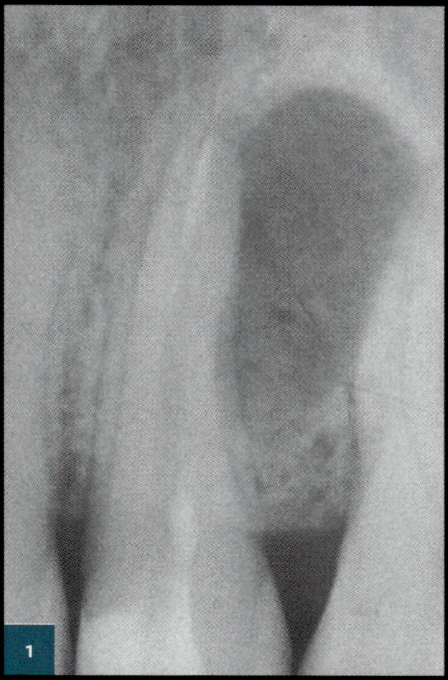

Fig. 1 ■ The radiological aspect indicate a widespread distribution of the septic process within the root.

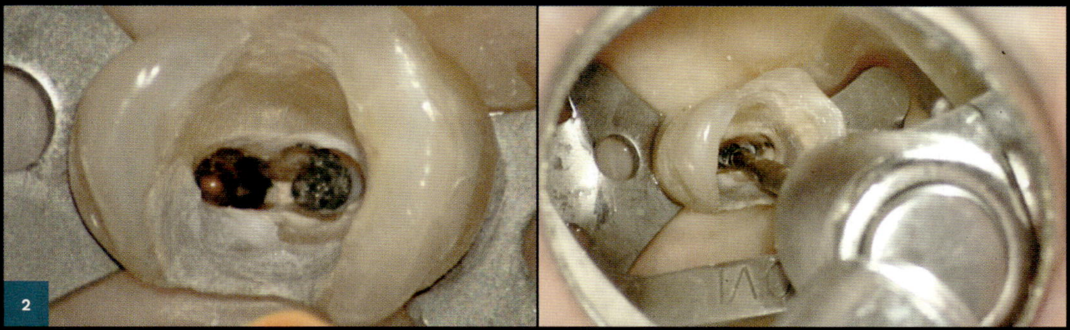

Fig. 2 ■ The clinical examination highlights the presence of posts in both roots.

> CONT'D

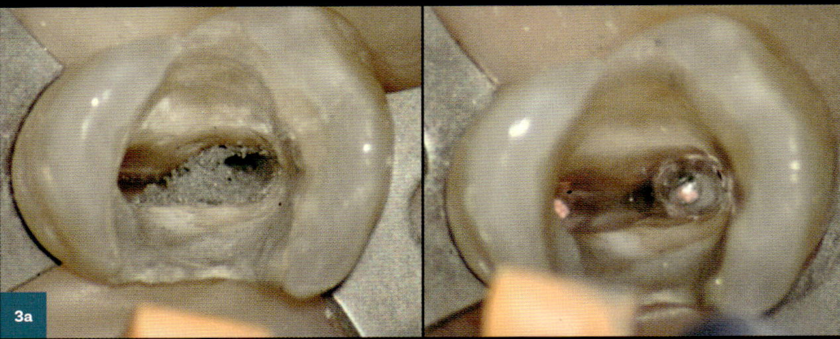

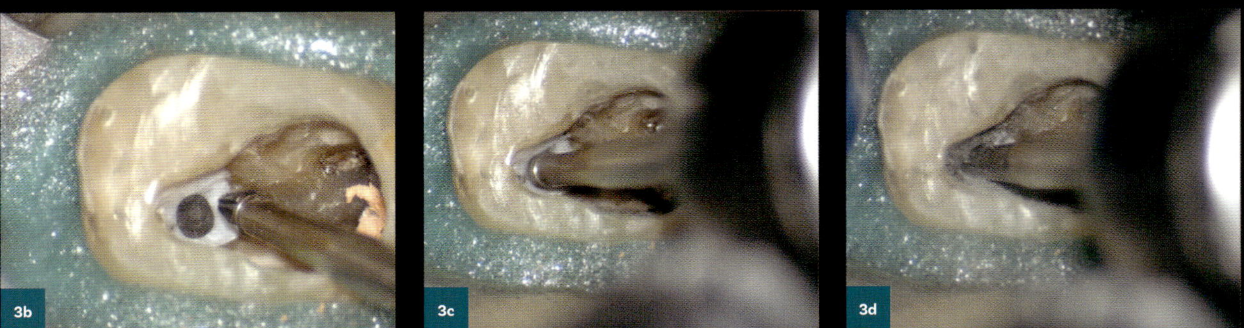

Figs. 3a-d ■ The use of burs and, most importantly, ultrasonic instruments with microscopic magnification should facilitate the effective removal of the posts.

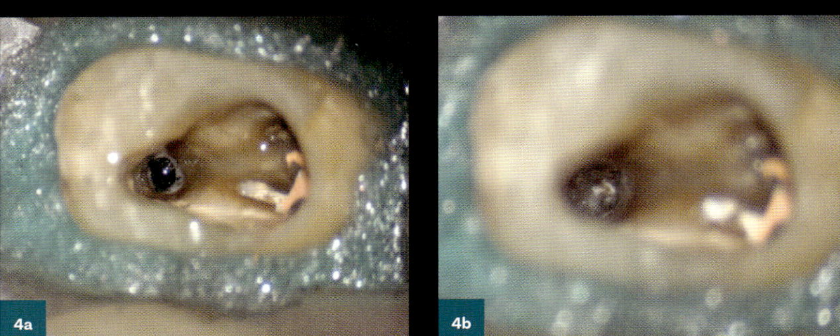

Figs. 4a,b ■ The empty canal is thoroughly irrigated to ensure optimal disinfection.

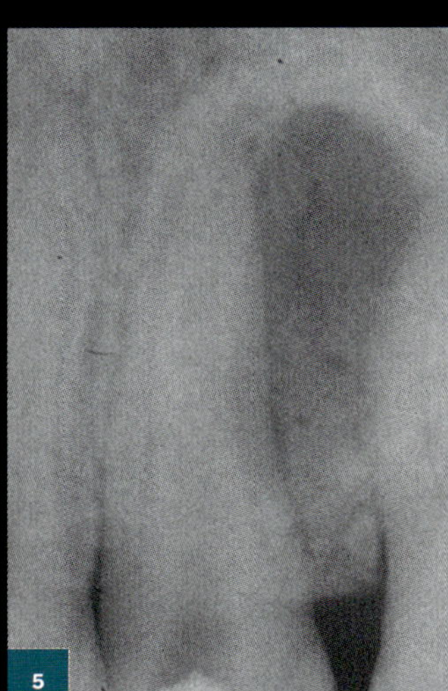

Fig. 5 ■ Radiographic valuation confirms the complete elimination of the intracanal materials.

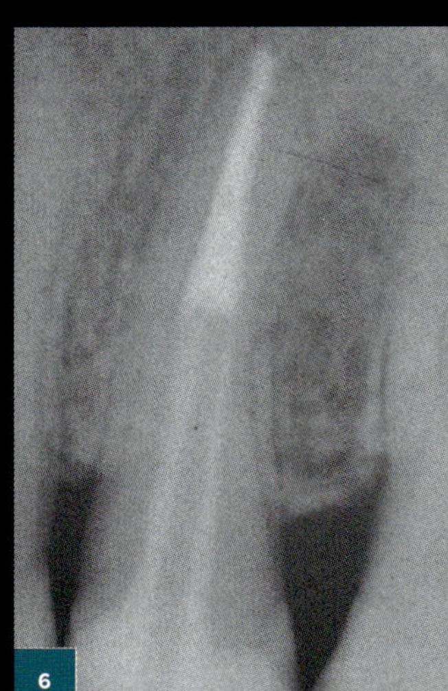

Fig. 6 ■ The case was resolved with a new reconstruction using a fibre post.

Therefore, re-establishing a durable and resilient structure will be crucial in repairing the tooth involved in the retreatment.
The key aspects of the tooth highlighted thus far include the following:

- Its clinical condition
- Its periapical state
- Its macroscopic and microscopic anatomy
- Its fate.

Moreover, it is crucial to consider operator-related factors, including their experience and the available instruments. These elements are crucial in determining whether teeth that would otherwise be extracted can be saved.
The decision-making algorithm is summarised in **Box 5.1** for easier understanding.
Additionally, it is worth noting that dentists must thoroughly assess their skills and the material and instruments required to address the challenges that retreatments inevitably pose to the clinician. Subsequently, Chapters 6, 7 and the final part of Chapter 8 describe the necessary steps to undertake this therapy safely.

Box 5.1 ■ Decisional algorithms in retreatments

When considering whether to perform a retreatment, a systematic approach is essential. This involves transitioning from general considerations to specific details in a consistent sequence that begins with the patient and progresses to the individual tooth. To ensure clarity, we present a scale of values arranged in descending order of importance without any rhetoric.

Sequence of factors to be evaluated

1. **Patients**
2. **Oral cavity**
3. **Quadrants**
4. **Teeth**

Pre-treatment considerations

Factors to consider in deciding whether to perform a new endodontic treatment include the following:

- **Asymptomatic patients**
- **Strategic importance of the tooth to be treated**
- **Real efficacy of the retreatment**
  - Chairside time and relative cost
  - Removal and fabrication of new prosthetic item
  - Technical difficulty
  - Hypothetical quality of the future result

Orthograde treatment

As mentioned earlier, the success rate of orthograde retreatments is highly dependent on multiple factors, with the first being the impact of previous treatment[7] on the root canal anatomy.
Chapter 6 will discuss root perforations and cases where treatment was interrupted due to a fractured root canal instrument.
Although cases where the root canal appears relatively normal will be focused upon, their previous treatment has left radiographical evidence of free space, either laterally to the closure or apically to the root canal obturation.
These cases are typical examples of root canal underfilling, leading to significant bacterial growth and an equally significant periapical reaction. Paradoxically, despite the microbiological challenges, these cases tend to exhibit the highest success rates. The consistent inflammatory reaction is often associated with root resorption, which ultimately enlarges the canal lumen. This event is significant due to the complexity of the shaping and disinfection phase and the challenging obturation stage. Detailed examination

CONT'D ON PAGE 48 >

Orthograde repair: Perforation + apical plug in MTA

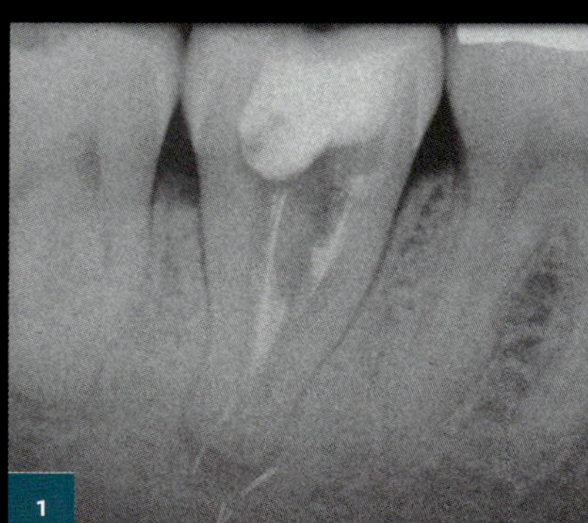

Fig. 1 ■ The patient attending our clinic presented with pain during chewing following a recent unsuccessful root canal treatment. The X-ray shows inconsistent and incomplete therapy and root canal fragments outside the root apex.

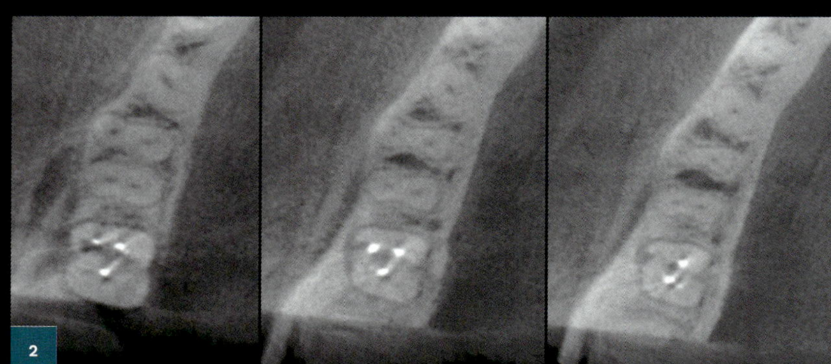

Fig. 2 ■ Axial CBCT images confirm a perforation in the middle third of the buccal aspect of the root, which necessitates orthograde retreatment and consequent repair of the perforation.

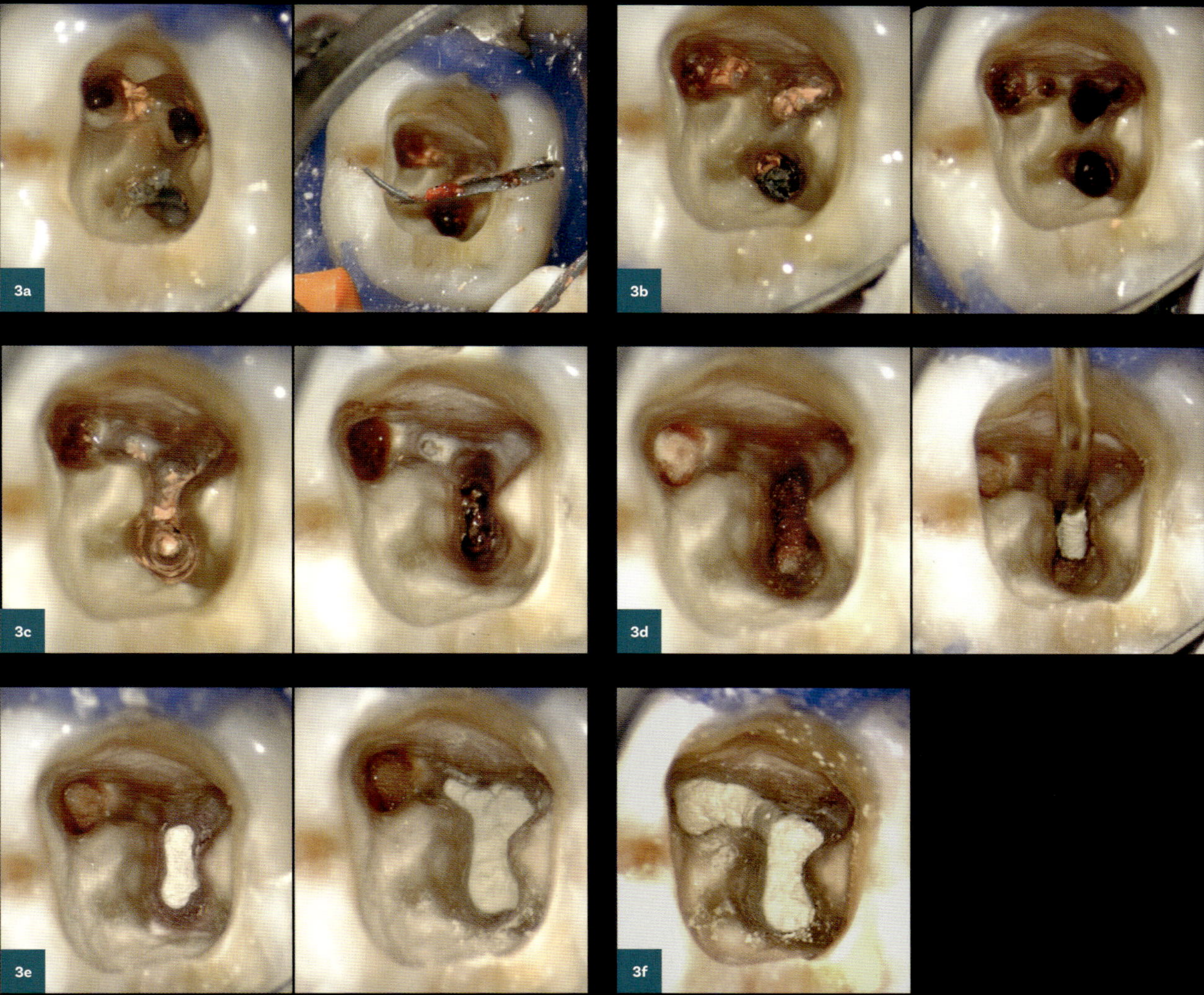

Figs. 3a-f ■ Intraoperative phases of the cleaning of the root system, where distinct anatomy is progressively revealed, indicating tap-root anatomy. The previous treatment's perforation is clearly visible on the vestibular wall. After thoroughly cleaning the root system, both the canal and the perforation are filled using the same material, MTA.

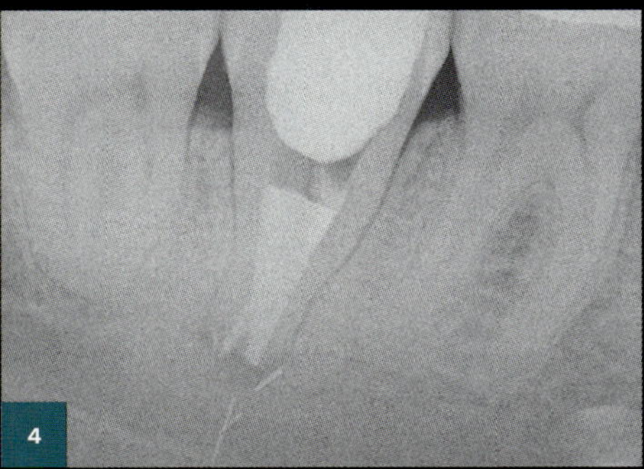

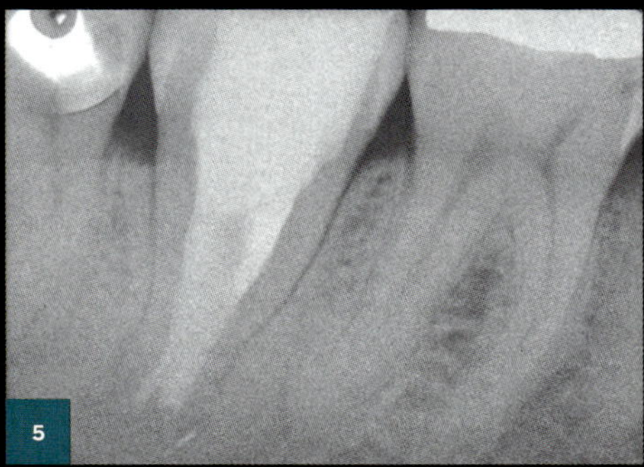

of these situations will be covered in the book's dedicated section on apical root resorption (see pages 81-94). For ease of reading, some contraindications for retreatment are summarised below:

- Unavailability of the patient for treatment
- Clinical history of repeated septic situations
- Presence of an extensive true periodontal lesion
- Presence of adjacent teeth in eruption
- Occlusal trauma
- Unfavourable crown-root ratio
- Complex root canal anatomy
- External root resorption
- Root fractures
- Previous root canal filling quality
- Relationship between lesion size and root canal obturation quality
- Overfilling or excessive material.

Removing posts from the endodontic canal, regardless of their type, may not seem overly complex. In teeth with periapical pathologies, these posts will have non-contiguous areas with the root canal wall. Here, appropriate instrumentation allows for creating space for post removal. Even fibre posts that can be removed using sonic or ultrasonic instruments pose challenges when resinous cements are involved. However, magnification greatly enhances the safety of this procedure.

Root canals can be shaped much better after removing the previous filling material from the endodontic space, preferably mostly without solvents. During this process, non-instrumented spaces or forgotten root canals are discovered, contributing significantly to the pathology.

In fact, the use of solvents has been extensively studied. In some cases, Dotto et al.[21] concluded that solvents offer limited advantages and should only be used in the initial stages of retreatment. Conversely, Chatchawanwirote et al.[22] reported positive results, including a higher probability of removing the intracanal gutta-percha and potential fracture of retreatment instruments with solvent use. Upon examining how laser affects the dissolution of cements and gutta-percha regardless of solvent involvement, Bago et al.[23] found that synergistic solvent use could improve all methods compared in the study, including laser treatment. However, Salgado et al.[24] did not observe significant utility in solvents.

As always, the clinician is crucial in deciding the relevance and methods of use in endodontic therapy. Disinfection plays a fundamental role, with numerous studies confirming that high concentrations of sodium hypochlorite and ultrasound[25] are effective in disinfection. Furthermore, recent advancements like heat carriers for gutta-percha condensation are particularly effective in microbiological control and debris removal within root canals.[26] Although extensive literature supports the synergistic use of a laser for disinfection,[27,28] there is no irrefutable evidence of real efficacy due to heterogeneous study designs and different clinical conditions of application.

The age-old debate on single or multiple-session treatments appears to be definitively resolved, as there are no contraindications in choosing between modalities.[29-31] As highlighted in several systematic reviews, the patient's clinical condition should guide the operator's choice, which does not impact the final treatment outcome.

The advent of bioactive cements, i.e., antibacterial cements that promote the healing of periapical pathologies, has altered the landscape of obturation methods. Although multiple laboratory studies have confirmed these cements' clinical and biological value, there is limited clinical evidence. Recently, Kim et al.[32] demonstrated successful treatments using calcium-silicate cements with the mono-cone technique, with post-operative complications in bioactive cement-filled teeth not being much lower than those with traditional cement based on zinc oxide and eugenol. However, a closer examination of the published works suggests a significant improvement in success rates recorded in teeth treated with bioactive cement. Ricucci et al.[33] recently reported highly biocompatible and bioactive characteristics of tricalcium silicate-based materials used in the obturation treatment of root canals based on the histological results from clinical cases.

Ultimately, each well-applied filling technique can fulfil the essential requirements for the body to start a healing process.

Upper molar with silver cones perforating the maxillary sinus

The presented case is particularly interesting due to its implications for endodontics and ear-nose-throat complications. Specifically, it involves a sinus reaction associated with the presence of silver cones used as filling material that protrudes into the maxillary sinus. The decision-making process for orthograde retreatment took considerable time, with the surgical option posing complexities and associated risks. The orthograde approach presented a two-fold challenge: 1) the removal of the silver cones entailed inherent risks and 2) the subsequent filling needed to be confined strictly within the endodontic space. To address the latter concern, a bioactive material was chosen, which can be carefully delivered into the root canals with a special syringe, followed by the insertion of a gutta-percha cone without vertical compaction to prevent cement extrusion beyond the canal boundaries

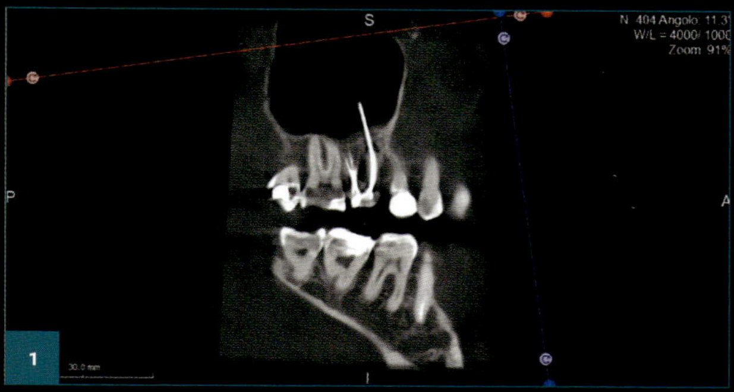

Fig. 1 ■ The CBCT imaging shows the silver cone intrusion inside the maxillary sinus.

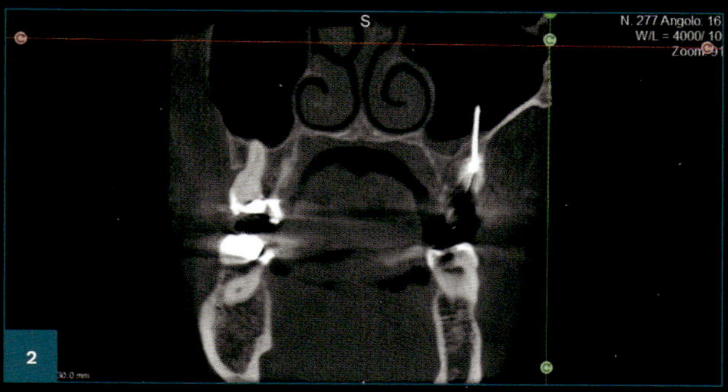

Fig. 2 ■ A different projection of the CBCT confirms the silver cone encroachment inside the maxillary sinus.

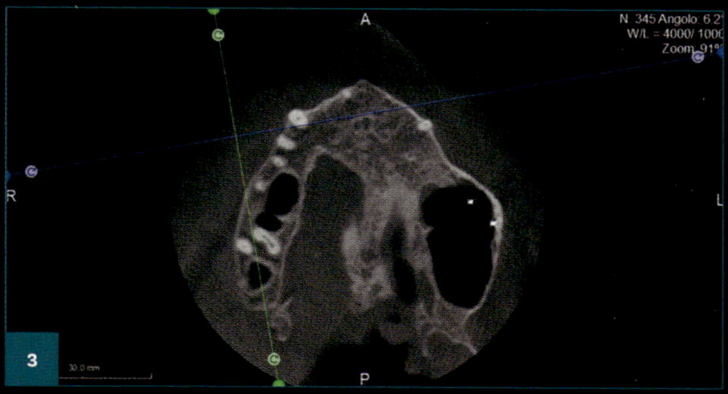

Fig. 3 ■ The axial view confirms the presence of the silver cones in the maxillary sinus.

CONT'D >

> *CONT'D*

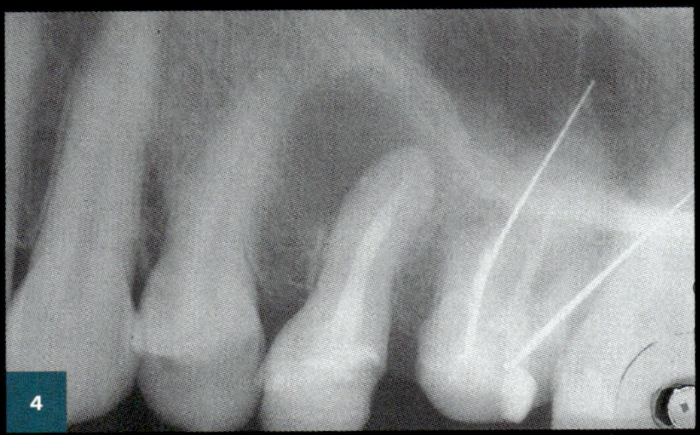

Fig. 4 ■ The intraoral radiograph serves as a valuable dimensional aid in dealing with the case.

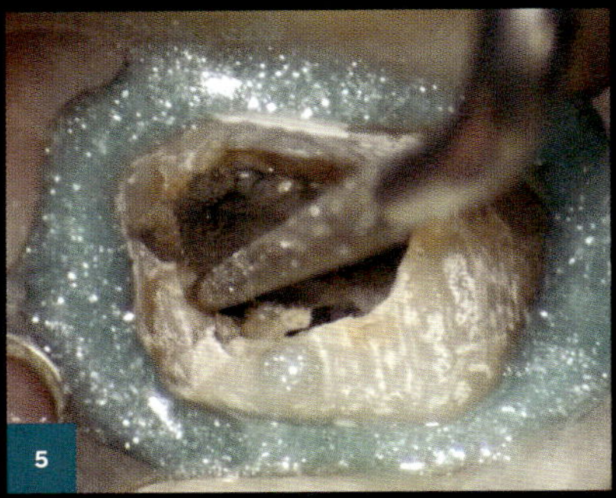

Fig. 5 ■ The cautious use of the ultrasonic tip allows isolation of the occlusal part of the cone.

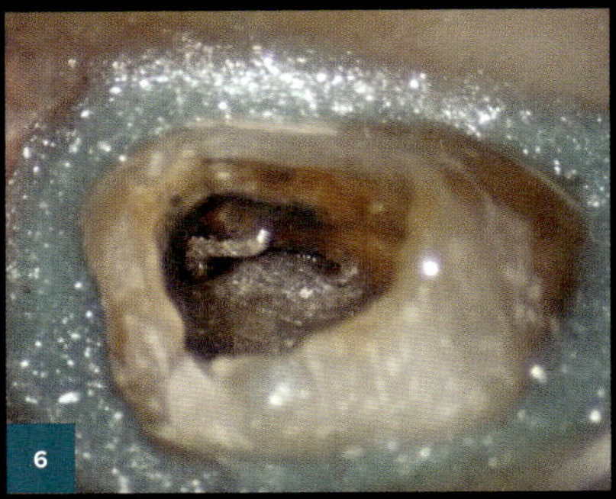

Fig. 6 ■ The silver cone is ready to be grasped with a Stieglitz-type forceps.

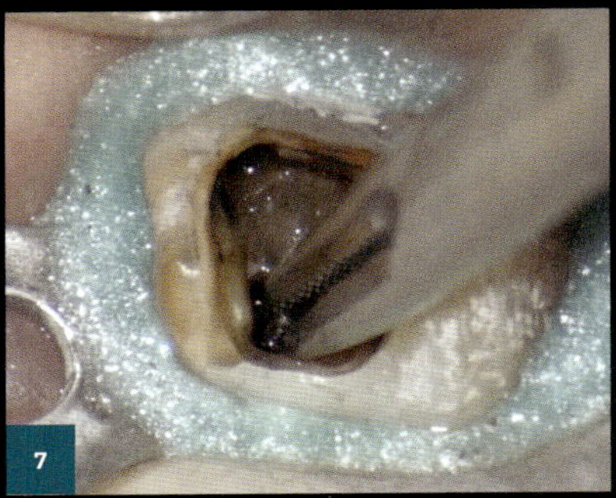

Fig. 7 ■ A phase of the cone extraction process.

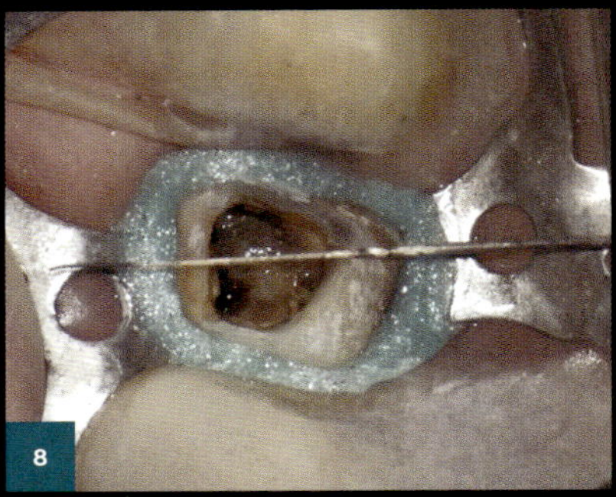

Fig. 8 ■ Extracted cone.

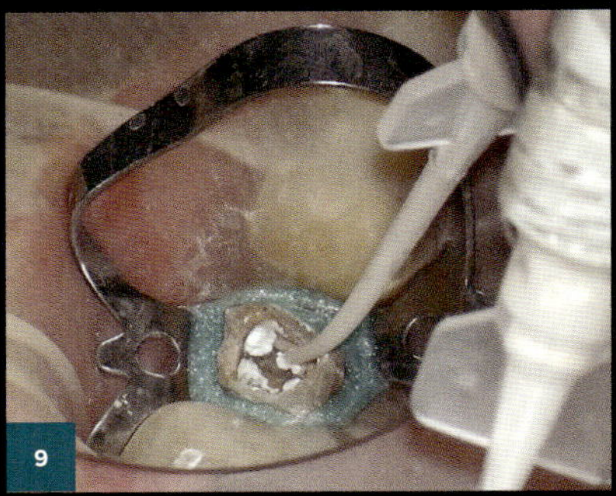

Fig. 9 ■ After being adequately shaped, the canal is filled with bioactive cement.

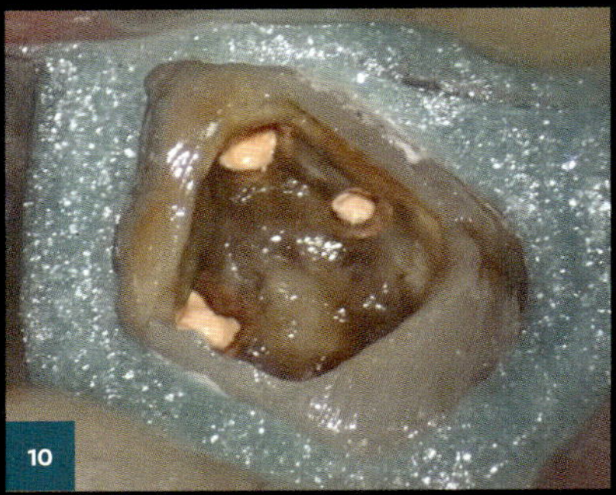

Fig. 10 ■ Root canal closure is completed with gutta-percha cones.

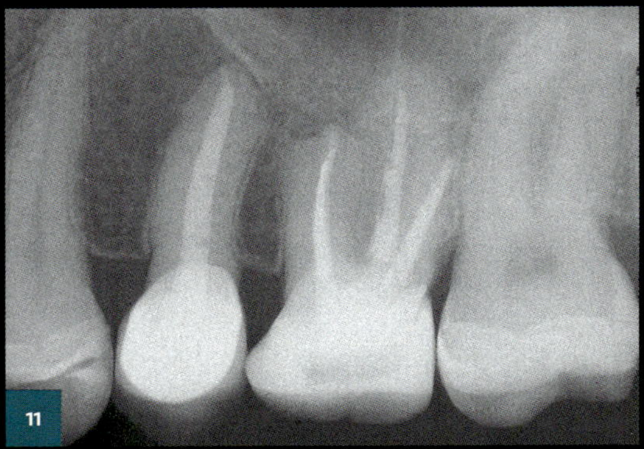

Fig. 11 ■ The radiographic image at the end of therapy.

In general, considering the individual items, we can easily understand how variables unrelated to endodontic therapy and those influenced by clinician's treatments intertwine in a list of possibilities which, when adhered to, can tip the balance towards either success or failure of the case as specified in **Table 5.4**.

Table 5.4 ■ The determininants of success or failure of a retreatment.

Factors that do not determine the failure of retreatment	Factors that lead to the failure of retreatment
■ Type of tooth ■ Tooth position ■ Age and sex of patient ■ Number of appointments required to do the treatment ■ Type of obturation material ■ Pre- or post-operative pain	■ Persistence of the infection ■ Incorrect shaping-canal transportation (haemorrhage) ■ Irritation of the periapical tissues by chemical agents ■ Minor and major iatrogenic errors (blockages and/or perforations)

Retrograde Treatment

Periapical lesions of endodontic origin can be treated through surgery, provided that established criteria are followed and performed with excellence. However, these findings are now widely accepted. In a systematic review, Del Fabbro et al.[34,35] emphasised various variables and found that surgical treatment is equivalent, if not slightly superior, to orthograde treatment in the short term. Microscopy has been considered a determining factor in achieving favourable results in 90% of cases. In fact, studies conducted by specialists equipped with operating microscopes and appropriate instruments have yielded encouraging results, suggesting that a well-performed surgery is usually simpler yet equally effective as a similar orthograde procedure.[36]

Setzer et al.[37] compiled data from the literature and concluded that endodontic surgery using traditional systems evidently yields favourable outcomes in 59% of cases, whereas microsurgical techniques can approach an overwhelming 94%.

The choice of retrograde sealing materials has been a long standing dispute, which, according to the Authors, would have clinically similar results.

Large radiolucent lesion on a lower molar resolved with immediate endodontic surgery

An emblematic case in endodontic surgery is encountered when a molar that does not heal despite a discreet root canal treatment must always lead one to suspect an extraradicular infection, which is far from infrequent

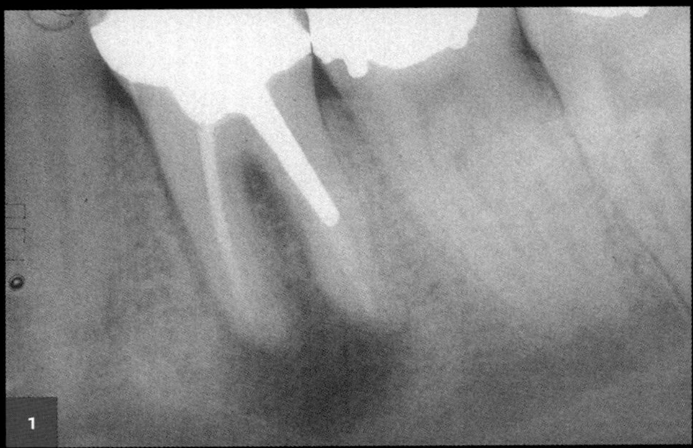

Fig. 1 ■ The pre-operative radiograph and the clinical examination strongly indicate the presence of an extraradicular infection.

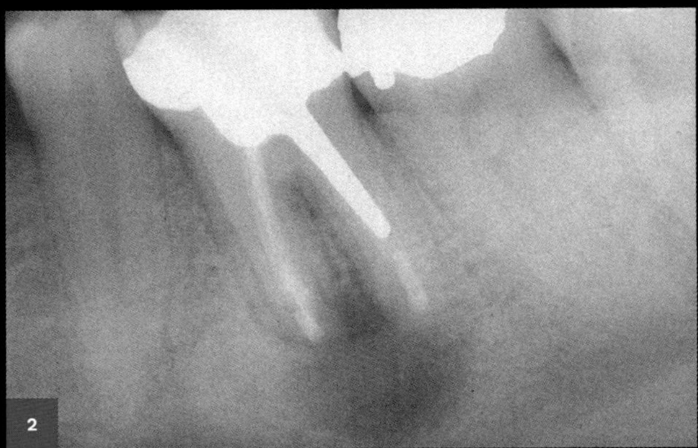

Fig. 2 ■ The apical resection with generous ostectomy enabled the effective sealing of the root apices possible using zinc oxide eugenol cement supplement with ethoxybenzoic acid.

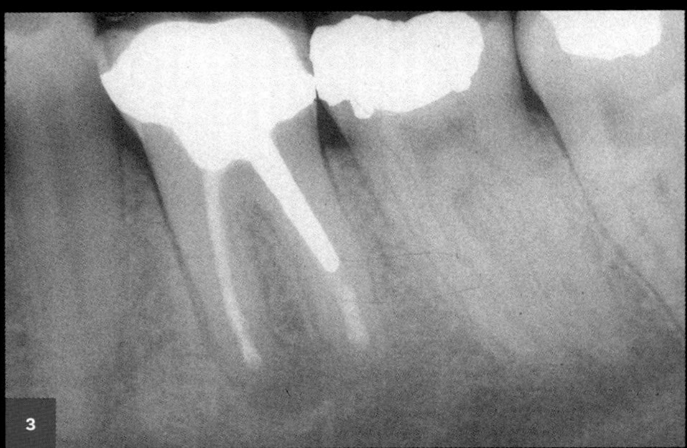

Fig. 3 ■ The case was resolved after a year of careful management.

Fracture initiating apically

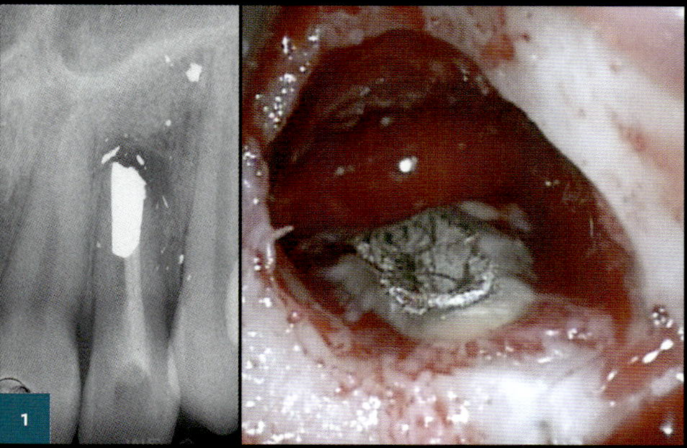

1

Fig. 1 ■ Pre-operative X-ray and intraoperative photo reveal the consequences of previous unsuitable root canal therapy due to past trauma and an even more incongruous surgical endodontic intervention with silver amalgam. These therapies led to the formation of an apical lesion, clinically presenting with pain and evident soft tissue swelling in the fornix region.

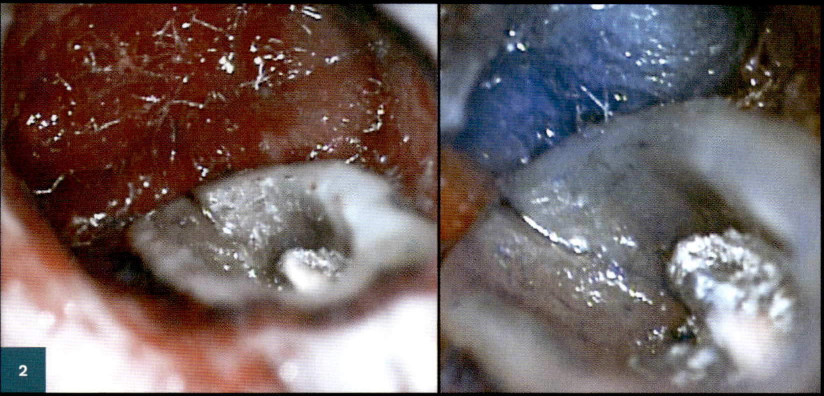

2

Fig. 2 ■ During intraoperative phases, the thin root walls and the improper use of the filling material led to the identification of an apical fracture line.

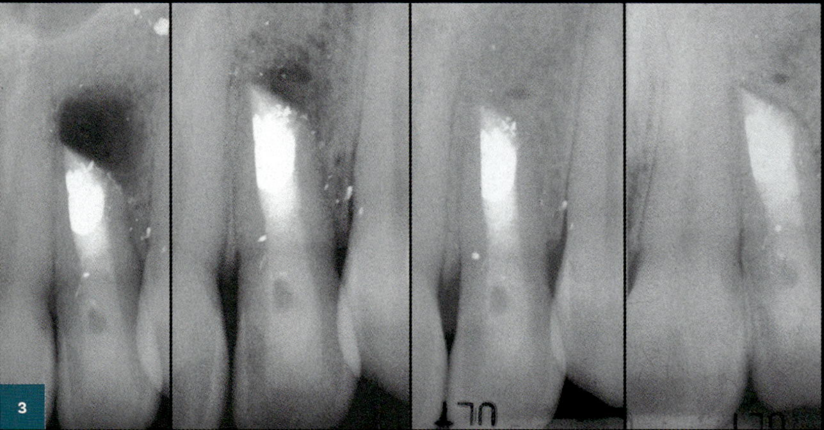

3

Fig. 3 ■ Post-operative radiograph and subsequent radiographic assessment. The radiological images clearly show an intriguing bone healing despite the fracture. During surgical re-entry, mineral trioxide aggregate (MTA) was used, a more appropriate material compared to amalgam, especially considering the size of the foramen and the thickness of the root margins. The wound has fully healed, and the radiolucent area away from the apex and centre of the lesion represents a typical apical scar characterized bynon-mineralized fibrous tissue.

Although mineral trioxide aggregate (MTA) appears to be the best choice, a review by Tang et al.[38] clearly indicates that it is not superior to zinc oxide eugenol cement (IRM). The meta-analysis by Kohli et al.[39] found no differences in positive outcomes when comparing cases treated with zinc oxide-eugenol cement with or without adding ethoxybenzoic acid and calcium-silicate cements.
Other clinical recommendations are related to handling the materials during delicate surgical phases. Materials that exhibit sufficient stability for introduction and compaction into retrograde cavities, produced by sonic or ultrasonic instrumentation, are equally effective as compared with materials with higher biocompatibility and a slightly stronger antibacterial potency. However, the latter materials are difficult to handle and risk altering their composition (ratio between powder and liquid) during the setting phase due to the effect of periradicular fluids.

Combined orthograde-retrograde treatment

The combined orthograde-retrograde treatment[40-43] (ORT) is worth mentioning, as it is not uncommon but is well-suited for situations where a significant but not complete portion of the root canal system can be easily instrumented and disinfected. In contrast, the apical portion requires a different approach.
This treatment is especially useful when the instruments separated at the apical level cannot be retrieved without compromising the canal walls.

Orthograde perforation repair with surgical removal of the fractured instrument

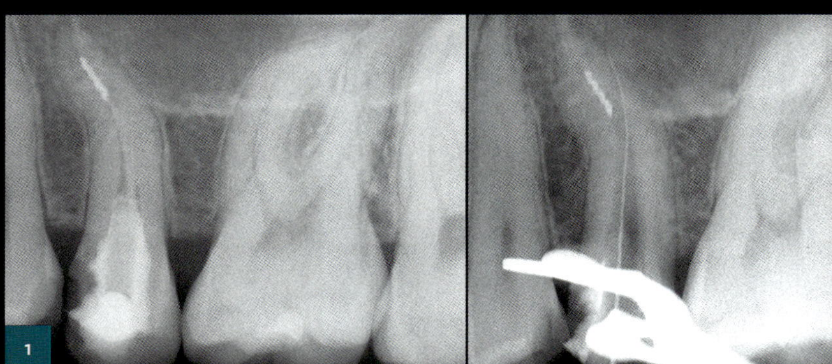

Fig. 1 ■ Pre-op Rx. The patient was referred for the removal of an instrument fragment in the apical third of the root, which is causing spontaneous pain and discomfort during chewing. The root exhibits an important buccolingual curvature, obstructing the visibility of the fragment and contributing to the pain. In fact, the previous treatment created a perforation in the curvature area. Considering the unique anatomy, the plan is to repair the perforation using an orthograde approach to salvage a considerable portion of the root with the subsequent endodontic surgery. Since the root defect has already been sealed with the orthograde obturation, the surgical approach is sufficient for fragment removal and subsequent retrograde filling to complete the case.

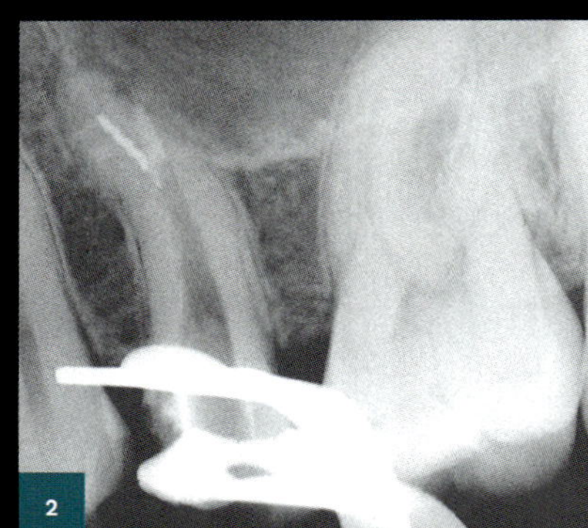

Fig. 2 ■ Post-op Rx of orthograde perforation repair.

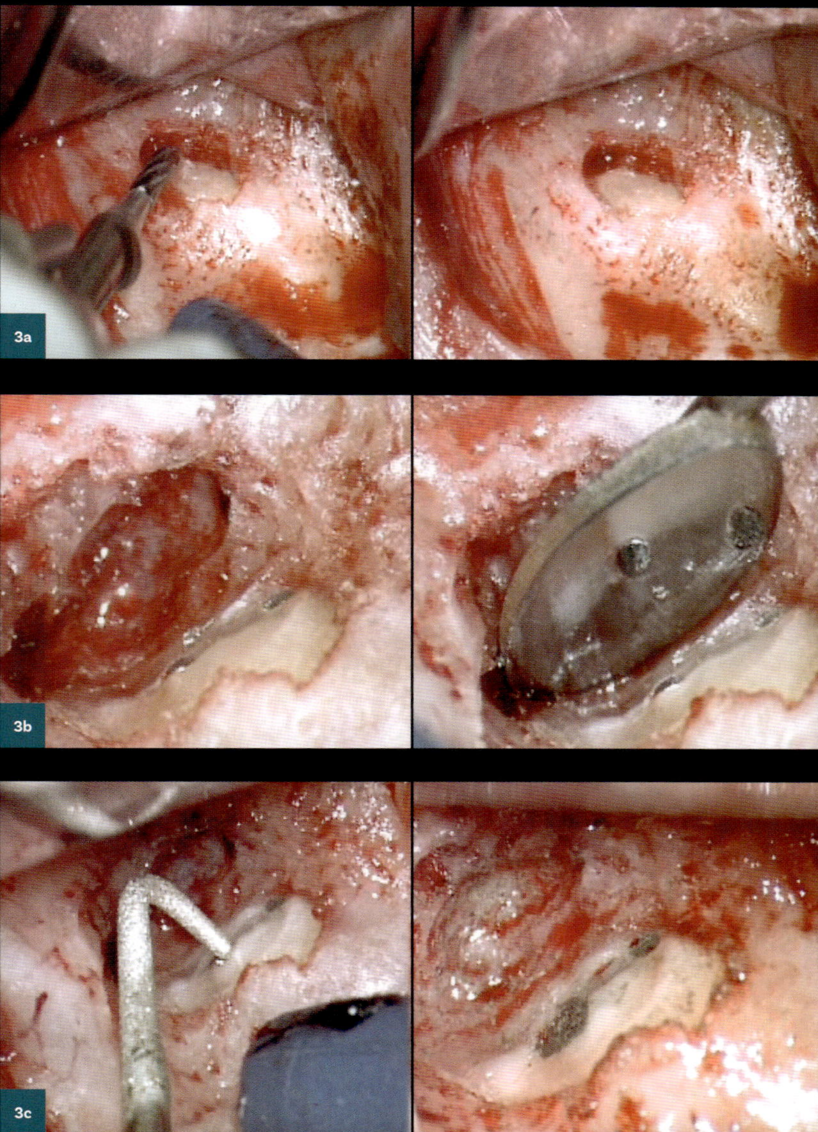

Figs. 3a-c ■ Intraoperative p
surgical endodontics: The fragn
successfully removed using a re
approach, followed by the appli
the retrograde MTA (mineral tri
gregate) seal. The photos show,
the maxillary sinus membrane
to the surgical cavity, the fractur
ment, the seal of the perforatio
retrograde root canal filling.

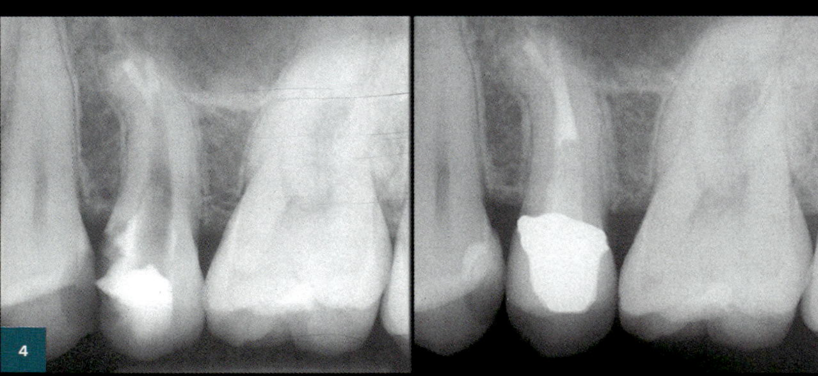

Fig. 4 ■ Post-operative Rx an
at 17 years. The final X-ray and l
follow-up demonstrate comple
graphic healing of the clinical cas
preservation of an important pa
root tissue, achieved through a
tion of orthograde and surgical e
tic strategies.

Opting for this dual approach (ORT) ensures an incomparable antegrade and retrograde seal, with minimal damage to both the root canal and the root components. Despite limited publications on this topic,[44] the success rate appears to be quite high based on the Authors' experience, with a positive result rate of 95-98% of treatments carried out with follow-up of over ten years. However, it is important to acknowledge the uncertainties associated with both methods, and they cannot guarantee absolute success rates.

Additionally, the treatment choice must consider the presence of extraradicular bacteria in selected microbiological niches, which are well-documented for fuelling inflammatory reactions. When endodontic treatment or retreatment fails to eradicate this septic component, periapical surgery becomes the only viable solution for these pathologies.

Double perforation and salvage with endodontic surgery

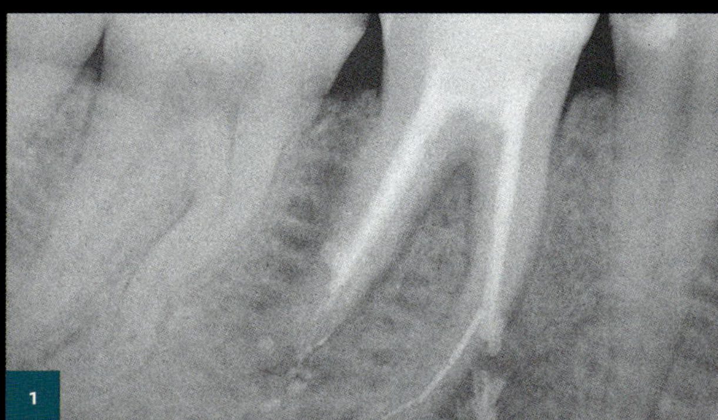

Fig. 1 ■ The patient initially received a significantly flawed root canal treatment, followed by an even more erroneous retreatment. During an attempt to remove a broken instrument, the colleague unintentionally caused two perforations: one in the mesial root and another in the middle third of the distal root.

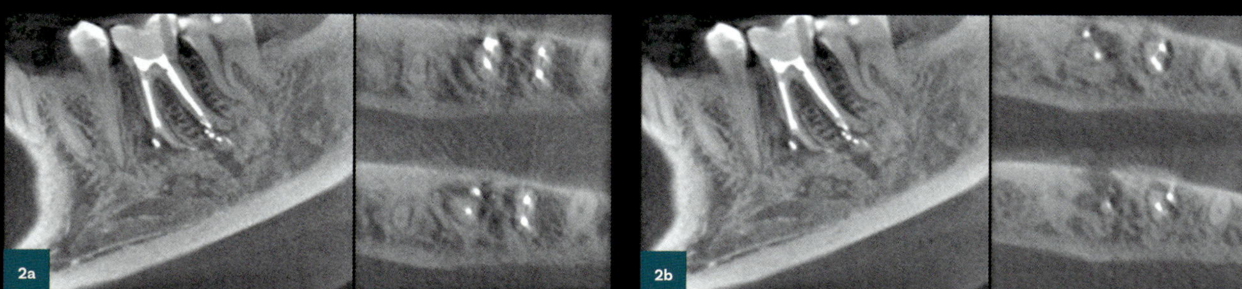

Figs. 2a,b ■ The CBCT check-up revealed no formation lesions, leading to the decision of attempting surgical recovery due to the excellent periodontal support.

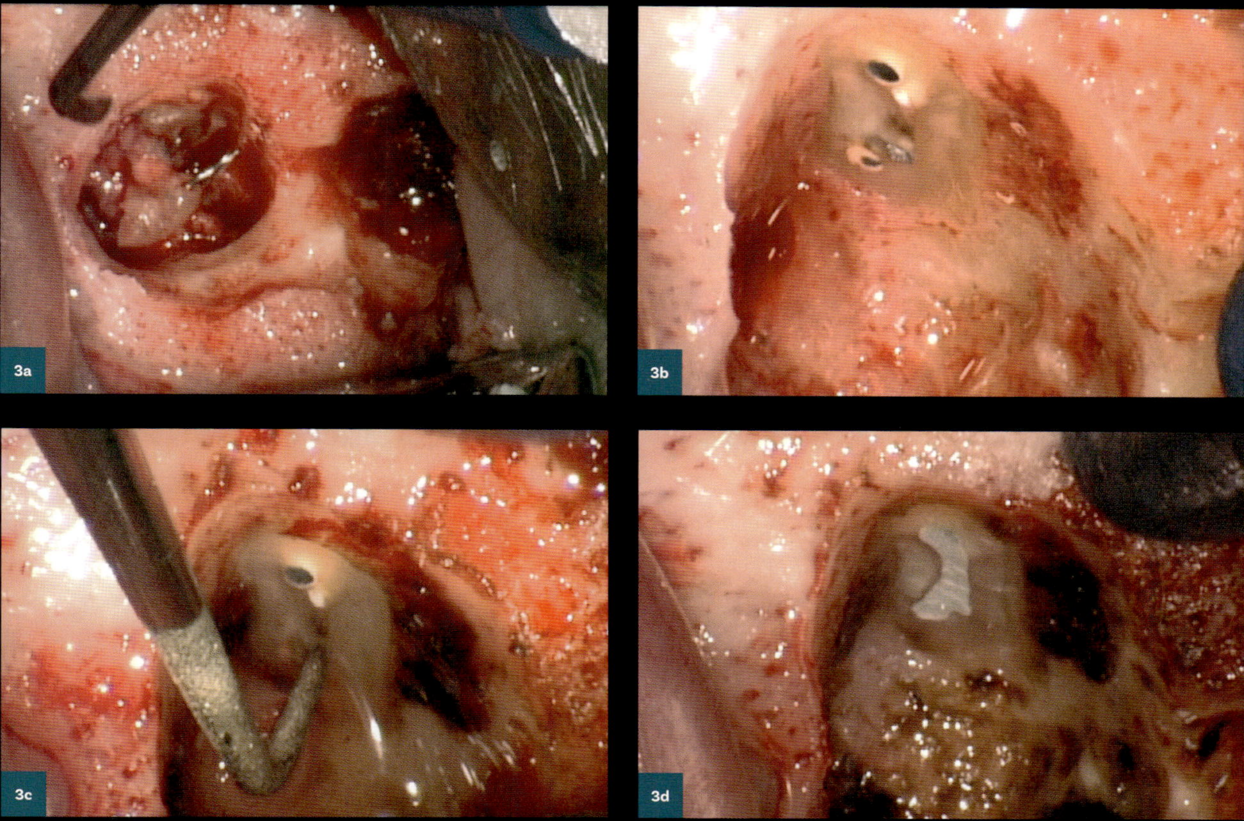

Figs. 3a-d ■ Intraoperative images of the mesial root show the different stages of apex removal, including the endodontic instrument fragment and the preparation of the apical foramen, which also involves addressing the isthmus between the two canals. Retrograde filling is carried out using Super EBA cement.

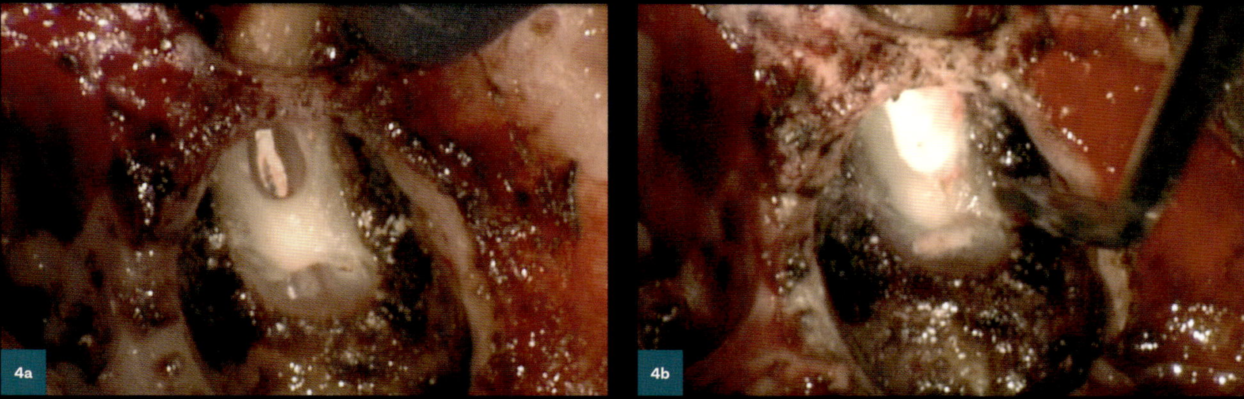

> *CONT'D*

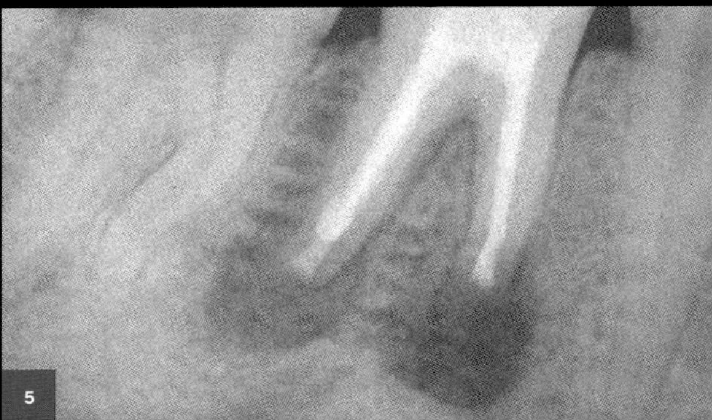

Fig. 5 ■ Post-op Rx.

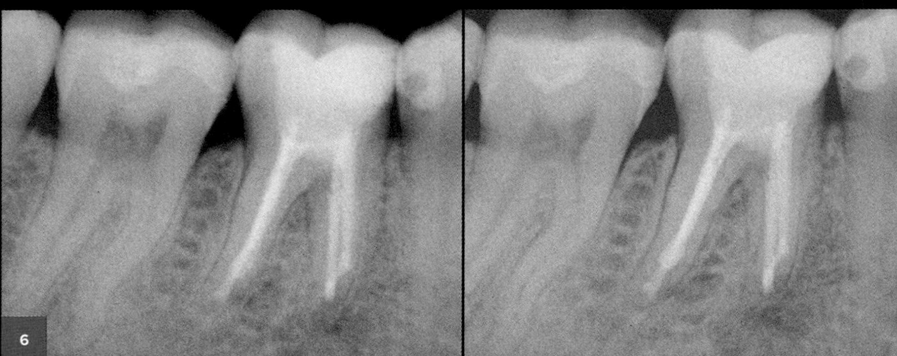

Fig. 6 ■ Check-up at 6 months and one year: the lesion appears completely healed.

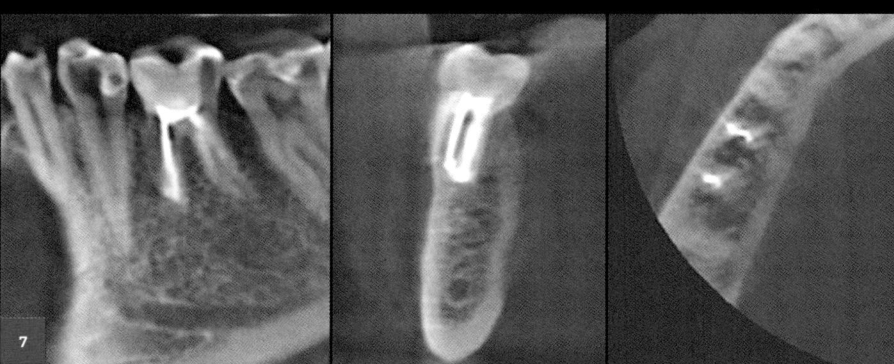

Fig. 7 ■ Radiographic control with a CBCT examination 5 years after surgery. Note the complete restitution ad integrum of the mandibular cortex, particularly visible especially in the axial and coronal sections of the examination.

Surgical repair of a buccal perforation

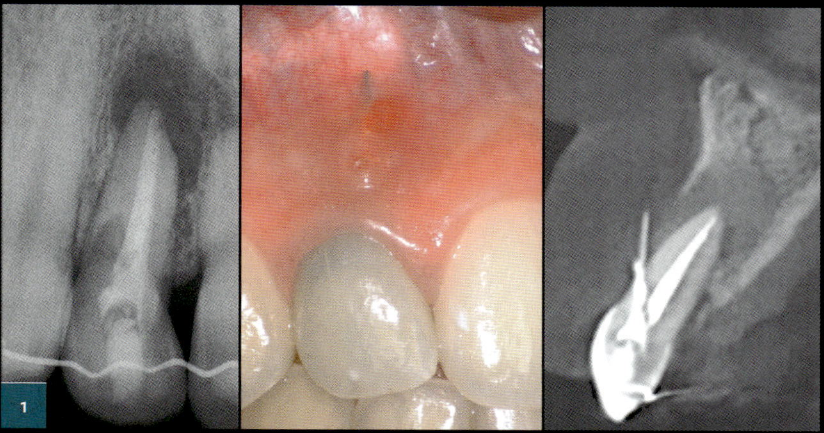

Fig. 1 ■ The pre-operative radiograph does not provide a clear interpretation of the problem with this right lateral incisor. However, clinically, the young patient exhibits redness of the fornix with tenderness upon palpation. Upon closer examination, a dark-coloured mass is visible in the transparency, emerging from the root. A CBCT scan confirms the diagnosis: a large lesion affecting nearly the entire root, both buccally and apically. The perforation contains a core of Thermafil that extends several millimetres into the periodontal tissues.

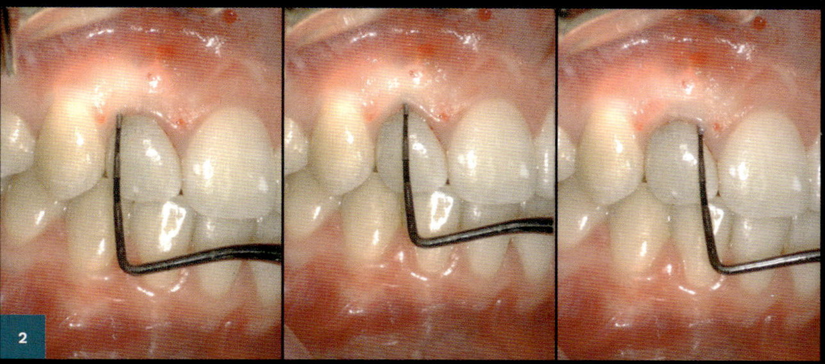

Fig. 2 ■ Clinical images show the absence of probing.

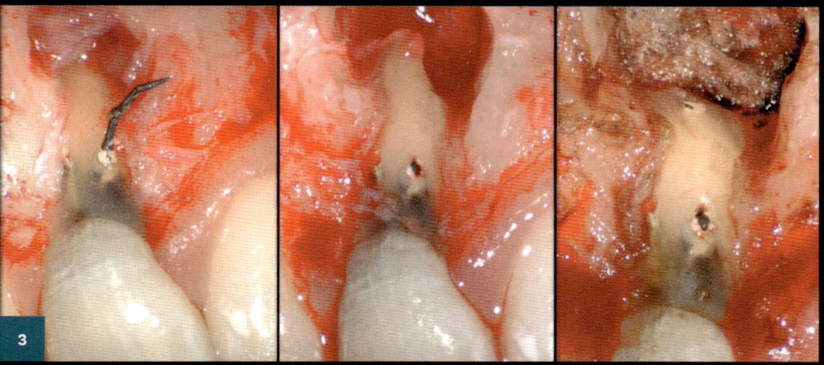

Fig. 3 ■ Photos after flap elevation show two perforations, a buccal bone dehiscence, and a periapical lesion.

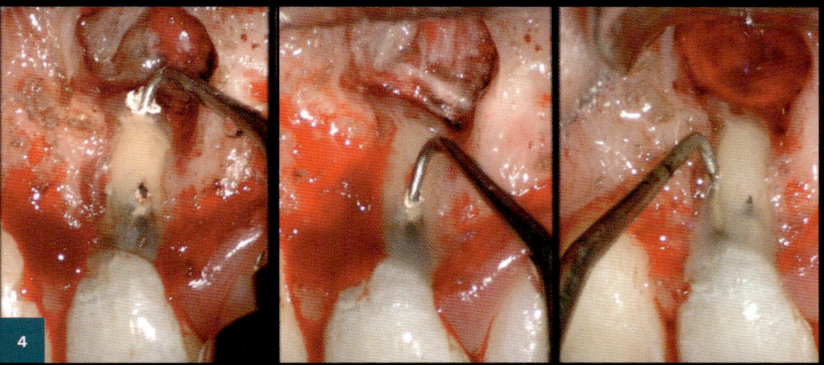

Fig. 4 ■ Resection of the apex and retrograde and buccal perforations are prepared.

CONT'D >

> CONT'D

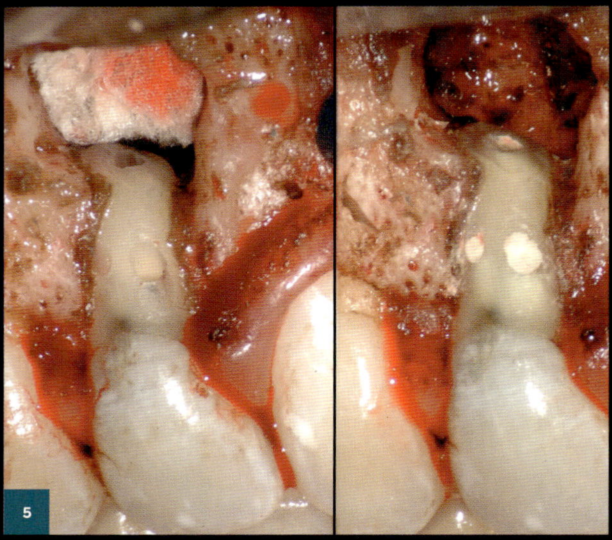

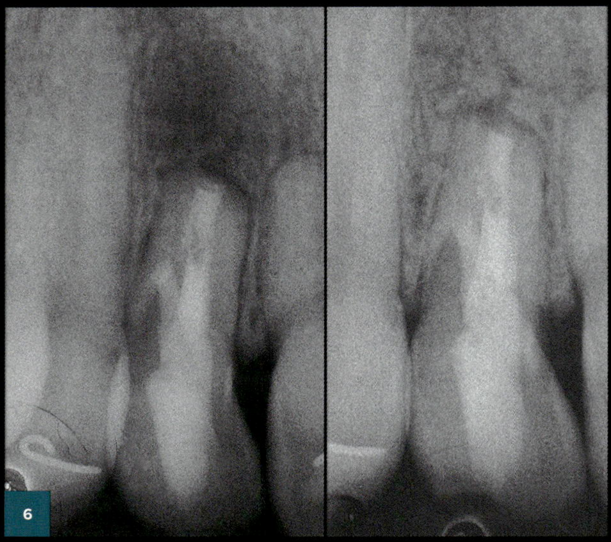

Fig. 5 ■ Perforations were repaired using MTA, which was also used for the retrograde filling.

Fig. 6 ■ Post-operative X-ray and 12-month follow-up. Radiographically demonstrates complete healing of the apical and periradicular tissues.

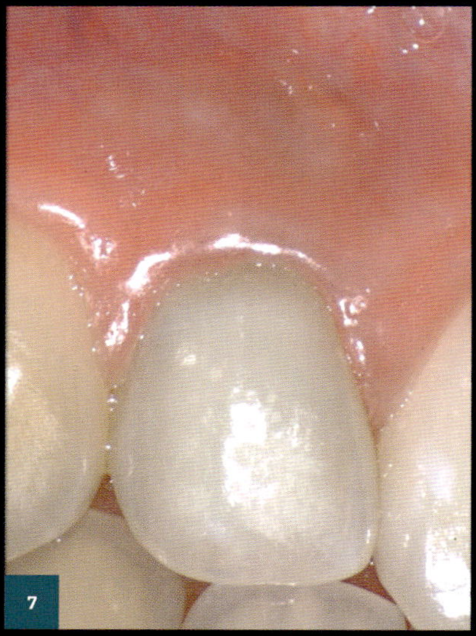

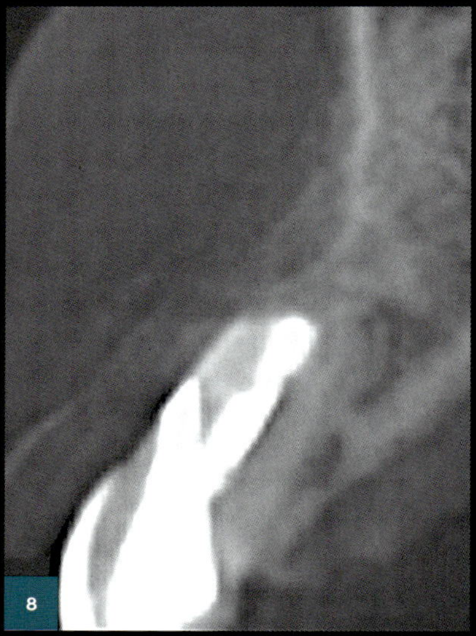

Fig. 7 ■ The clinical photo shows complete healing of the soft tissues, with complete resolution of the symptoms.

Fig. 8 ■ The control CBCT allows us to evaluate the *restitution ad integrum* of the alveolar process, ensuring compatible clinical healing for the young patient and preparing the area for a possible future implant-prosthetic solution for the replacement of this tooth.

Bibliography

1. Tiburcio-Machado CS, Michelon C, Zanatta FB, Gomes MS, Marin JA, Bier CA. The global prevalence of apical periodontitis: a systematic review and meta-analysis. *Int Endod J.* 2021;54(5):712-735.
2. Wigsten E, Jonasson P, EndoReCo, Kvist T. Indications for root canal treatment in a Swedish county dental service: patient- and tooth-specific characteristics. *Int Endod J.* 2019;52(2):158-168.
3. Boreak N. Effectiveness of Artificial Intelligence Applications Designed for Endodontic Diagnosis, Decision-making, and Prediction of Prognosis: A Systematic Review. *J Contemp Dent Pract.* 2020;21(8):926-934.
4. Herbst CS, Schwendicke F, Krois J, Herbst SR. Association between patient-, tooth- and treatment-level factors and root canal treatment failure: A retrospective longitudinal and machine learning study. *J Dent.* 2022;117:103937.
5. Liew J, Zainal Abidin I, Cook N, Kanagasingam S. Clinical decision-making in complex endodontic cases between postgraduate students across dental specialties at a UK dental school: A pilot study. *Eur J Dent Educ.* 2022;26(4):707-716.
6. Taha NA, Albashaireh ZS, Alfied RG. Endodontic decision making for asymptomatic root-filled teeth with apical periodontitis. A radiographic survey. *Aust Endod J.* 2019;45(1):40-45.
7. Gorni FG, Gagliani MM. The outcome of endodontic retreatment: a 2-yr follow-up. *J Endod.* 2004;30(1):1-4.
8. Tosun S, Karataslioglu E, Tulgar MM, Derindag G. Fractal analysis and periapical index evaluation of multivisit nonsurgical endodontic retreatment: A retrospective study. *Oral Surg Oral Med Oral Pathol Oral Radiol.* 2022;133(2):245-251.
9. Yamaguchi M, Noiri Y, Itoh Y, et al. Factors that cause endodontic failures in general practices in Japan. *BMC Oral Health.* 2018;18(1):70.
10. Tifooni A, Al-Nuaimi N, Dawood A, Mannocci F, Patel S. Validation of the effectiveness of the Dental Practicality Index in predicting the outcome of root canal retreatments. *Int Endod J.* 2019;52(10):1403-1409.
11. Santos-Junior AO, De Castro Pinto L, Mateo-Castillo JF, Pinheiro CR. Success or failure of endodontic treatments: A retrospective study. *J Conserv Dent.* 2019;22(2):129-132.
12. Cujé J, Bargholz C, Hülsmann M. The outcome of retained instrument removal in a specialist practice. *Int Endod J.* 2010;43(7):545-554.
13. Madarati AA, Qualtrough AJ, Watts DC. Endodontists experience using ultrasonics for removal of intra-canal fractured instruments. *Int Endod J.* 2010;43(4):301-305.
14. Terauchi Y, Sexton C, Bakland LK, Bogen G. Factors Affecting the Removal Time of Separated Instruments. *J Endod.* 2021;47(8):1245-1252.
15. Laukkanen E, Vehkalahti MM, Kotiranta AK. Impact of type of tooth on outcome of non-surgical root canal treatment. *Clin Oral Investig.* 2019;23(11):4011-4018.
16. Gudac J, Hellén-Halme K, Machiulskiene V. Prognostic validity of the Periapical and Endodontic Status Scale for the radiographically assessed 2-year treatment outcomes in teeth with apical periodontitis: a prospective clinical study. *BMC Oral Health.* 2021;21(1):354.
17. Bhagavatula P, Moore A, Rein L, Szabo A, Ibrahim M. Multi-state outcome analysis of treatment interventions after failure of non-surgical root canal treatment: a 13-year retrospective study. *J Appl Oral Sci.* 2021;29:e20201079.
18. Olcay K, Ataoglu H, Belli S. Evaluation of Related Factors in the Failure of Endodontically Treated Teeth: A Cross-sectional Study. *J Endod.* 2018;44(1):38-45.
19. Riis A, Taschieri S, Del Fabbro M, Kvist T. Tooth Survival after Surgical or Nonsurgical Endodontic Retreatment: Long-term Follow-up of a Randomized Clinical Trial. *J Endod.* 2018;44(10):1480-1486.
20. Al-Nuaimi N, Ciapryna S, Chia M, Patel S, Mannocci F. A prospective study on the effect of coronal tooth structure loss on the 4-year clinical survival of root canal retreated teeth and retrospective validation of the Dental Practicality Index. *Int Endod J.* 2020;53(8):1040-1049.
21. Dotto L, Sarkis-Onofre R, Bacchi A, Pereira GKR. The use of solvents for gutta-percha dissolution/removal during endodontic retreatments: A scoping review. *J Biomed Mater Res B Appl Biomater.* 2021;109(6):890-901.
22. Chatchawanwirote Y, Yanpiset K, Jantarat J. Effect of solvent on root canal filling material removal by two different rotary file systems in C-shaped root canals. *Aust Endod J.* 2022;48(3):487-493.
23. Bago I, Plotino G, Katić M, et al. Effect of a novel laser-initiated photoacoustic activation of a solvent or sodium hypochlorite in the removal of filling remnants after retreatment of curved root canals. *Photodiagnosis Photodyn Ther.* 2021;36:102535.
24. Salgado KR, de Castro RF, Prado MC, Brandão GA, da Silva JM, da Silva EJNL. Cleaning Ability of Irrigants and Orange Oil Solvent Combination in the Removal of Root Canal Filling Materials. *Eur Endod J.* 2019;4(1):33-37.
25. Crozeta BM, Chaves de Souza L, Correa Silva-Sousa YT, Sousa-Neto MD, Jaramillo DE, Silva RM. Evaluation of Passive Ultrasonic Irrigation and GentleWave System as Adjuvants in Endodontic Retreatment. *J Endod.* 2020;46(9):1279-1285.
26. Iandolo A, Abdellatif D, Amato M, et al. Dentinal tubule penetration and root canal cleanliness following ultrasonic activation of intracanal-heated sodium hypochlorite. *Aust Endod J.* 2020;46(2):204-209.
27. Genc Sen O, Kaya M. Effect of Root Canal Disinfection with a Diode Laser on Postoperative Pain After Endodontic Retreatment. *Photobiomodul Photomed Laser Surg.* 2019;37(2):85-90.
28. Chen Y, Chen XL, Zou XL, Chen SZ, Zou J, Wang Y. Efficacy of low-level laser therapy in pain management after root canal treatment or retreatment: a systematic review. *Lasers Med Sci.* 2019;34(7):1305-1316.
29. Figini L, Lodi G, Gorni F, Gagliani M. Single versus multiple visits for endodontic treatment of permanent teeth. *Cochrane Database Syst Rev.* 2007(4):CD005296.

30. Figini L, Lodi G, Gorni F, Gagliani M. Single versus multiple visits for endodontic treatment of permanent teeth: a Cochrane systematic review. *J Endod.* 2008;34(9):1041-1047.

31. Santos-Junior AO, De Castro Pinto L, Mateo-Castillo JF, Pinheiro CR. Success or failure of endodontic treatments: A retrospective study. *J Conserv Dent.* 2019;22(2):129-132.

32. Kim JH, Cho SY, Choi Y, Kim DH, Shin SJ, Jung IY. Clinical Efficacy of Sealer-based Obturation Using Calcium Silicate Sealers: A Randomized Clinical Trial. *J Endod.* 2022;48(2):144-151.

33. Ricucci D, Grande NM, Plotino G, Tay FR. Histologic Response of Human Pulp and Periapical Tissues to Tricalcium Silicate-based Materials: A Series of Successfully Treated Cases. *J Endod.* 2020;46(2):307-317.

34. Del Fabbro M, Taschieri S, Testori T, Francetti L, Weinstein RL. Surgical versus non-surgical endodontic re-treatment for periradicular lesions. *Cochrane Database Syst Rev.* 2007;(3):CD005511.

35. Taschieri S, Del Fabbro M, Testori T, Weinstein RL. Endodontic reoperation using an endoscope and microsurgical instruments: One year follow-up. *Br J Oral Maxillofac Surg.* 2007;45(7):582-585.

36. Tsesis I, Faivishevsky V, Kfir A, Rosen E. Outcome of surgical endodontic treatment performed by a modern technique: a meta-analysis of literature. *J Endod.* 2009;35(11):1505-1511.

37. Setzer FC, Kohli MR, Shah SB, Karabucak B, Kim S. Outcome of endodontic surgery: a meta-analysis of the literature--Part 2: Comparison of endodontic microsurgical techniques with and without the use of higher magnification. *J Endod.* 2012;38(1):1-10.

38. Tang Y, Li X, Yin S. Outcomes of MTA as root-end filling in endodontic surgery: a systematic review. *Quintessence Int.* 2010;41(7):557-566.

39. Kohli MR, Berenji H, Setzer FC, et al. Outcome of Endodontic Surgery: A Meta-analysis of the Literature-Part 3: Comparison of Endodontic Microsurgical Techniques with 2 Different Root-end Filling Materials. *J Endod.* 2018;44(6):923-931.

40. Evans M. Combined endodontic and surgical treatment of a three-rooted maxillary first premolar. *Aust Endod J.* 2004;30(2):53-55.

41. Ozçakir Tomruk C, Tanalp J, Yurdagüven H, Ersev H. Endodontic and surgical management of a maxillary lateral incisor with type III dens invaginatus: a 12-month follow-up. *Oral Surg Oral Med Oral Pathol Oral Radiol Endod.* 2008;106(3):e84-e87.

42. Karabucak B, Setzer FC. Conventional and surgical retreatment of complex periradicular lesions with periodontal involvement. *J Endod.* 2009;35(9):1310-1315.

43. Del Fabbro M, Corbella S, Sequeira-Byron P, et al. Endodontic procedures for retreatment of periapical lesions. *Cochrane Database Syst Rev.* 2016;10(10):CD005511.

44. Dudeja PG, Dudeja KK, Garg A, Srivastava D, Grover S. Management of a Previously Treated, Calcified, and Dilacerated Maxillary Lateral Incisor: A Combined Nonsurgical/Surgical Approach Assisted by Cone-beam Computed Tomography. *J Endod.* 2016;42(6):984-988.

6

Managing endodontic complications: perforations, stripping, and removal of fractured instrument fragments

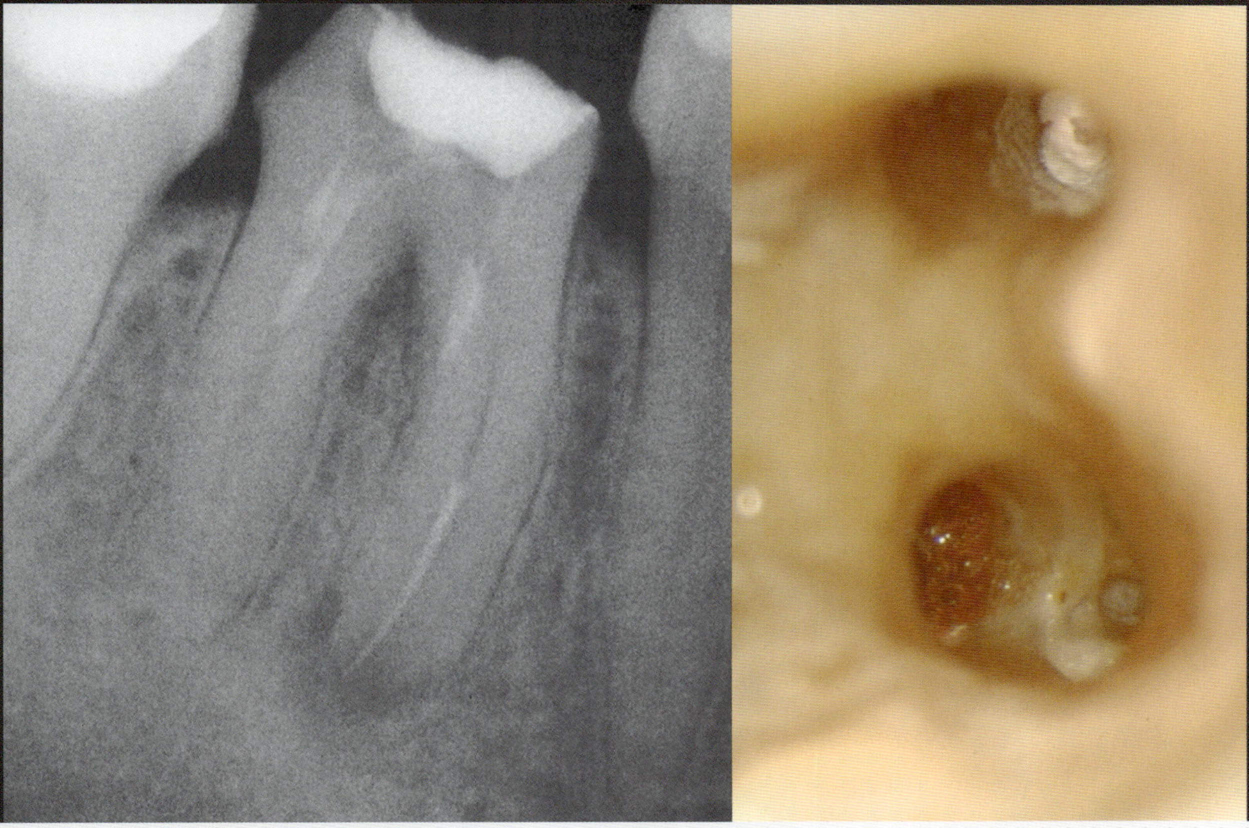

We will dedicate a chapter to these unique aspects by summarizing the possible iatrogenic errors during endodontic treatments.

Once an error occurs, the clinician has two options: resolve the problem independently to minimize side effects or refer the case to a more experienced clinician. Since both options usually yield favourable outcomes, further dwelling is unnecessary. However, if these errors go unidentified and are "buried" underneath other endodontic procedures, they can lead to irreparable consequences or temporary solutions with limited survival rates (maximum of ten years).

Perforations

Perforations are intriguing in endodontic retreatments due to their challenging nature and uncertain long-term prognosis despite the constant advancements in treatment techniques.

A previous study by the authors of this book[1-2] highlighted several prognostic factors that could guide various phases of retreatment, including a periodontal probing depth exceeding 5 mm as a very unfavourable prognostic indicator for any periradicular problems linked to perforations. Recent 14-year-old survey data suggests plateaued success rates of 50% for treating dento-radicular perforations, with teeth displaying a periodontal probing depth of over 5 mm having a survival rate below 20% after 14 years, a relatively low percentage. However, tooth extraction should not be immediately considered while exploring other available options. Opting to repair a perforation should be viewed as a bone-saving measure, especially when there is a desire to delay the implant placement until it becomes the only viable option. Accurate identification and subsequent sealing of these pathological communications between the endodontic space and periodontium with suitable materials are crucial.

As mentioned in other chapters of this book, using an operating microscope is essential for precisely performing these procedures. Additionally, using sonic or ultrasonic sources further enhances the clinical phases of debridement and demarcation of the iatrogenic dentinal defects.

Mineral trioxide aggregate (MTA) is universally considered the ideal obturation material, a highly biocompatible compound of calcium silicates with strong antibacterial and excellent osteo-conductive qualities. In various working conditions, fibrin glues, collagen or haemostatic gels can be a valuable option[3,4] for controlling bleeding control in tissues surrounding the perforation and creating a solid base for sealing.

The success of the endo-periodontic communication's obturation phase depends on its localization, accessibility and the extent of residual root canal space, which may require shaping if needed.

The following series of clinical cases describes the operative sequences. Employing magnifying systems and an adequate array of instruments is crucial for positive treatment outcomes.

However, the long-term prognosis for these cases seems unfavourable. In a recent article,[2] this book's authors highlighted that periradicular probing depths exceeding 5 mm and radiographic lesion dimensions exceeding 3 mm might impact treatment success. Nevertheless, beyond the ten-year mark, a significant number of teeth experience recurrence or fractures, leading to subsequent extraction.

In summary, this treatment can maintain a tooth only for a few years.

External invasive root resorption

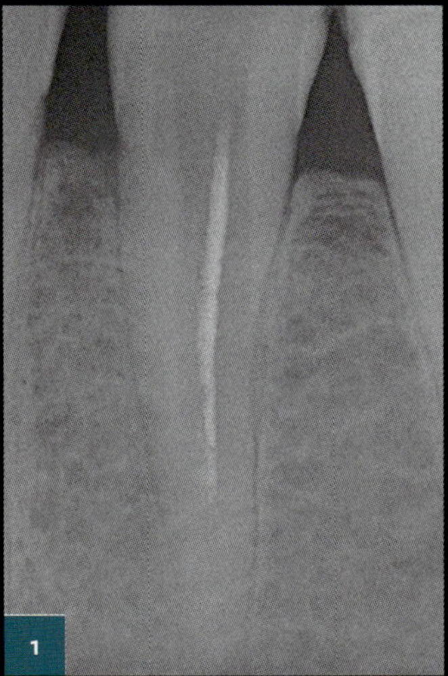

Fig. 1 ■ The patient, who is a colleague, unfortunately undergoes an endodontic treatment with an unfortunate outcome on one of his teeth. A macroscopic error occurs during cavity opening, resulting in a large perforation at the middle third of the root.

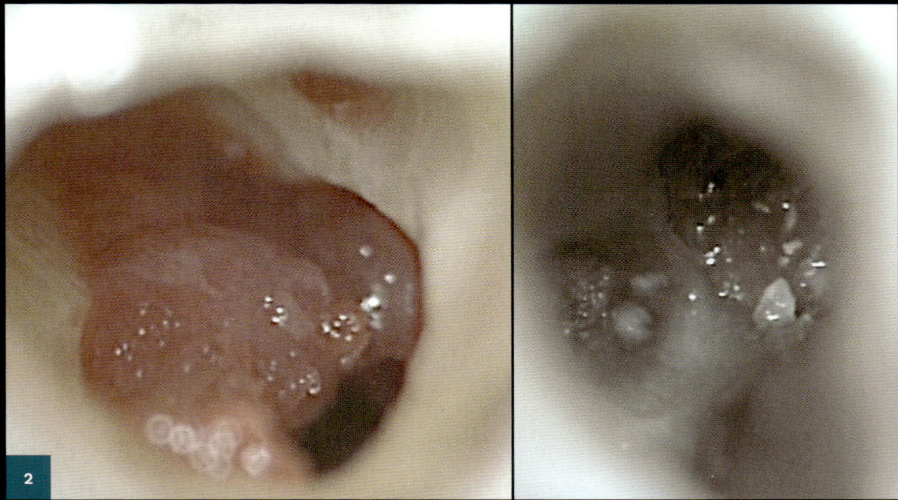

Fig. 2 ■ The intraoperative images clearly show a large defect that has been invaded by granulation tissue. After tissue removal, one can see how irregular the perforation is, with parts of the bone marrow visible through the opening.

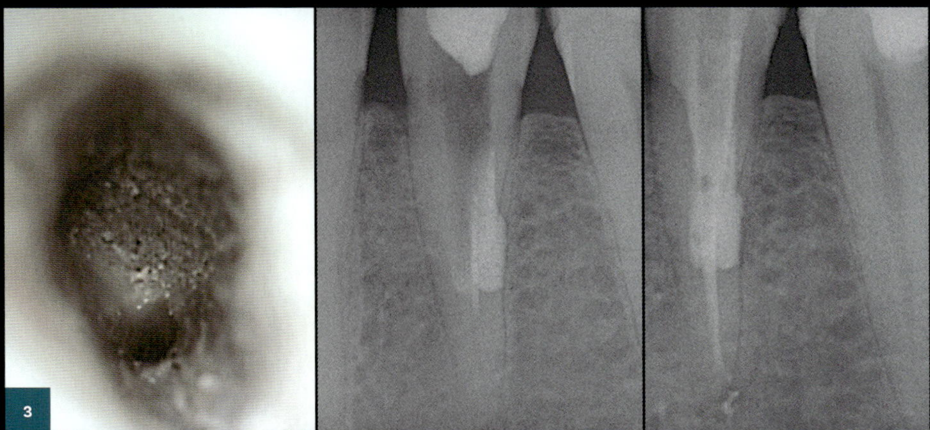

Fig. 3 ■ The perforation is sealed with MTA while maintaining canal patency. This will allow us to successively perform an endodontic treatment.

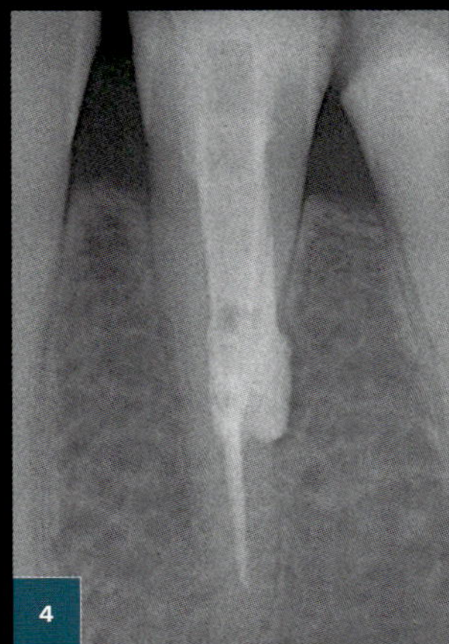

Fig. 4 ■ A follow-up period of 16 years demonstrates the

Root stripping

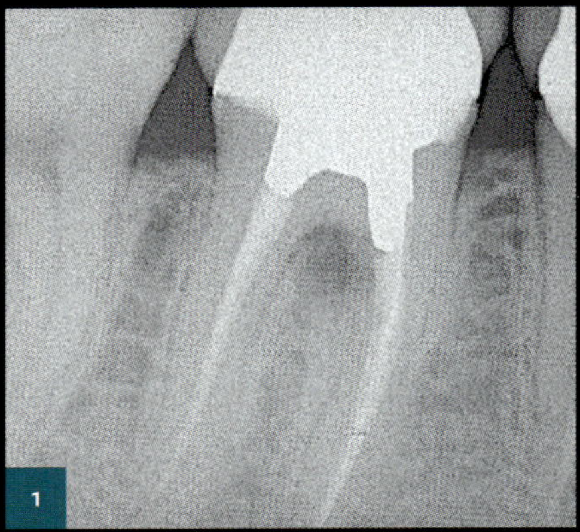

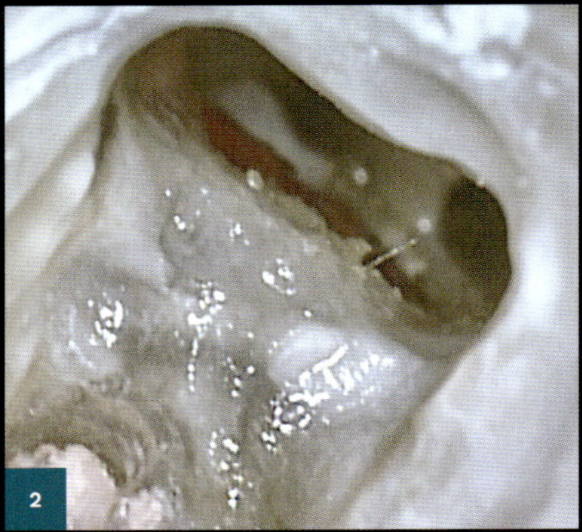

Fig. 1 ■ Several months after endodontic treatment and subsequent restoration, the tooth shows clinical and radiographic indications of root stripping-induced damage.

Fig. 2 ■ The photograph shows the wide defect present at the furcation level.

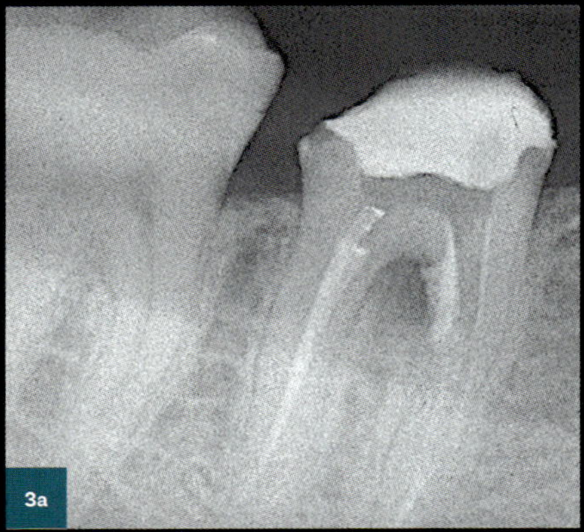

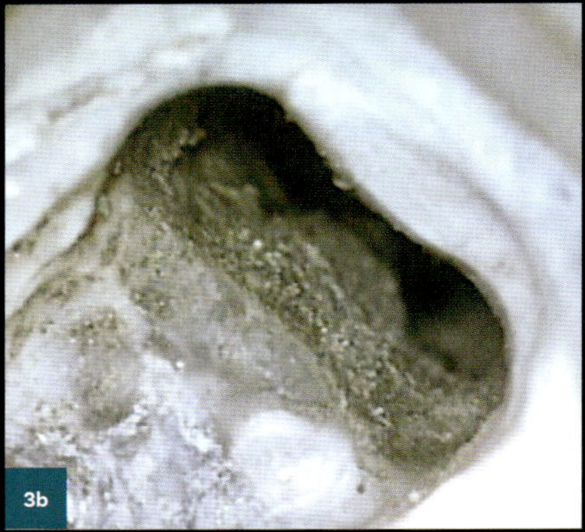

Figs. 3a,b ■ Repair performed using MTA.

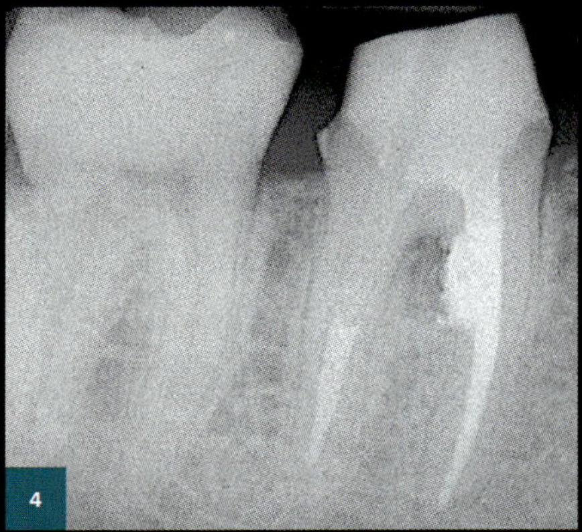

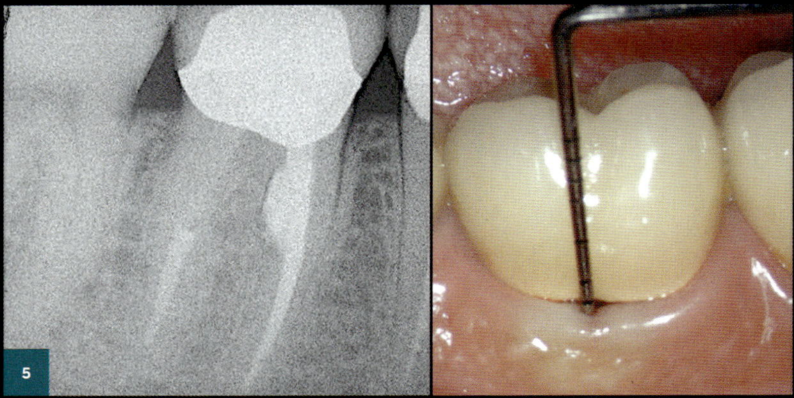

Fig. 4 ■ Post-operative radiographic image.

Fig. 5 ■ A 14-year-old radiographic follow up revealed the absence of probing and perfect soft tissue adaptation around the prosthetic crown.

Sandwich technique – apical third perforation – upper lateral incisor

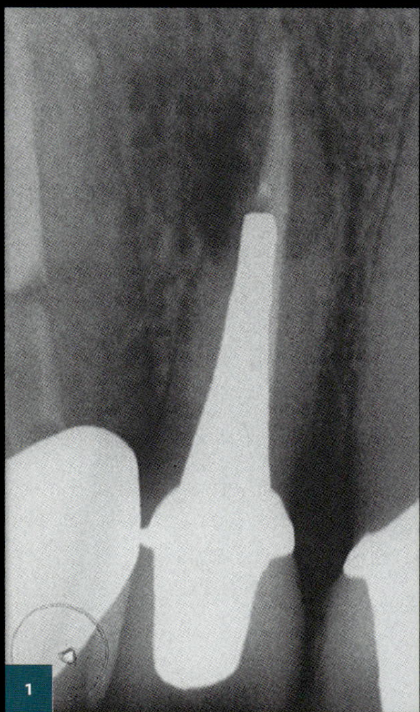

Fig. 1 ■ The tooth exhibits swelling and pain attributed to a buccal perforation caused by a poorly executed and inaccurately inclined cast post.

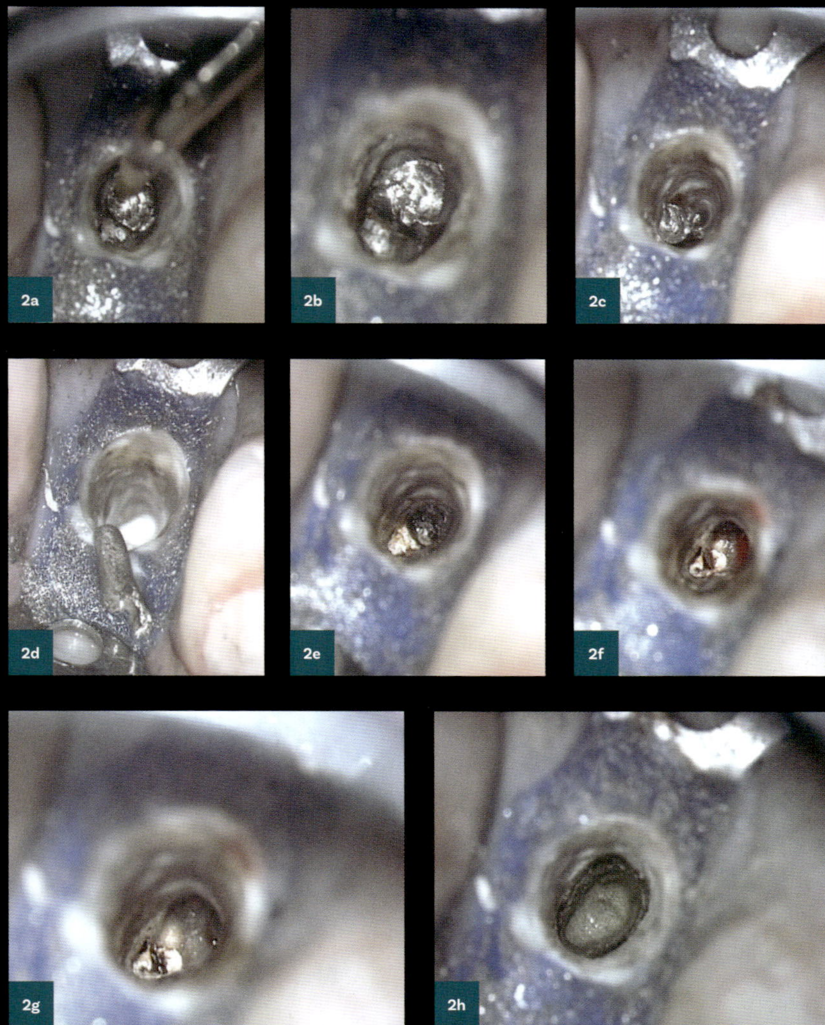

Figs. 2a-h ■ Photographic sequence illustrating the systematic removal of the post's apical fragment, meticulous cleansingof the perforation site, and successive repair procedure.

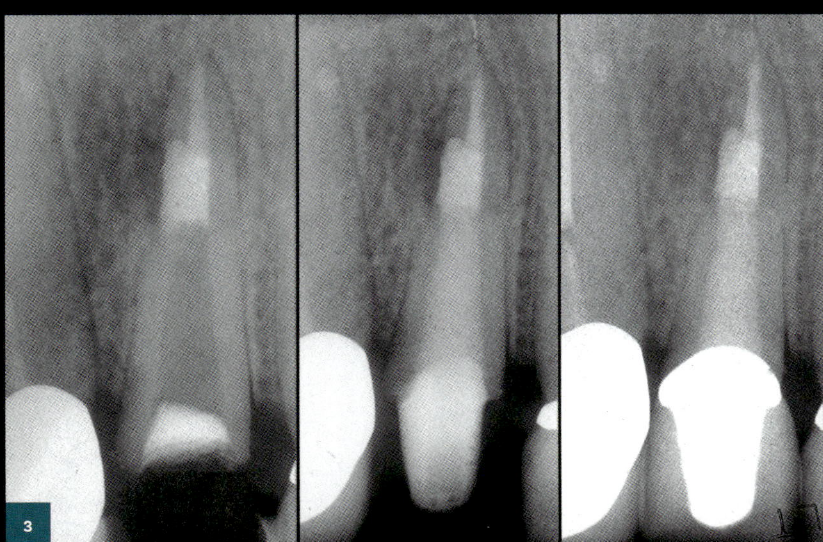

Fig. 3 ■ Post-operative radiograph after the successful repair with MTA and the application of a fibre post for endodontic build up. A follow-up radiographic captured after 10 years demonstrates an evident recovery of the periapical tissue.

Broken Instruments

A broken instrument in the endodontic space is not difficult, and its occurrence is decreasing due to the growing material control and handling methods.[5] In fact, about 87% of broken instruments may be removed successfully. An intraoperative microscope is essential for proper operation.[6] Literature analysis has demonstrated that a broken instrument does not adversely affect the prognosis if the case is treated properly without signs of periapical pathology. Therefore, file removal may not be necessary in such cases, and the fragment can be incorporated into the obturation or bypassed. However, if a periapical lesion is present, the prognosis is found to be significantly compromised, and any method of instrument removal is justified (orthograde or retrograde approach).

Various highly effective methods for fragment removal are available, requiring an operating microscope and specialist expertise. Recent literature shows us a less than 1% incidence of these complications. Ruivo et al.[7] found 0.27% and 0.26% fracture rates in shaped canals and endodontically treated teeth, respectively. Most fractures (71.43%) occurred at the apical third, while only 28.57% happened at the middle third ($p<0.01$). In the same study, only one file was removed and one bypassed, while the fragment was left inside the canal in five cases. Therefore, from a therapeutic point of view, the choice is very simple. The broken instruments left in the canals[8] do not compromise the prognosis of endodontically treated teeth without apical periodontitis. However, if apical periodontitis is present, healing is significantly reduced.

In conclusion, a broken instrument in the canals can have three outcomes: removal, bypass, or incorporation inside the obturation. There are two approaches for fragment removal: orthograde or surgical removal. The crucial determinant for fragment removal is the pre-operatory pathological condition. If an endodontic-related periapical lesion is present, the only choice is that leaving the fragment in the canal would significantly reduce medium-term success rates. Another important factor is the fragment's localisation. Managing a fragment broken off beyond a curve is more challenging than one broken in the coronal third.

A study verifying the possibility of fragment removal up to the middle third showed that overall removal success rates were 90% with ultrasonic equipment and 95% with a dedicated file-removal system.[9] However, the group using ultrasonic tips had a longer average time of removal. The authors of this book, in agreement with many other authors, would again like to emphasise the operative implications of instrument breakage in the canals. This often requires treatment suspension and subsequent patient referral to an expert or immediate fragment removal if adequate instruments are available. This approach has clear advantages for the potential treatment outcome, considering the favourable microbiological and anatomical conditions of the root canals at this stage. Therefore, three approaches are viable depending on the fragment's position: fragment removal when possible, fragment bypass or endodontic surgery.

Fractured instrument and perforation at the root's medium third

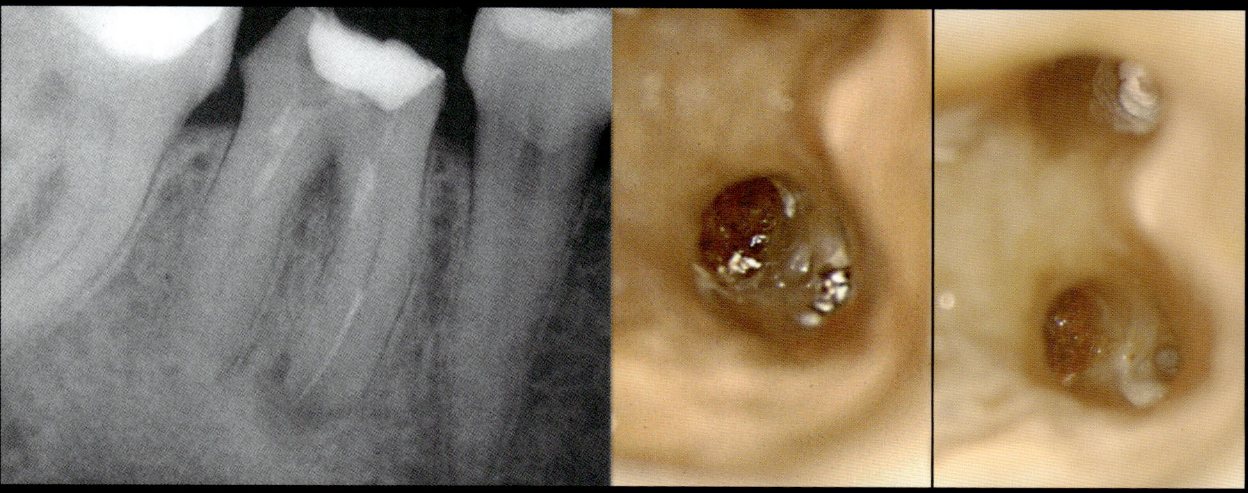

Fig. 1 ■ During the procedure, the colleague inadvertently broke an instrument inside the canal, which created a perforation at the root's medium third while trying to remove the fragment. The intraoperative image shows the fragment in the canal and the adjacent perforation.

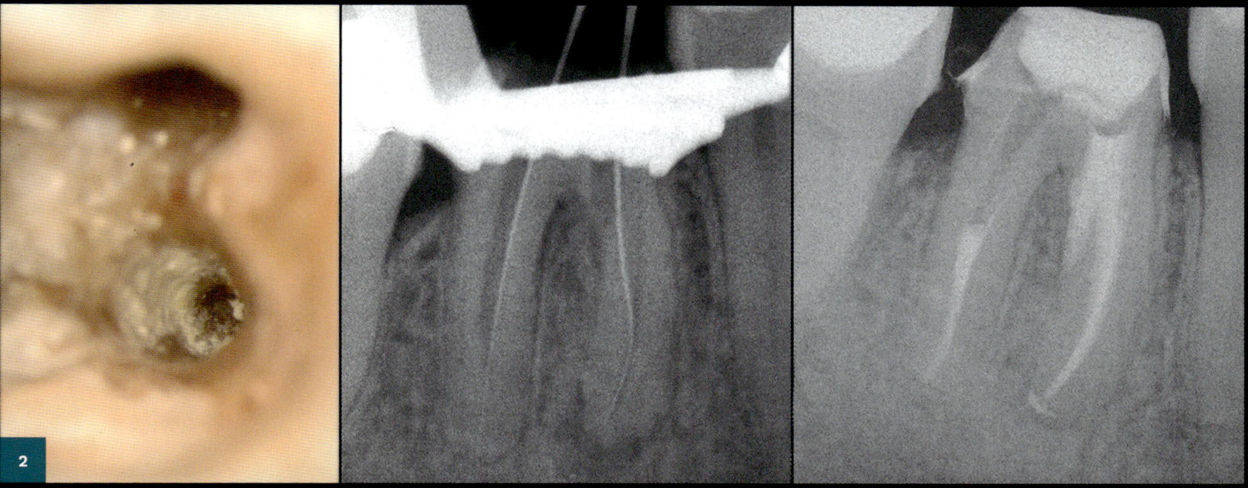

Fig. 2 ■ Perforation sealing with MTA. Intraoperative radiograph for accurately measuring the working length and post-operative radiograph to assess the treatment outcome.

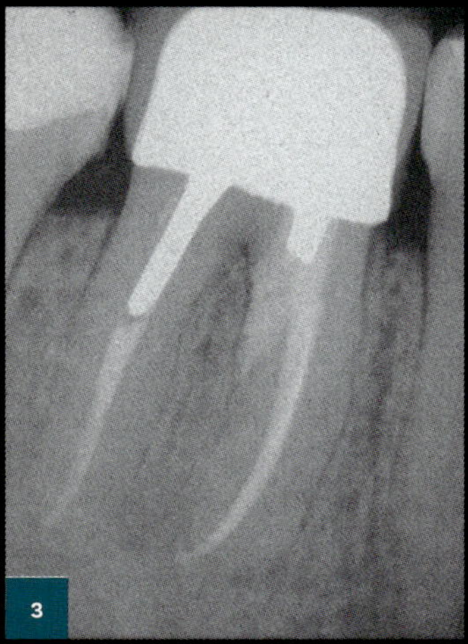

Fig. 3 ■ 13-year follow up after the operation.

Bibliography

1. Gorni FG, Andreano A, Ambrogi F, Brambilla E, Gagliani M. Patient and Clinical Characteristics Associated with Primary Healing of Iatrogenic Perforations after Root Canal Treatment: Results of a Long-term Italian Study. *J Endod.* 2016;42(2):211-215.
2. Gorni FG, Ionescu AC, Ambrogi F, Brambilla E, Gagliani M. Prognostic factors and primary healing on root perforation repaired with MTA: a 14-year longitudinal study. *J Endod.* 2022;48(9):1092-1099.
3. Mente J, Hage N, Pfefferle T, et al. Treatment outcome of mineral trioxide aggregate: repair of root perforations. *J Endod.* 2010;36(2):208-213.
4. Pontius V, Pontius O, Braun A, Frankenberger R, Roggendorf MJ. Retrospective evaluation of perforation repairs in 6 private practices. *J Endod.* 2013;39(11):1346-1358.
5. Suter B, Lussi A, Sequeira P. Probability of removing fractured instruments from root canals. *Int Endod J.* 2005;38(2):112-123.
6. McGuigan MB, Louca C, Duncan HF. Endodontic instrument fracture: causes and prevention. *Br Dent J.* 2013;214(7):341-348.
7. Ruivo LM, Rios MA, Villela AM, et al. Fracture incidence of Reciproc instruments during root canal retreatment performed by postgraduate students: a cross-sectional retrospective clinical study. *Restor Dent Endod.* 2021;46(4):e49.
8. Pruthi PJ, Nawal RR, Talwar S, Verma M. Comparative evaluation of the effectiveness of ultrasonic tips versus the Terauchi file retrieval kit for the removal of separated endodontic instruments. *Restor Dent Endod.* 2020;45(2):e14.
9. Terauchi Y, O'Leary L, Suda H. Removal of separated files from root canals with a new file-removal system: Case reports. *J Endod.* 2006;32(8):789-797.

7

Resorbed apices

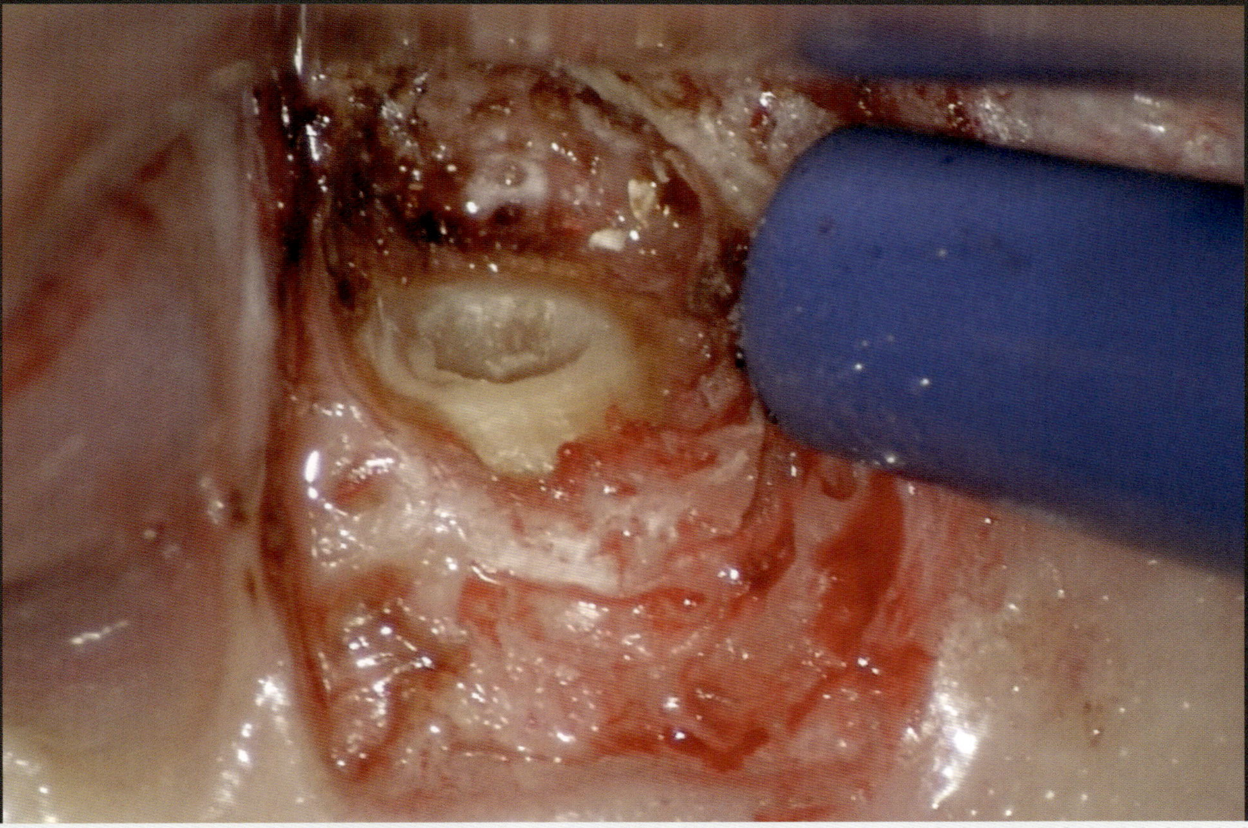

Apical resorption is one of the most common features of severely compromised teeth. The periapical osteolytic area often shows elevated resorption (**Figs. 7.1 a, b**). The inflammatory tissue enables clastic cells to cause both bone and root surface damage.

Histopathological changes in the periapical area can range from minor effects on the dental component to significant structural repercussions. Cementitious reactions sometimes result in roots with a club-shaped appearance.

All these alterations in the root area, particularly the terminal part, affect the neuralgic area of the root canal. The apical zone is crucial for correctly sealing the thoroughly cleaned and disinfected endodontic space.

These technical implications are significant. Improved disinfection procedures with well-proven products, such as using sodium hypochlorite concentrations above 2.5%, maybe more effective with techniques like heating or employing irrigation systems triggered by ultrasonic, subsonic or other technologies, as discussed in Part II of this volume.

A more cylindrical appearance in the root canal's terminal part is desired to preserve the intracanal dentin and tooth strength when shaping root canals,[1] especially when the apical diameters exceed ISO 60. However, as supported by several studies,[2,3] in cases with high septic content that may have gone unnoticed for a long time, enlarging the root canal becomes crucial for successful treatment.

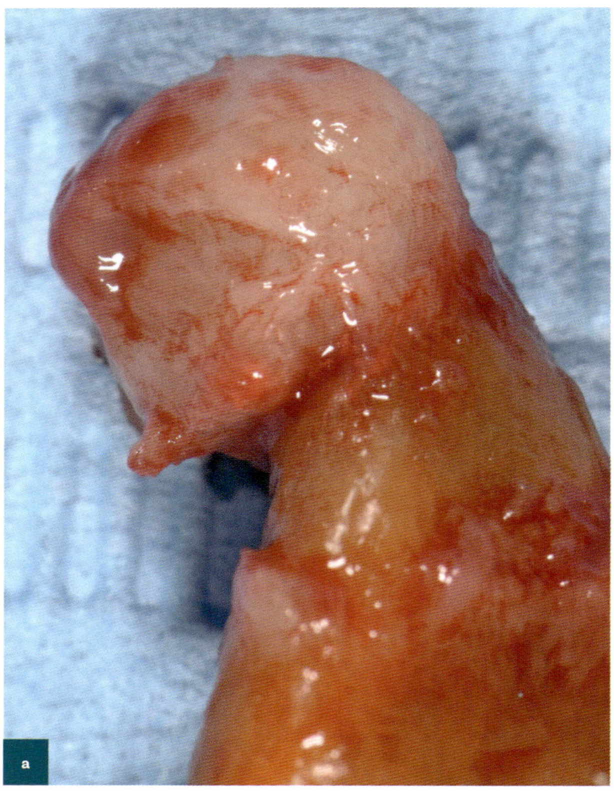

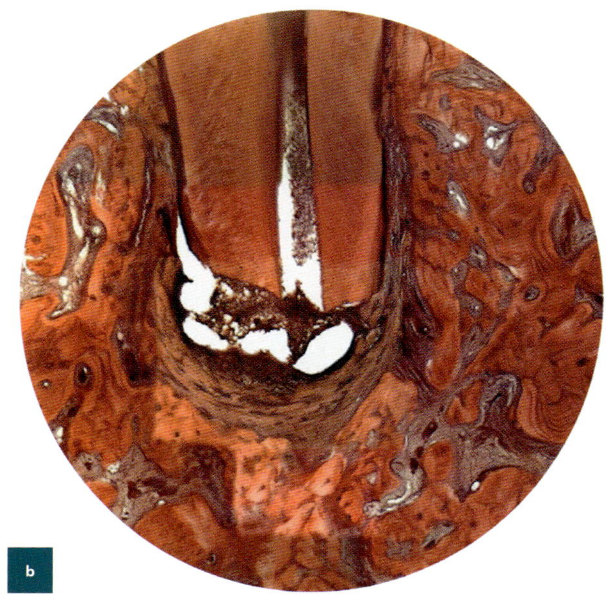

Fig. 7.1a ▪ Clinical appearance of a periapical lesion.

Fig. 7.1b ▪ Histologically, it is evident that the lytic process affecting the periapical tissues involved the root surface (courtesy of Dr. Nicola Perrini).

Finally, choosing the correct root canal obturation system is crucial. Bioactive cements are well-documented for sealing the apical area. The "apical-plug" method is preferred in clinical situations where the estimated root apex size exceeds ISO 70.

Figure 7.2 clearly shows that achieving significant conicity obtainable is challenging with large apices. Techniques like gutta-percha condensation or pre-heated gutta-percha (Thermafil Technique, to name the most popular example) are not recommended due to limited control over the filling material's termination point. Additionally, calcium silicate-based materials (e.g., MTA) offer superior sealing capacities in these situations because accurately drying the apical third becomes difficult.[4-6]

Since the aforementioned moisture-responsive materials have excellent hardening capacities, it makes them the most preferable. Finally, in cases involving these dental elements, a combined intervention, i.e., an intervention involving retrograde completion, should not be excluded.

If this scenario arises, a second retrograde closure would be unnecessary, as the antegrade seal with bioactive materials can easily substitute the closure of the endodontic space via the posterior route.

CONT'D ON PAGE 76 >

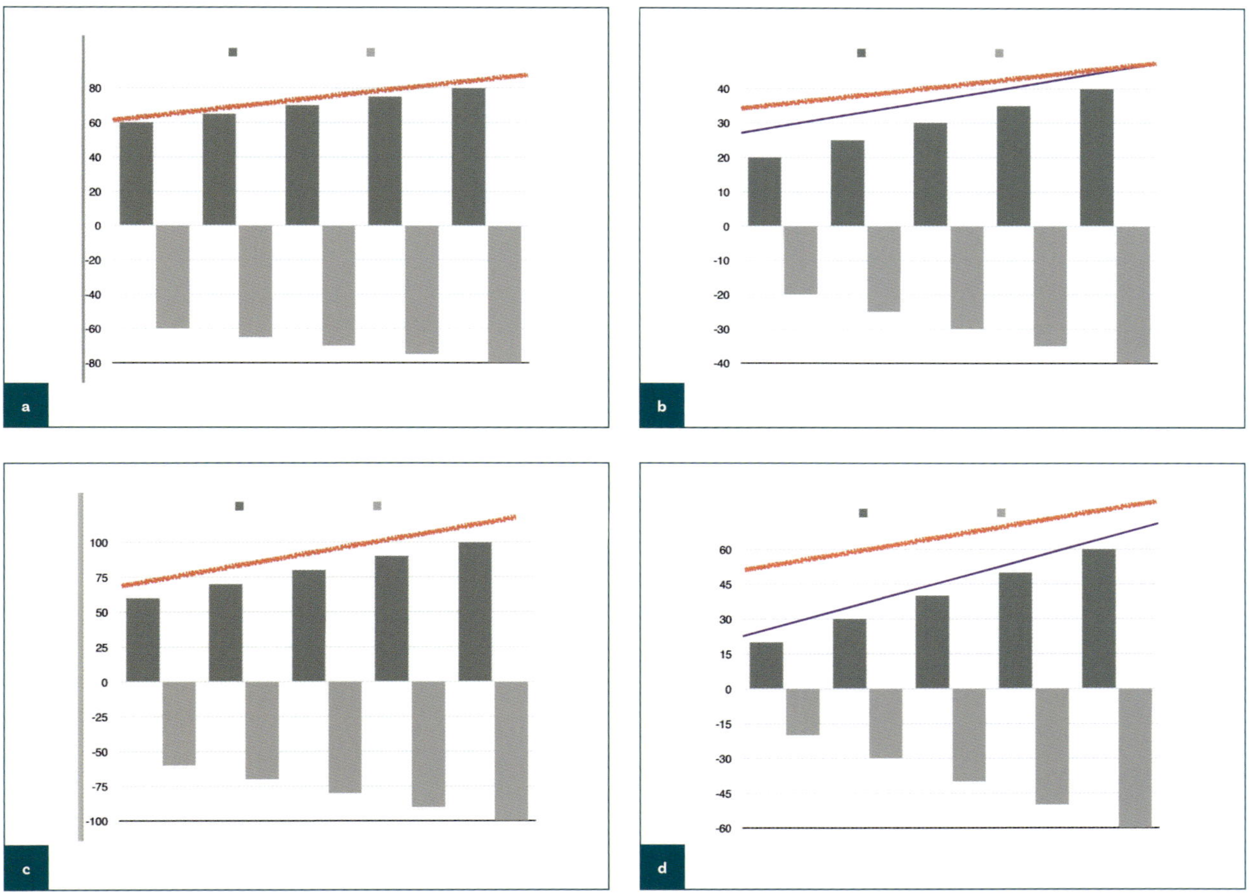

Fig. 7.2 ■
a) A taper of ISO 5 with a starting diameter of ISO 60.
b) A taper of ISO 5 with a starting diameter of ISO 20.
c) A taper of ISO 10 with a starting diameter of ISO 60.
d) A taper of ISO 10 with a starting diameter of ISO 20.

Retreatment with apical plug in the palatal root

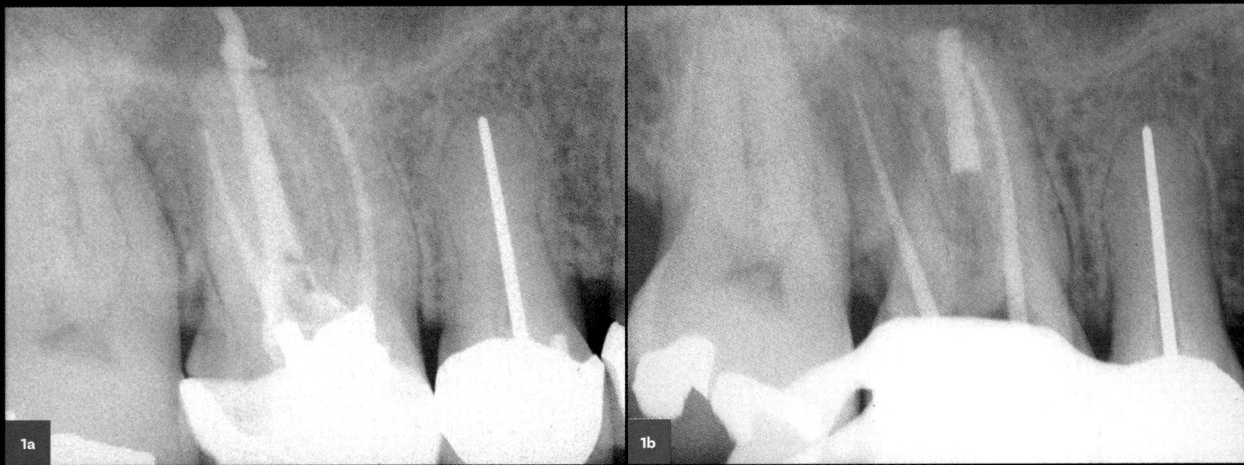

Fig. 1a ■ Pre-op: periapical lesion involving the palatal and distal root of the upper first molar. Previous root canal therapy created obvious overfilling due to a technical problem with the retreatment.

Fig. 1b ■ Post-op: thanks to the use of the operating-microscope it was possible to remove the gutta-percha beyond the apex, guaranteeing the best conditions for cleansing and filling the foramen using an apical plug in MTA.

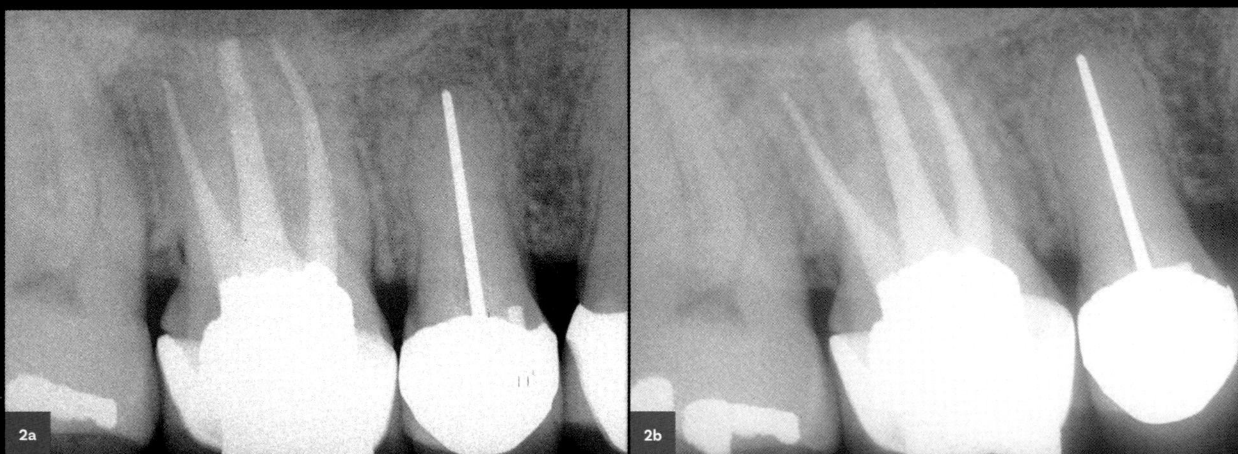

Figs. 2a,b ■ Check-up 6 months and 10 years after treatment with complete healing of the periapical tissues.

Retreatment with removal of the metal post abutment and apical plug with MTA

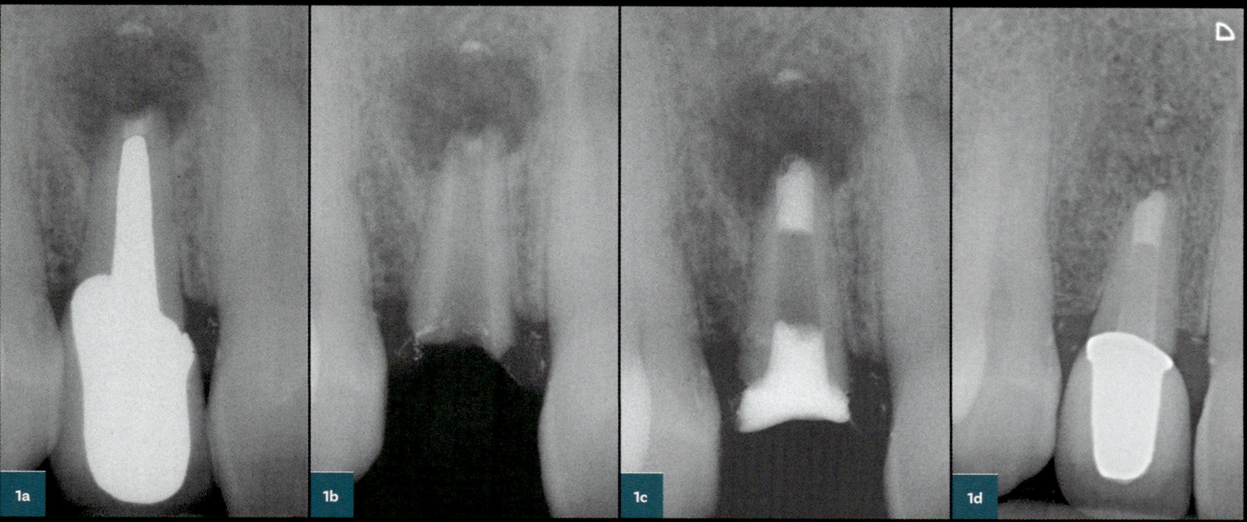

Fig. 1a ■ Pre-op. The patient who refused extraction and an implant in the aesthetic zone requested further endodontic surgery due to previous failure. After a careful clinical examination, it became evident that performing further surgery was unfeasible due to the insufficient space for the retrograde filling and subsequent sealing. Therefore, the decision was made to remove the abutment post, followed by an apical plug using MTA to address the situation.

Fig. 1b ■ Intra-op. The radiograph shows the completely empty canal.

Fig. 1c ■ Post-op. Apical plug.

Fig. 1d ■ The 23-year follow-up shows a complete healing of the lesion from a radiological point of view with total absence of symptoms.

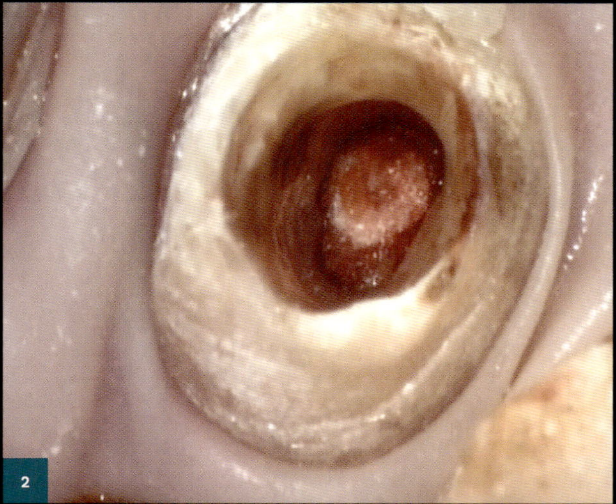

Fig. 2 ■ Intra-op photograph of the extra-apical collagen barrier used to contain the filling material. It was necessary to use this type of technique given the large size and irregularity of the apex.

In conclusion, we would like to present a diagram (**Table 7.1**) which summarises the variables and highlights the problems to be analysed before and during a reintervention procedure, whether orthograde or retrograde, to eliminate periapical pathology of endodontic origin. However, **Table 7.2** lists the essential tools to safely carry out all the procedures described in this part of the volume.

Table 7.1 ■ Elements to consider in a retreatment.

Factors that condition the prognosis	Iatrogenic errors that necessitate retreatment	General factors to consider with retreatments	Contraindications to retreatment
• Pre-operative state of the periapical tissues • Size of the periradicular lesion • Canal anatomy • Coronal or radicular fracture • Iatrogenic factors • Quality of the post endodontic restoration • Amount of time passed since first treatment • Microbiology • Observation period	• Separated instruments • Canal blockages-ledges or plugs • Perforations • Incomplete canal obturation due to length and quality • Missed canals • Extension of the obturation beyond the apex	• Patient's general health • Operator experience • Available instrumentation • Diagnosis and overall treatment plan • Radiographic interpretation • Canal anatomy • Quality and extension of the canal seal • Quality of the post endodontic retreatment restoration	• During the diagnostic phase, it is crucial to carefully consider the inevitable weakening of the tooth root caused by endodontic retreatment. Additionally, other factors must be taken into account. The use of burs or ultrasonic instruments during the procedure can cause heating of the root, potentially causing damage to the surrounding periodontium. This, in turn, weakens the support structure of the tooth itself

Table 7.2 ■ Instruments for retreatment.

■ Handpiece for Ni-Ti alloy instruments
■ Magnification
■ Operating microscope
■ Ultrasonic or sonic system with tips dedicated to endodontics
■ Instruments for the removal of endodontic posts
■ Instrument(s) for atraumatic bridge and/or crown removal
■ Endodontic instrument for the removal of root canal content
■ Instrument set for removal of root canal instruments
■ Solvents
■ Sonic and ultrasonic systems for activating sodium hypochlorite
■ Laser
■ Obturation materials: bioactive cements - calcium silicate

Retreatment in case of incorrect apical plug

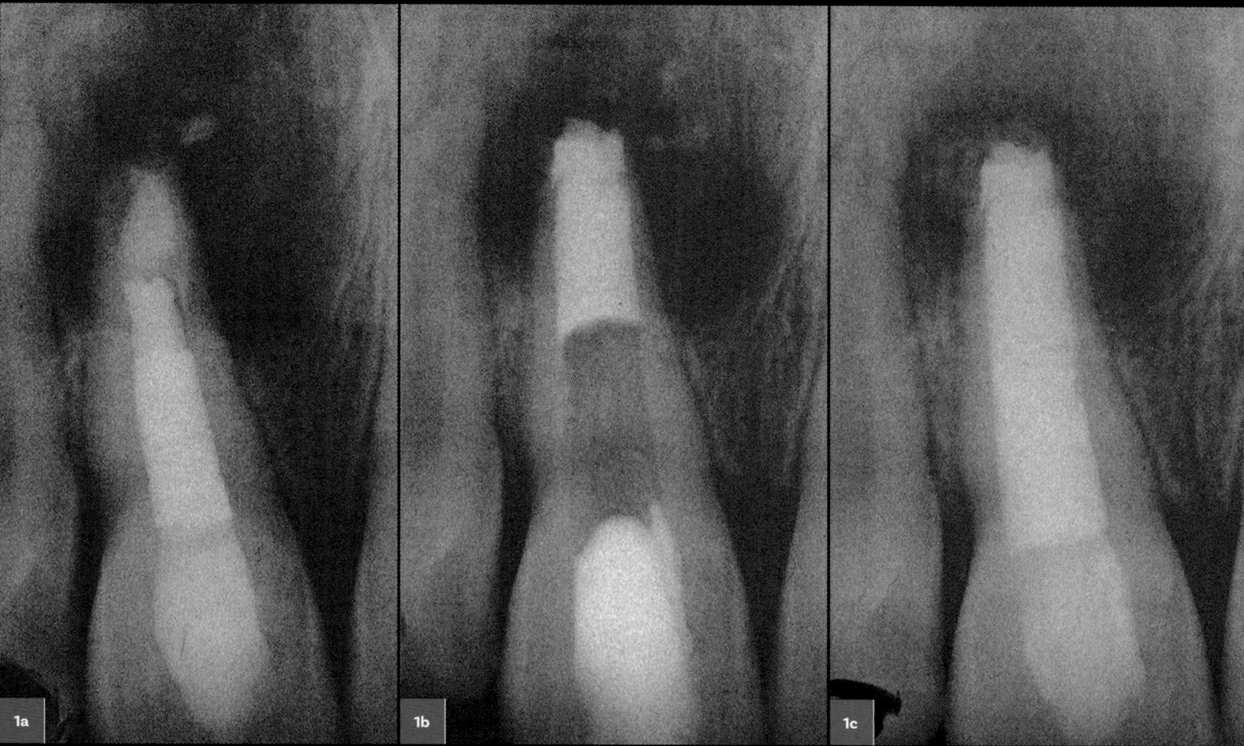

Fig. 1a ■ Pre-op. Large periapical lesion in an 11-year-old patient resulting from trauma to the right central incisor. The previous treatment shows an evident incongruity in the apical obturation. The lack of three-dimensionality in the MTA obturation increases the likelihood of future failure.

Fig. 1b ■ Intra-op. New MTA apical plug that ensures the three-dimensionality of the obturation.

Fig. 1c ■ Post-op.

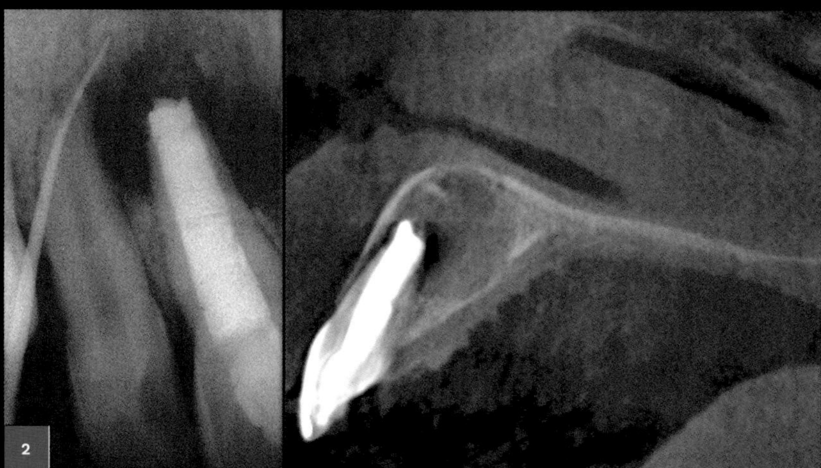

Fig. 2 ■ 18-month follow-up. Despite initial clinical and radiographic improvement, there is a recurrence of the pathology that manifests itself as a fistula in the fornix. CBCT shows a large lesion of probable cystic nature. Given the patient's young age, further clinical intervention is necessary to prolong the tooth's lifespan until a suitable age for implant replacement.

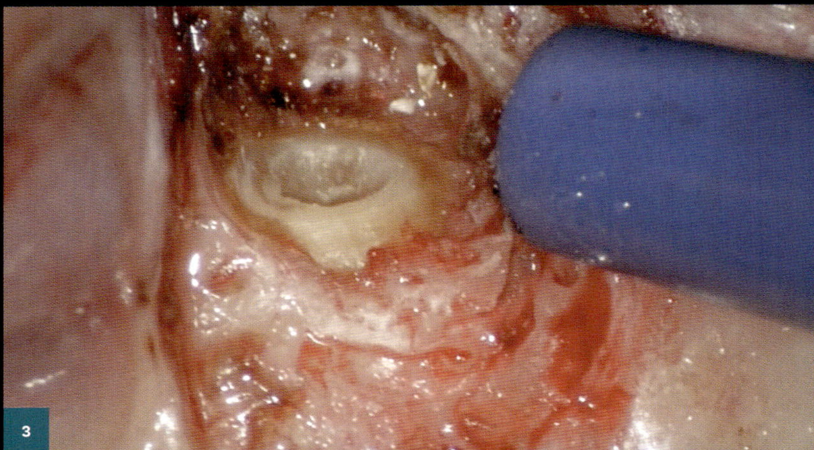

Fig. 3 ■ Intra-op photograph during the apical surgery.

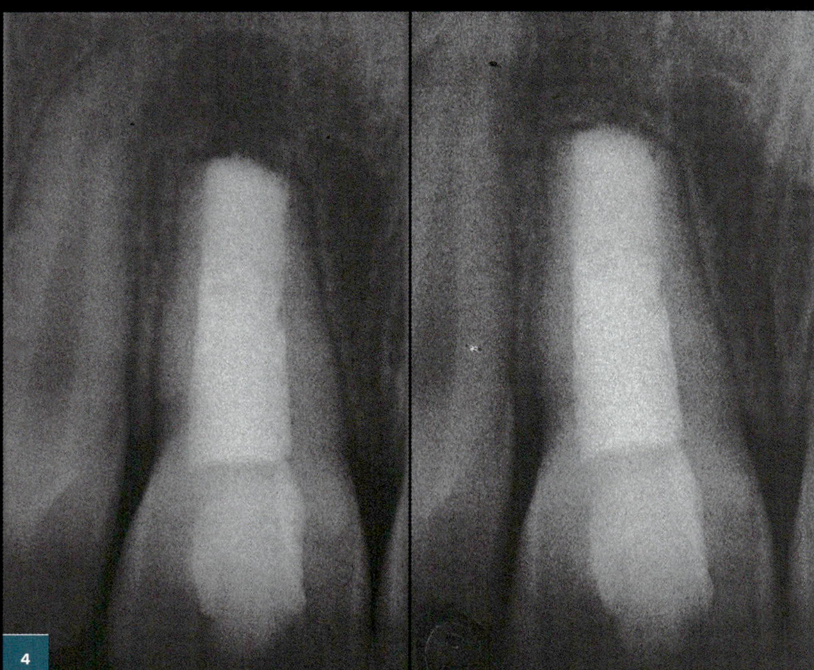

Fig. 4 ■ Post-op Rx and radiographic control eight years after the endodontic surgery where the cystic lesion was successfully removed and an apical seal was recreated using the same material used for the MTA orthograde apical plug.

A case of resorbed apex with periapical lesion of endodontic origin

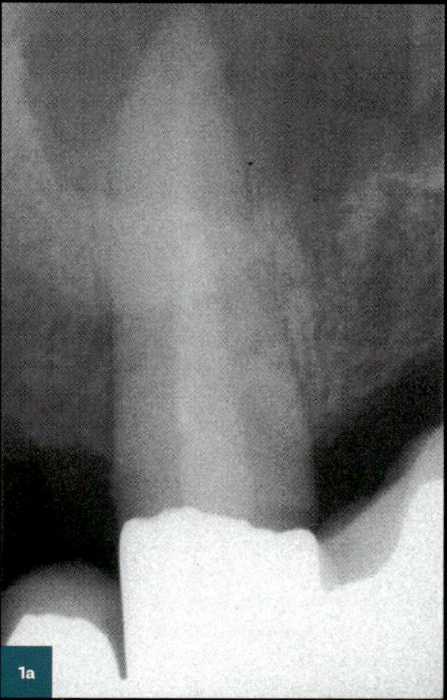

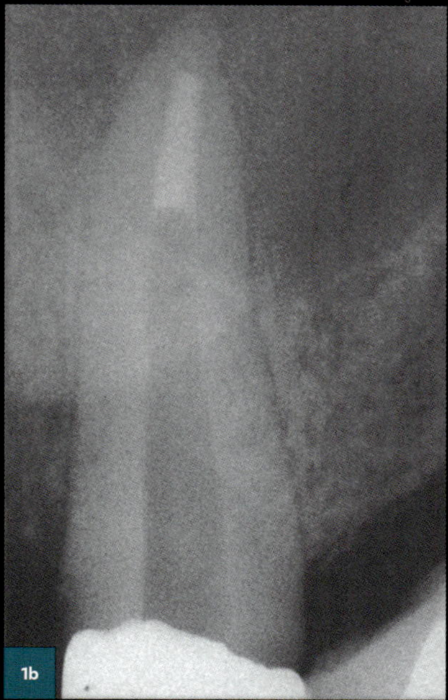

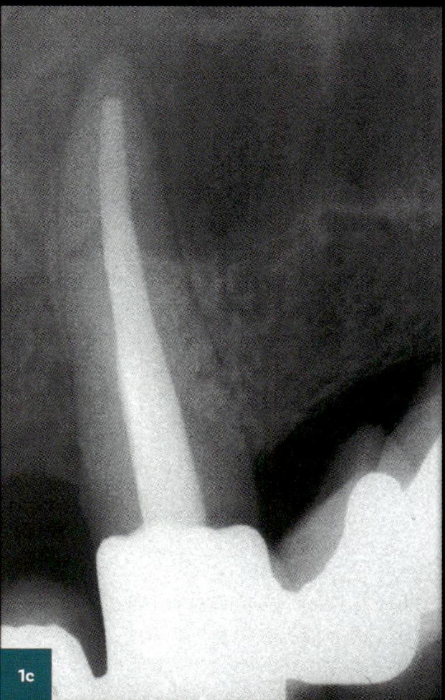

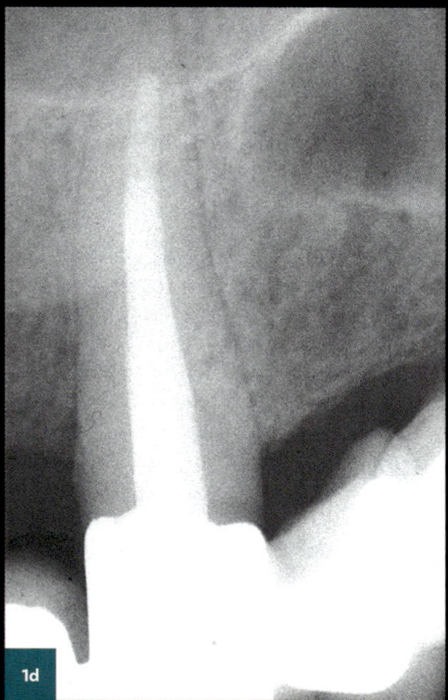

Fig. 1a ■ Periapical granulomatous lesions commonly lead to apical resorptions, resulting in challenges for the clinician to effectively manage the apical preparation and correctly seal the final area of the root canal. In this case, thorough instrumentation facilitated the removal of a large part of the residual pulp tissue and the previously incongruous root canal filling.

Fig. 1b ■ Once the root canal was properly shaped, an apical plug in mineral trioxide aggregate (MTA) was placed after completion of the procedure.

Fig. 1c ■ At the end of the hardening process, the remaining part of the root canal was filled with vertically condensed gutta-percha.

Fig. 1d ■ The case was resolved after about 9 months.

Bibliography

1. Albuquerque PP, Hungaro Duarte MA, Pelegrine RA, et al. Influence of foraminal enlargement on the apical extrusion of filling material: Volumetric analysis using micro-computed tomography. *Aust Endod J.* 2020;46(2):210-216.
2. Gesi A, Mareschi P, Doldo T, Ferrari M. Apical Dimension of Root Canal Clinically Assessed with and without Periapical Lesions. *Int J Dent.* 2014;2014:374971.
3. Wen C, Yan L, Kong Y, Zhao J, Li Y, Jiang Q. The antibacterial efficacy of photon-initiated photoacoustic streaming in root canals with different diameters or tapers. *BMC Oral Health.* 2021;21(1):542.
4. Ree MH, Schwartz RS. Long-term Success of Nonvital, Immature Permanent Incisors Treated With a Mineral Trioxide Aggregate Plug and Adhesive Restorations: A Case Series from a Private Endodontic Practice. *J Endod.* 2017;43(8):1370-1377.
5. Torabinejad M, Nosrat A, Verma P, Udochukwu O. Regenerative Endodontic Treatment or Mineral Trioxide Aggregate Apical Plug in Teeth with Necrotic Pulps and Open Apices: A Systematic Review and Meta-analysis. *J Endod.* 2017;43(11):1806-1820.
6. Torabinejad M, Parirokh M, Dummer PMH. Mineral trioxide aggregate and other bioactive endodontic cements: an updated overview - part II: other clinical applications and complications. *Int Endod J.* 2018;51(3):284-317.

8

Managing root resorption: internal, cervical invasive, and root replacement with ankylosis

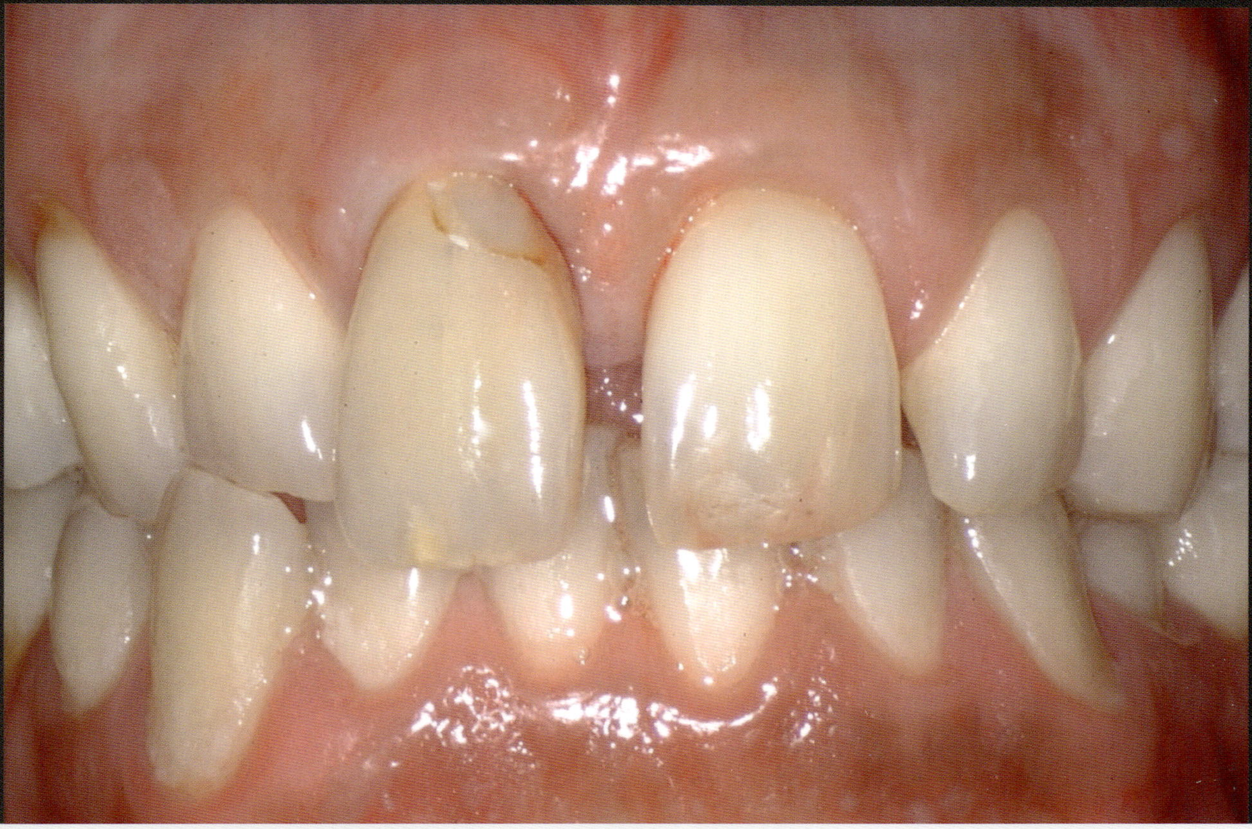

Root resorption is an uncommon pathology that involves resorption and replacement of dental tissue with different tissues. While it is natural and leads to exfoliation in deciduous teeth, it causes serious problems for permanent teeth.

Tissue resorption and apposition are normal biological mechanisms, particularly observed in bone tissue, where pressure leads to resorption and traction causes tissue apposition. Orthodontics utilizes this phenomenon. However, permanent teeth should not undergo resorption, except when apical remodelling may occur as an undesired consequence of prolonged and complex orthodontic treatments or possible genetic predisposition.[1]

Root resorption in permanent teeth involves the activation of clastic cellular activity, which may start internally or externally to the tooth. The dentine has a layer of odontoblasts and unmineralized pre-dentine internally, whereas externally, it has a layer of cementoblasts and cementoid tissue, the organic substance of cement. These unmineralized layers prevent the adhesion to and subsequent resorption of the tissue surface by odontoclasts. However, injury or infection of these barriers can expose mineralized dentine, leading to loss of pre-cement or pre-dentine and possible trauma to the dentine itself.[2-3] Therefore, tooth resorption may be self-limiting and clinically indistinguishable,[4] but if the noxious cause persists, resorption of the surrounding dental structures continues, causing a consistent loss of dental tissue.[5]

There are numerous classifications of root resorption, all based on histologic and etiopathogenetic criteria.[6] A literature review identified 15 classifications.[7] Among them, Patel and Saberi's recent classification is simple and clinically relevant,[8] and is shown in the following figure (**Fig. 8.1**).

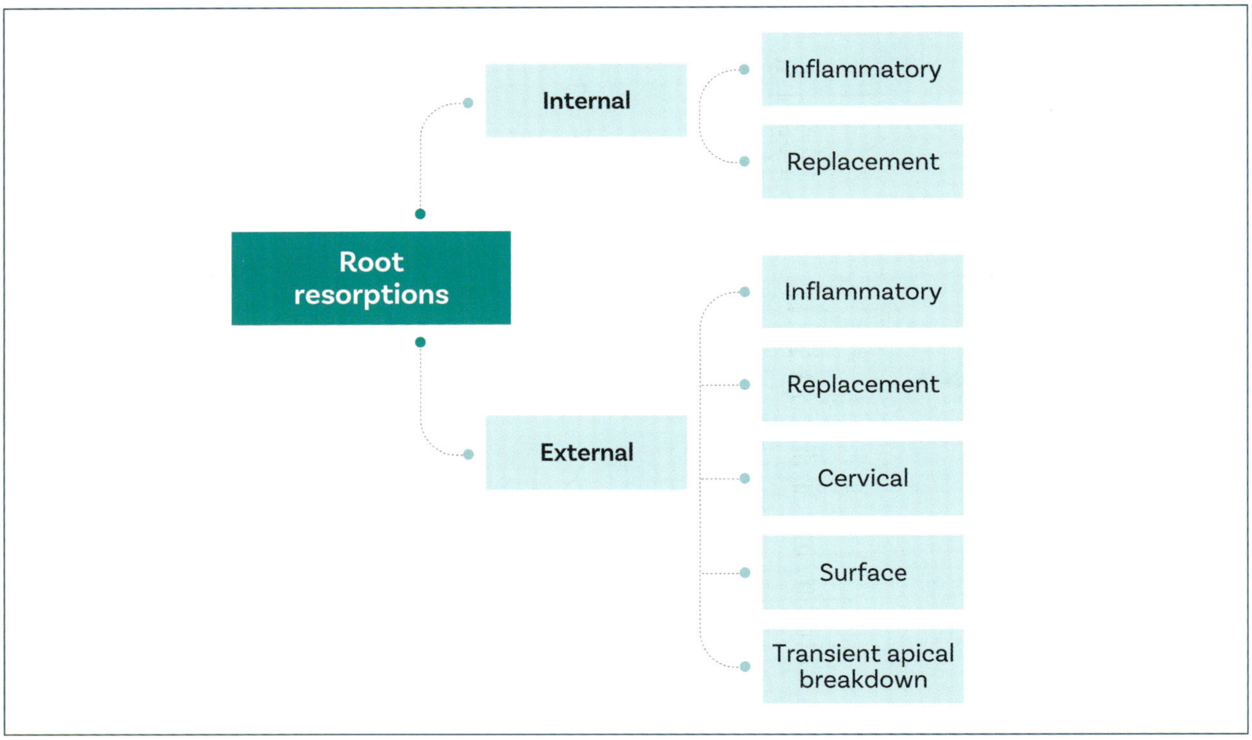

Fig. 8.1 ■ Patel and Saberi's classification.

Internal resorption

Internal inflammatory resorption

Internal inflammatory resorption may occur following acute or chronic pulp trauma,[9-10] autotransplantation, orthodontic treatment[11] or unknown causes.[12] It is characterized by an enlarging pulp space at various root canal levels. Normally, the pulp tissue above the resorption site becomes necrotic, while the apical pulp tissue remains vital, providing cells and nourishment for the resorption process progression.

Internal inflammatory resorption often goes unnoticed, being asymptomatic and is discovered incidentally on radiographic examinations. However, advanced stages may cause symptoms of pulpal or periapical origin after complete pulp necrosis. Additionally, the newly formed spaces may cause pink discolouration of the crown due to invasion by the resorbing dentin tissue. In cases where the lesions are not excessively large, endodontic treatment, possibly including intermediate medication with calcium hydroxide, can effectively resolve the condition. If a perforation is present, bio-ceramic materials are recommended for canal obturation.

Internal replacement resorption

This is a rare pathology of unknown aetiology, although its inflammatory form is associated with the abovementioned factors mentioned above. The resorbed dentine is replaced by metaplastic tissue with an osseous or cementitious nature. Although symptoms and treatment resemble its inflammatory variant, accessing the apical endodontic space becomes technically complex due to calcification.[13] Using fine ultrasonic tips together with an operating microscope may help overcome any difficulties.

External resorption

External inflammatory resorption

It commonly occurs in teeth with infected root canals, a prevalent characteristic of apical periodontitis.[14] It can result from severe trauma, such as tooth luxation or avulsion, where the primary cause is damage to the root surface and adjacent periodontal tissues. If the pulp remains vital, the consequences may be temporary remodelling. However, if pulp necrosis occurs, it promotes microbial contamination and subsequent involvement of the damaged surface by bacterial toxins through the canals. This causes progressive inflammatory resorption. It shows symptoms resembling chronic apical periodontitis, including pain upon biting and swelling. Furthermore, an oral examination may find clinical indicators like pain upon percussion, tooth mobility, and unresponsiveness to pulp sensitivity tests. Radiographically, we can observe the resorbed radicular areas and often noticeably enlarged neighbouring periodontal space. Therefore, to halt the resorption process, an endodontic treatment, potentially including intermediate phases of calcium hydroxide medication, can stop the process of resorption, provided sufficient root structure remains.

External replacement resorption

This is a pathological result of severe trauma, damaging the periodontal ligament. Osteoclastic resorption affects the ligament cells, cement, and dentine, followed by osteoblastic proliferation and alveolar bone deposition. Eventually, the entire root may be replaced by bone, although sometimes the process may spontaneously halt. Consequently, the affected tooth becomes ankylosed, losing its natural mobility and producing a unique, sharper sound to percussion. If the tooth is still erupting, it becomes trapped in infraocclusion and does not respond to orthodontic forces. Unfortunately, there are no viable treatment options, and the lesion's progression can cause complete root loss, especially quicker in younger individuals. To manage this condition in younger patients, elective decoronation of the affected tooth is a potential approach. It involves sectioning the tooth at the amelocemental junction and covering it with attached gingiva. This aims to preserve the alveolar bone until the patient is old enough for definitive treatment.[15-16]

Cervical resorption

It is a dangerous pathology that can occur in both vital and non-vital teeth. It starts as a small subgingival cavity, gradually leading to significant dentine resorption. Although its aetiology is unknown, the predisposing factors identified include previous orthodontic treatments, trauma, intra-coronal bleaching and periodontal therapy.[17] Furthermore, genetic factors[19] and varicella-zoster virus infection[18] have also been listed as possible causes. A rare variant, called multiple idiopathic cervical root resorption, affects multiple teeth in individual patients, potentially devastating their entire dentition.[20] Interestingly, this pathology strongly resembles odontoclastic resorption in domestic cats and other felines.[21]

The pathogenesis of these lesions is attributed to a defect in the sub-epithelial cement infiltrated by osteoclastic cells supported by fibrovascular tissue. The lesions are asymptomatic in the early stages and can be clinically identified after periodontal probing. This reveals a hyperaemic area where we will find a hard lesion instead of soft carious tissue. However, in the advanced stages, the affected tooth may appear pink due to the granulation tissue penetration within the crown. These lesions are often incidentally found after radiographic examination. Differentiating between internal and external resorption is possible due to a thin layer of dentine surrounding the pulp.

According to severity, the most cited Heitersay's[22] staging classification divides this pathology into four classes. With the advent of three-dimensional imaging techniques, this two-dimensional classification has been integrated with the three-dimensional classification of Patel et al.[23] The treatment options for cervical resorptions depend on the entity of the lesion. They may involve an external reconstruction of the defect with or without endodontic treatment, intentional re-implantation if feasible, or extraction of the affected tooth in cases of extensive defects.

External surface resorption

It is resorption induced by pressure and originating from external factors, such as orthodontic movements, impacted teeth, tumours or cysts. It is often asymptomatic and often incidentally discovered through radiographic examination. Treatment of the underlying cause of the pathology stops the progression of the resorption.[24]

Transient apical breakdown

First described by Andreasen in 1985,[25] refers to a temporary resorption of the tooth apex following an injury. It manifests as the emergence of a spontaneous radiolucency, potentially of significant dimensions, shortly after the traumatic event. However, the radiolucency disappears during follow-up, which typically spans less than 12 months. Additionally, it is also often associated with temporary alterations in tooth colour and sensitivity. This phenomenon is regarded as an outcome of the healing process during injured tissue removal.

Conclusions

Root resorptions are a group of pathologies with two main characteristics: they are initially asymptomatic and can severely damage affected teeth before their diagnosis. They can occur in the anterior teeth (due to trauma) and the posterior teeth (due to caries, occlusal trauma, or unknown causes). Once the resorption has been diagnosed and classified, prompt treatment is necessary when possible, or the patient should be informed about potential tooth loss if the affected tooth is too severely compromised.

For small affected areas, treatment options include exposing and filling external cervical resorption with composite resin after periodontal surgery or using orthodontic extrusion. For internal resorptions, effective endodontic treatment involves possible intermediate medication using calcium hydroxide and subsequent canal obturation with bio-ceramic materials if there is an endo-periodontal communication. Finally, if the lesion compromises the tooth's structure, tooth replacement techniques will be necessary, which will be discussed in the following chapters.

Double external root resorption

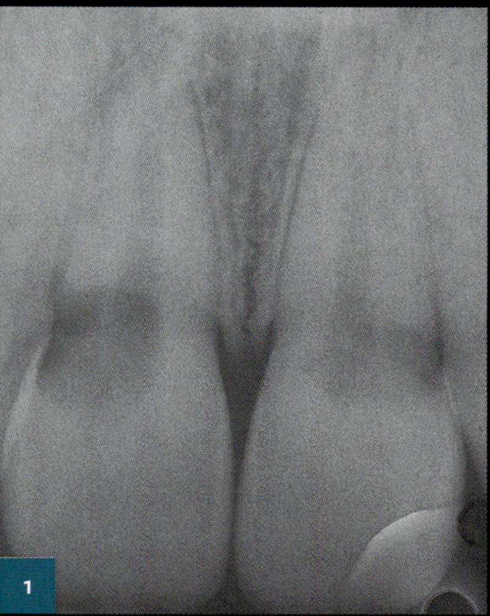

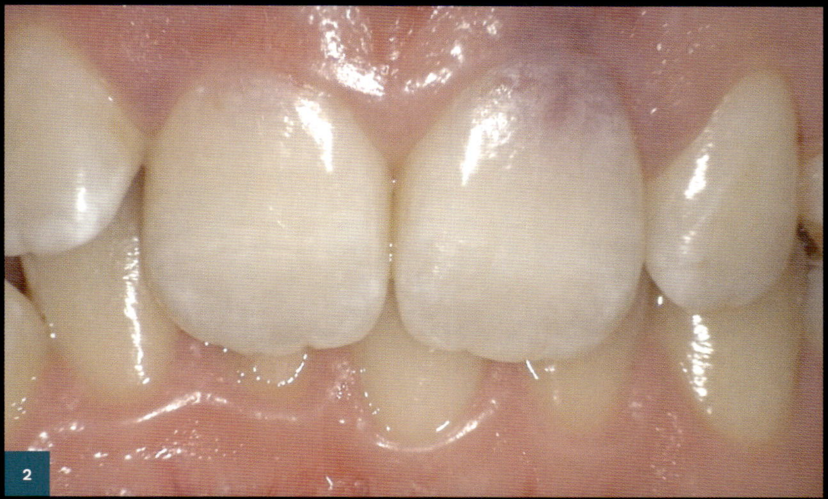

Fig. 1 ■ The radiographic image shows a case of double cervical resorption in a 17-year-old patient.

Fig. 2 ■ The patient is completely asymptomatic. The only observable sign of pathology is represented by the pink discolouration at the cervical portion of the teeth.

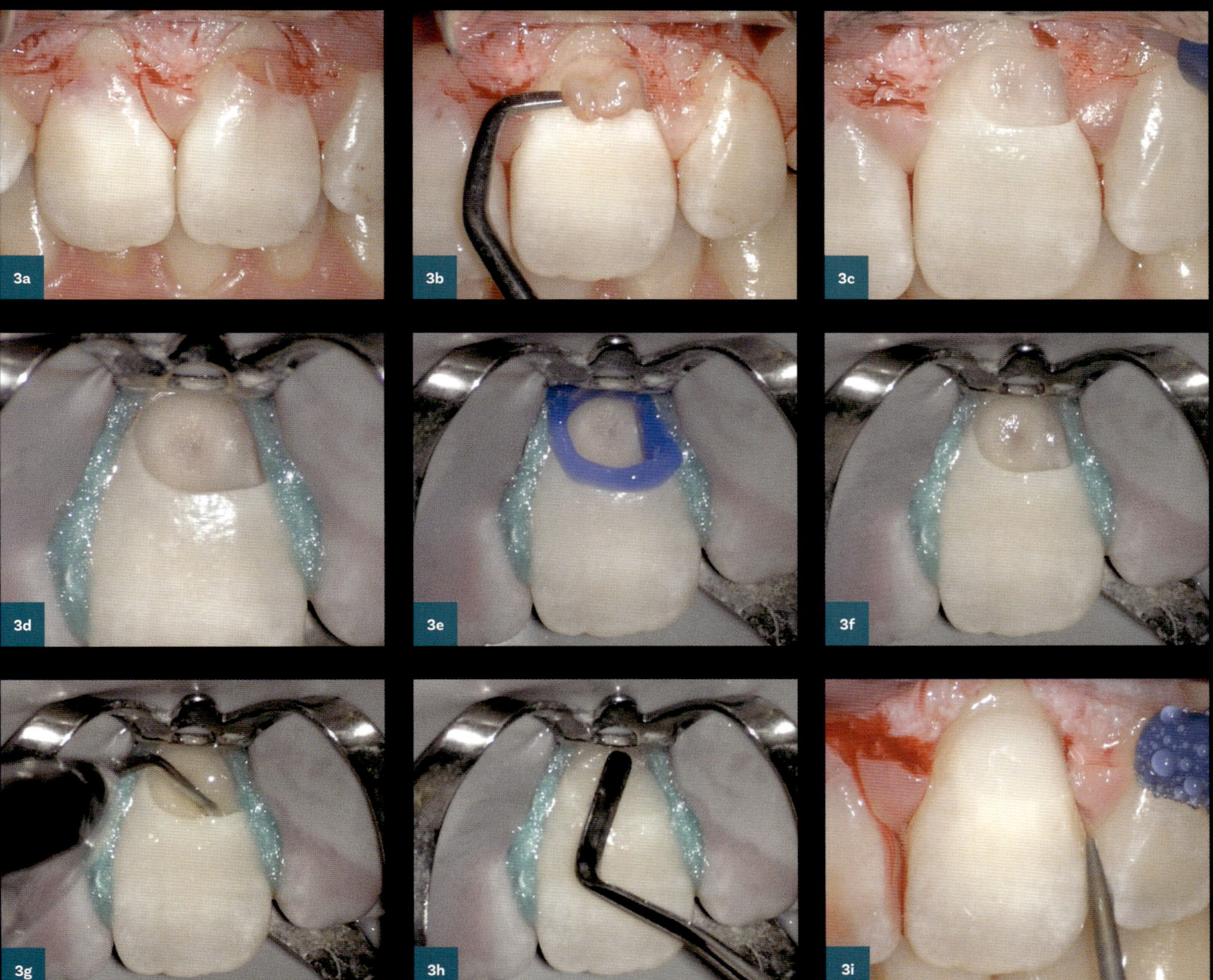

CONT'D >

> *CONT'D*

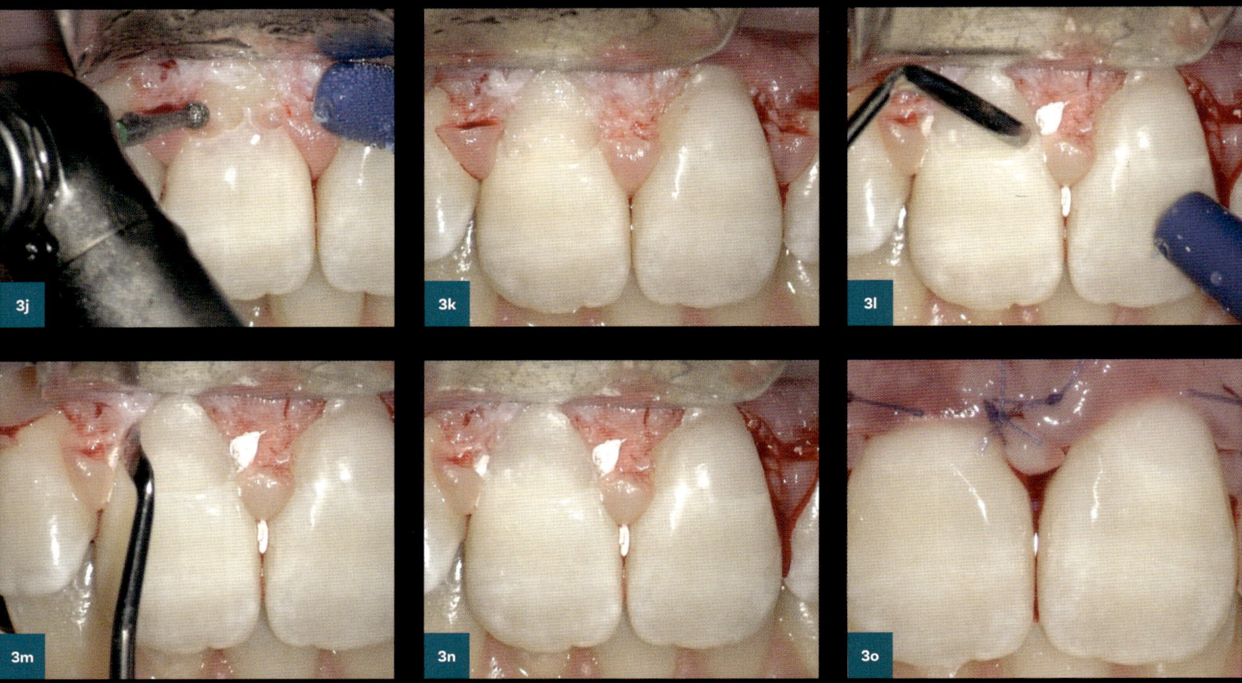

Figs. 3a-o ■ Intraoperative phases of the defect being repaired with composite material. A flap was created to facilitate the placement of a rubber dam under the open flap allowing for individual execution of procedures for each tooth. This approach aided in the isolation of the operating field. Considering the absence of the endodontic space invasion and lack of symptoms, a decision was made to preserve the vitality of the teeth.

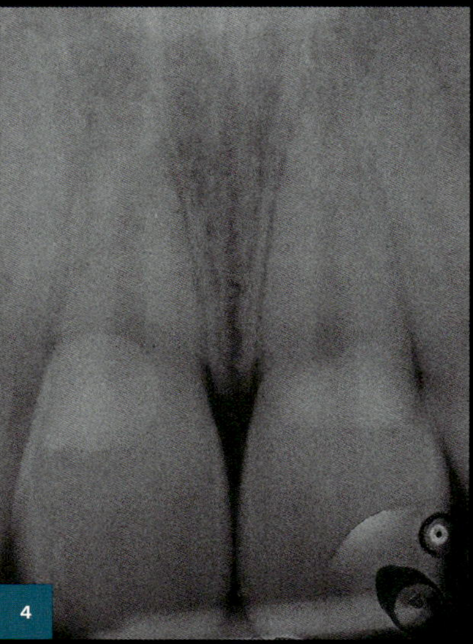

Fig. 4 ■ Post-operative radiograph.

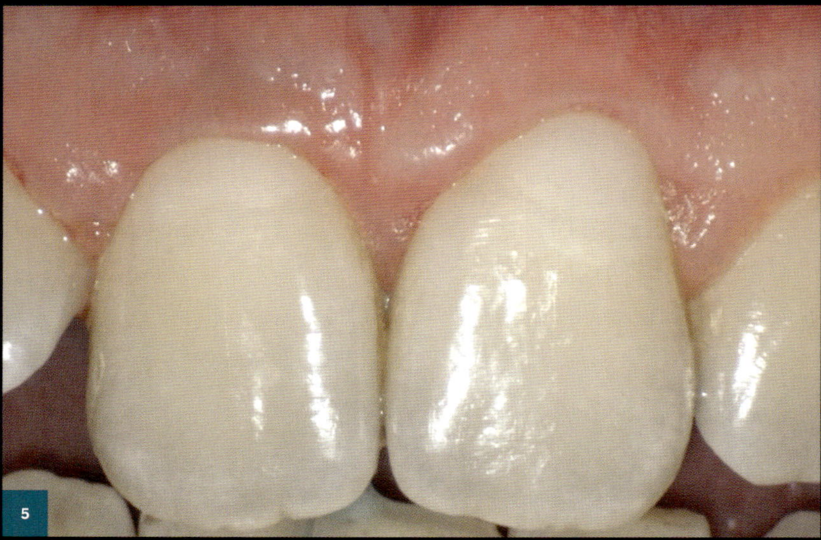

Fig. 5 ■ Soft tissue follow-up at 3 months shows good healing and adaptation to the intraoperative restorations that can now be improved and made completely mimetic.

External invasive root resorption

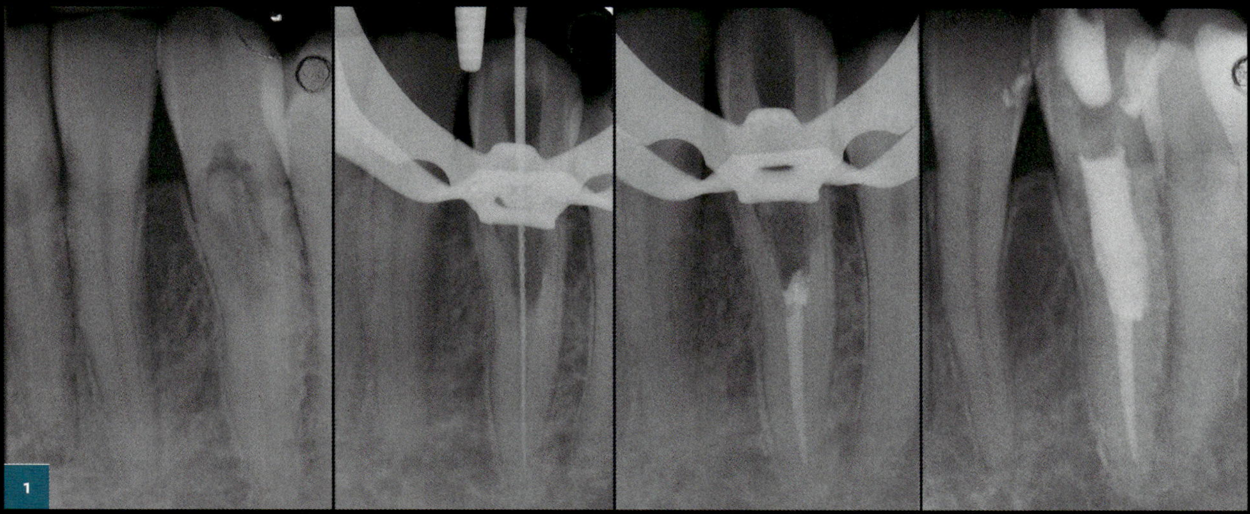

Fig. 1 ■ Radiographic history of a clinical case of external invasive cervical root resorption in a lower canine. After endodontic treatment, the tooth defect is then cleaned and sealed with MTA.

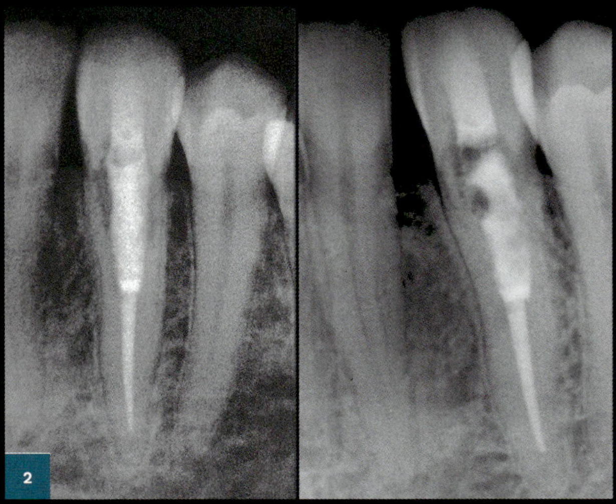

Fig. 2 ■ A radiographic follow-up at 13 and 15 years reveals the onset of a new inflammatory process, but the patient is asymptomatic.

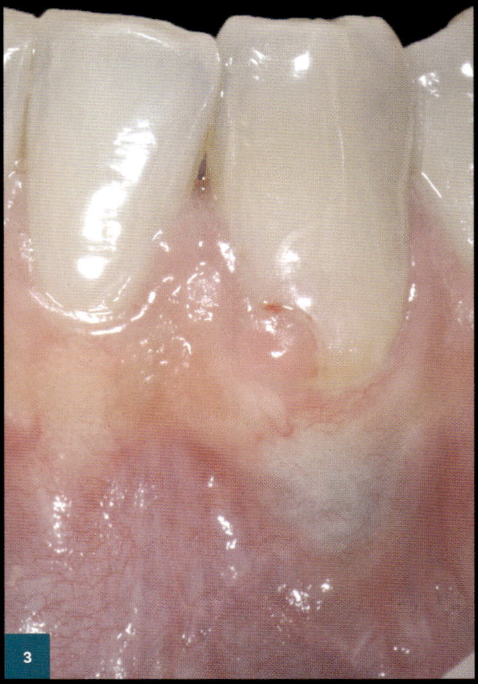

Fig. 3 ■ The patient is asymptomatic. The only sign of pathology is the presence of gingival hyperplasia surrounding the tooths cervical area.

CONT'D >

> CONT'D

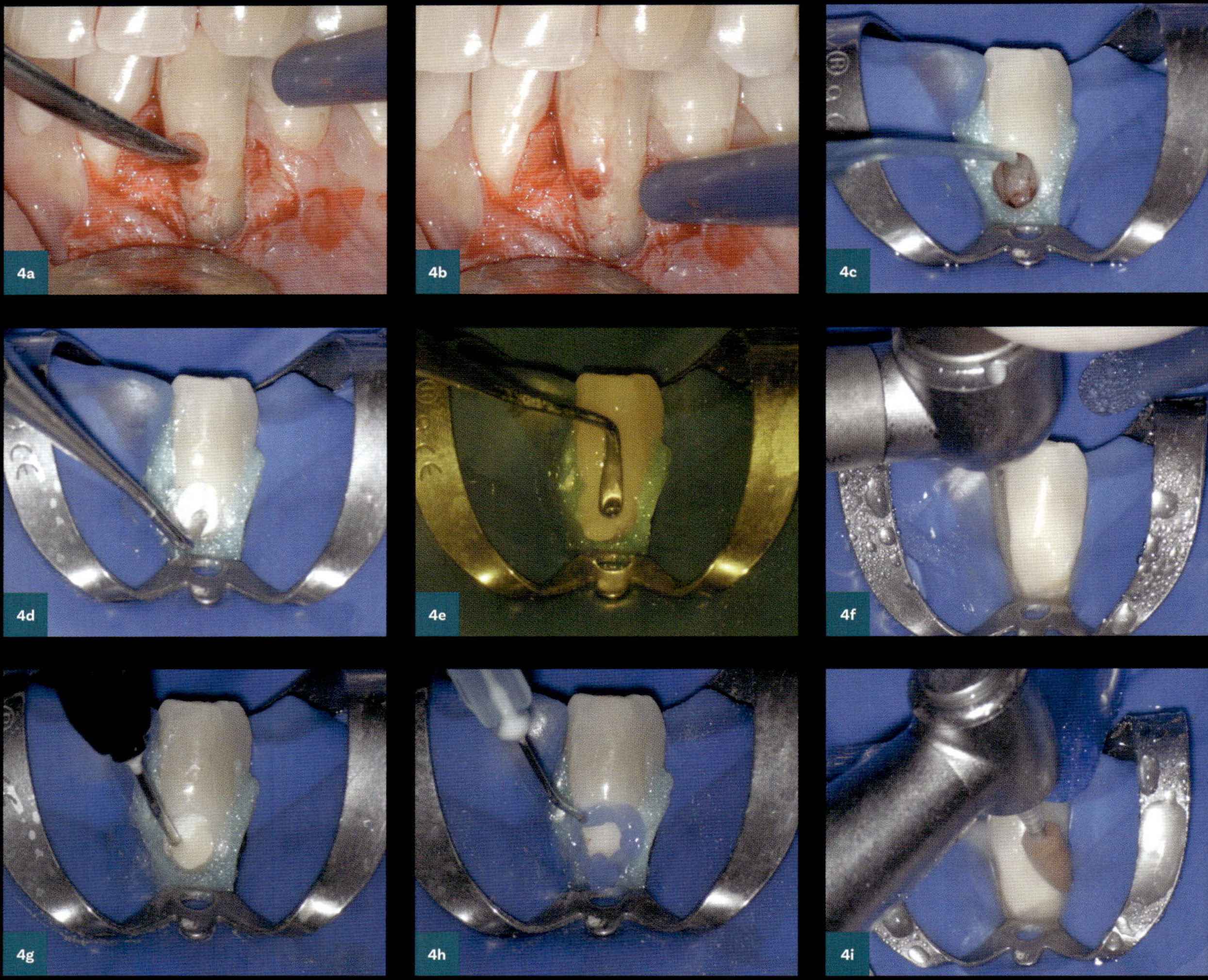

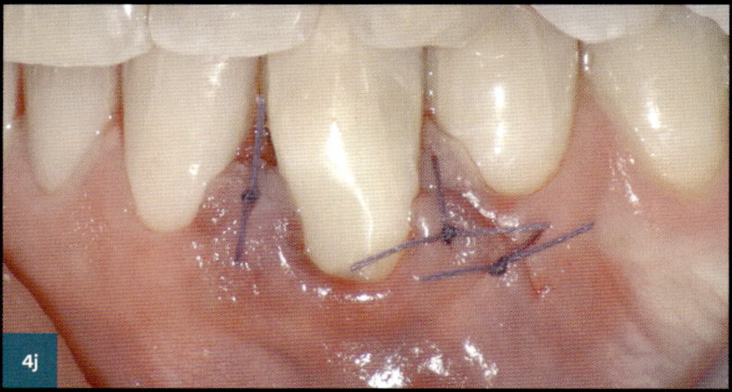

Figs. 4a-j ■ Intraoperative phases, from surgical access to rubber dam placement with open flaps and then complete treatment of the lesion. After pathological tissue removal, the affected area is repaired using bioceramic cement and then filled with a composite resin. Achieving high-quality polishing is crucial for the proper adaptation of the periodontal tissues around the composite filling.

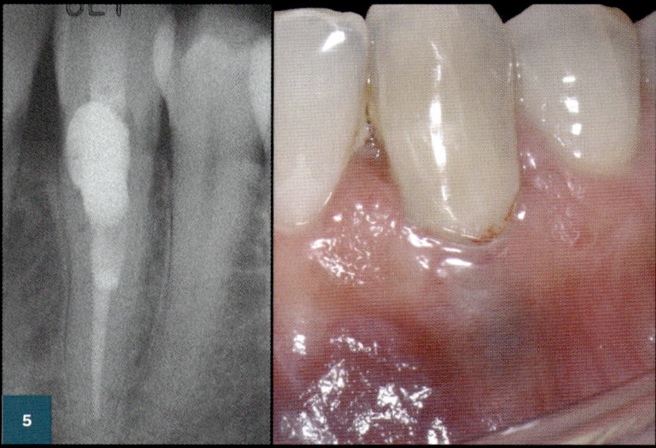

Fig. 5 ■ Post-operative radiograph and re-styling of the intraoperative filling is refined to improve the final aesthetics. Approximately a month later, a good soft tissue adaptation can be observed.

External resorption with intra-canal reparation in a single rooted tooth

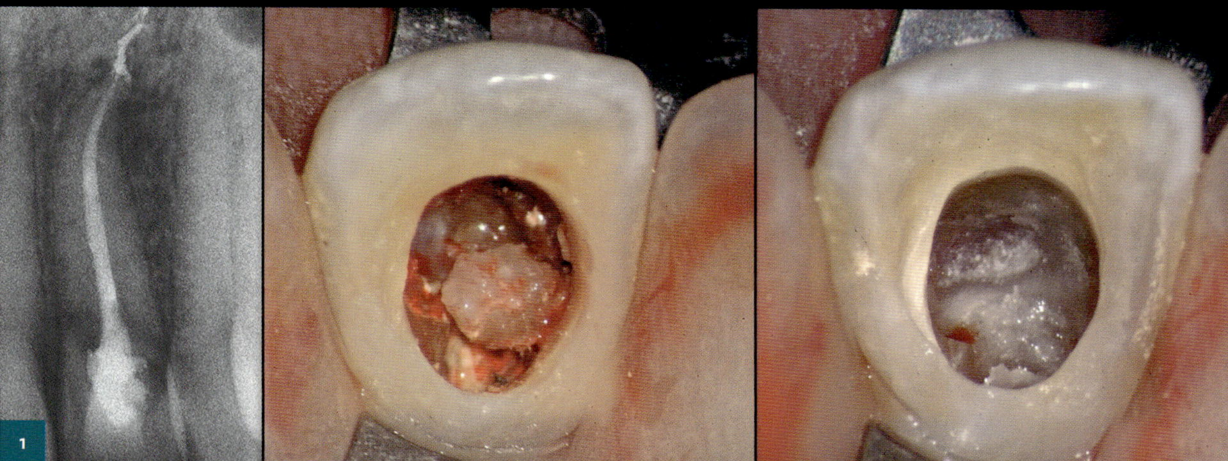

Fig. 1 ■ This 21-year-old patient had an endodontic treatment performed on an upper lateral incisor that was presenting spontaneous symptomatology. The cause was to be found in an undiagnosed external resorption. On re-opening the access-cavity we can appreciate how an inflammatory tissue has invaded large amounts of the pulp chamber.

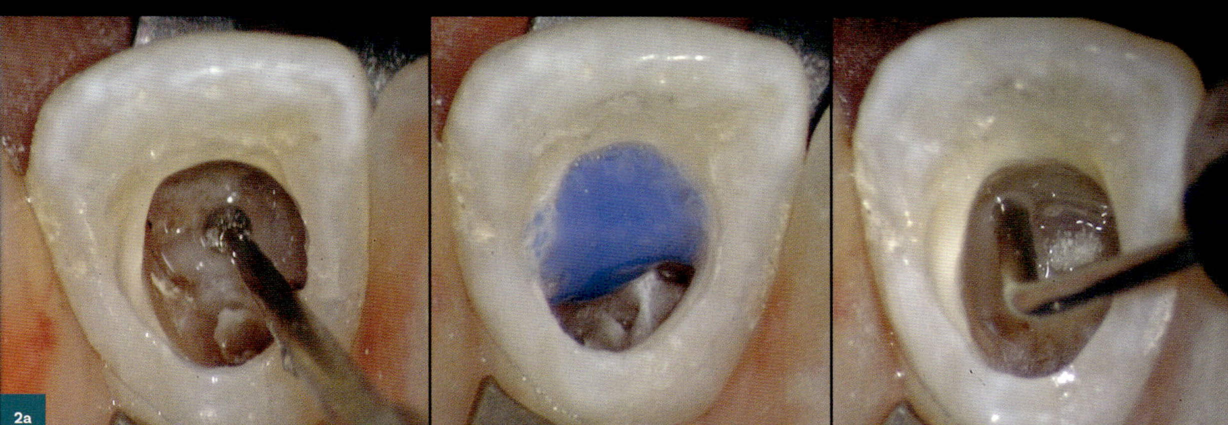

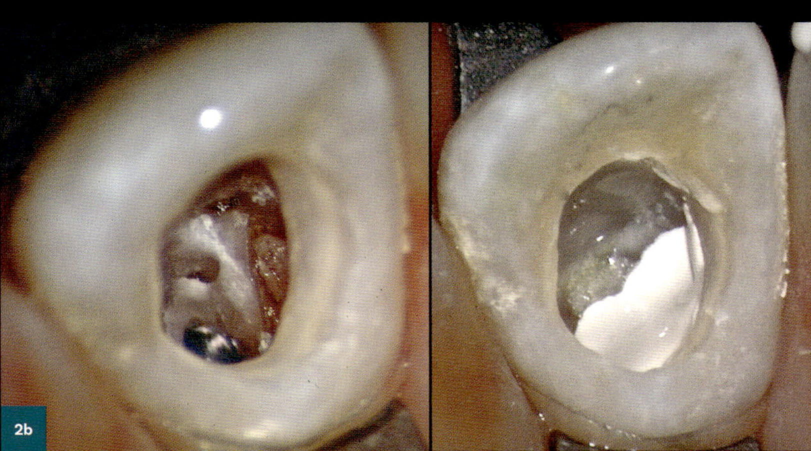

Figs. 2a,b ■ The intraoperative photos show various phases of the treatment and of the defect's repair from inside the pulp chamber. Part of the defect is just above gum level while the remaining portion is below the CEJ.

> CONT'D

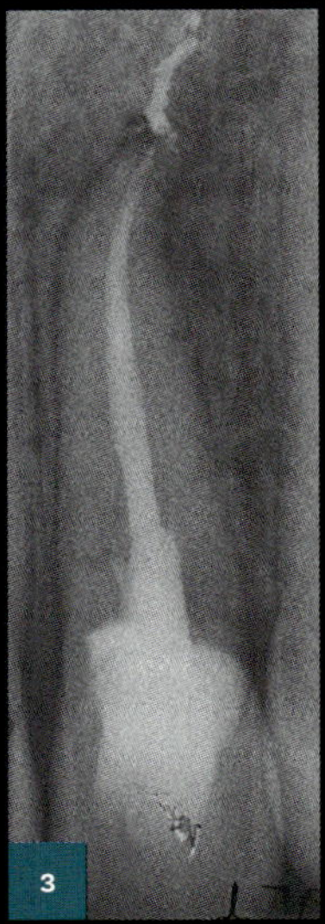
3

Fig. 3 ■ Post-operative radiograph.

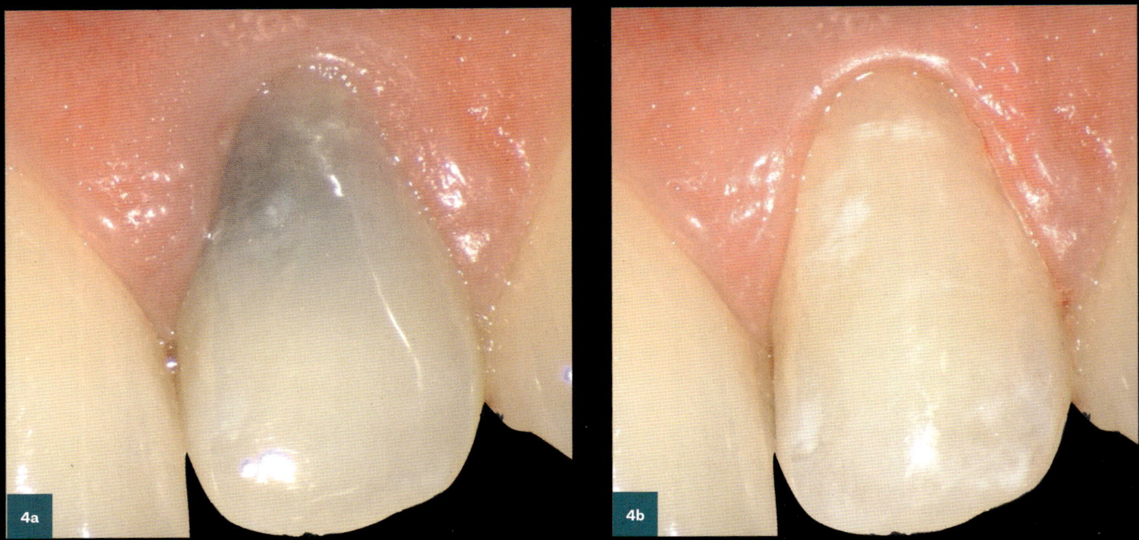
4a 4b

Figs. 4a,b ■ The two photographs show the before and after images of the defects repair.

CLINICAL CASES

External cervical resorption in an upper second molar

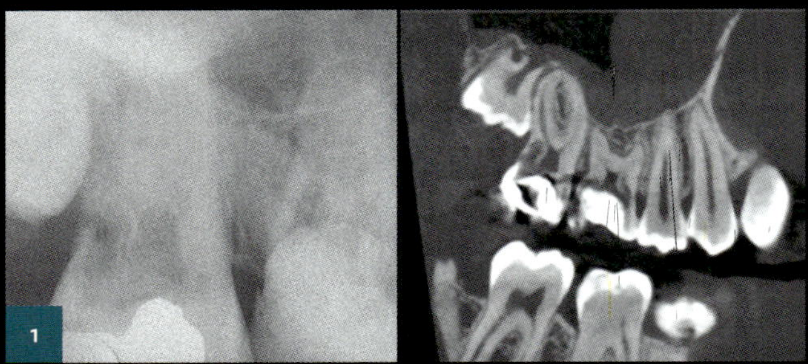
1

Fig. 1 ■ The evident external resorption noticeably affects the cervical area of this upper molar.

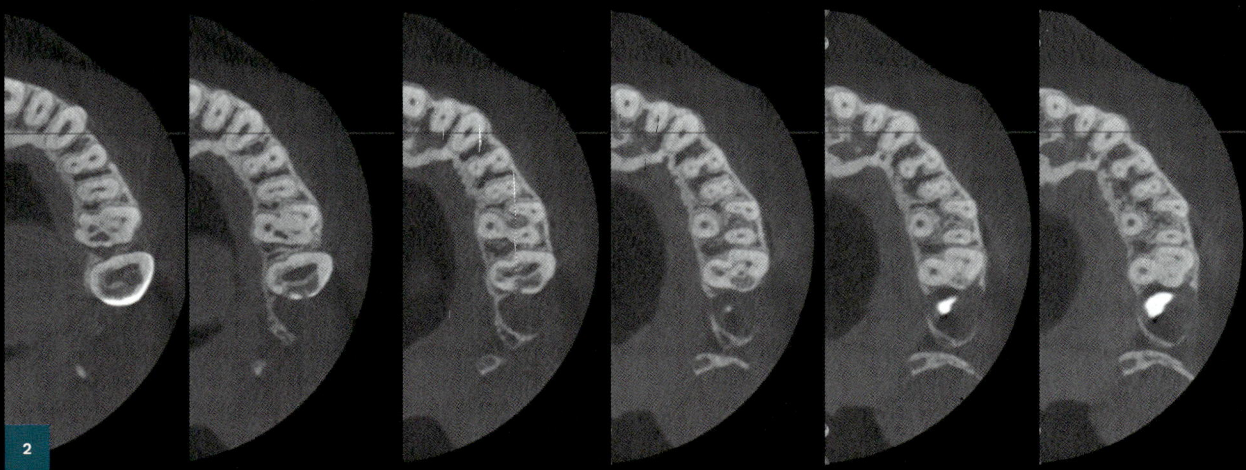
2

Fig. 2 ■ The pre-operative examination, conducted with cone beam computed tomography (CBCT) highlights the progressive expansion of the lesion from the coronal to apical regions, and ultimately stops at the cementoenamel junction (CEJ).

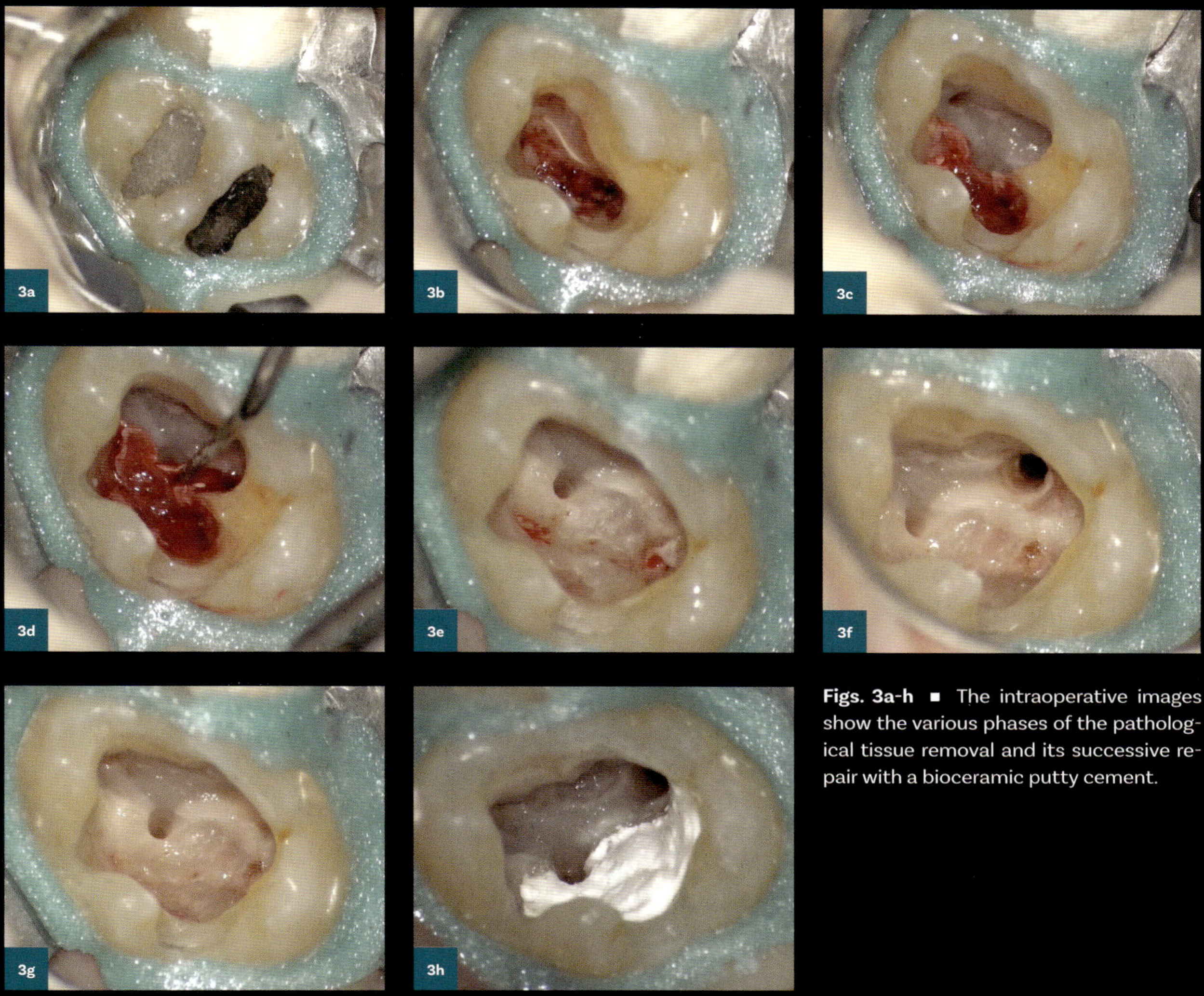

Figs. 3a-h ■ The intraoperative images show the various phases of the pathological tissue removal and its successive repair with a bioceramic putty cement.

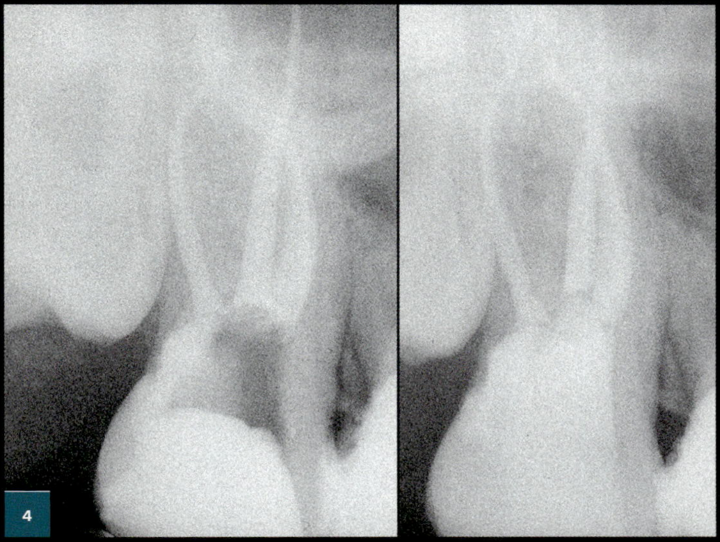

Fig. 4 ■ Post-operative radiograph and final radiograph after complete tooth restoration.

External invasive root resorption

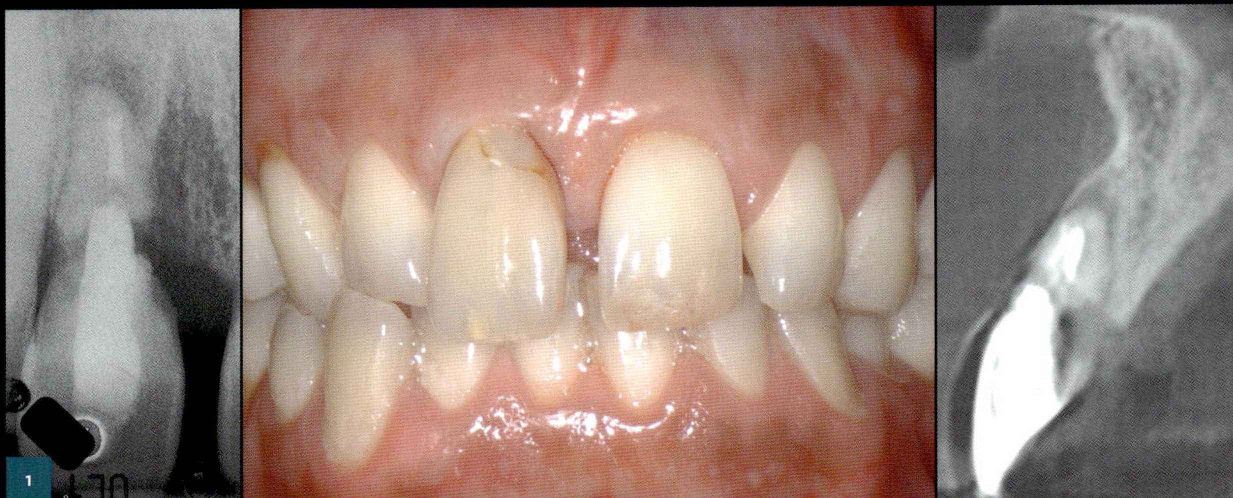

Fig. 1 ■ Pre-operative radiograph, CBCT and pre-operative photo. Since the tooth cannot be saved with a conservative approach, the decision was made to proceed with an immediate post-extraction loaded implant.

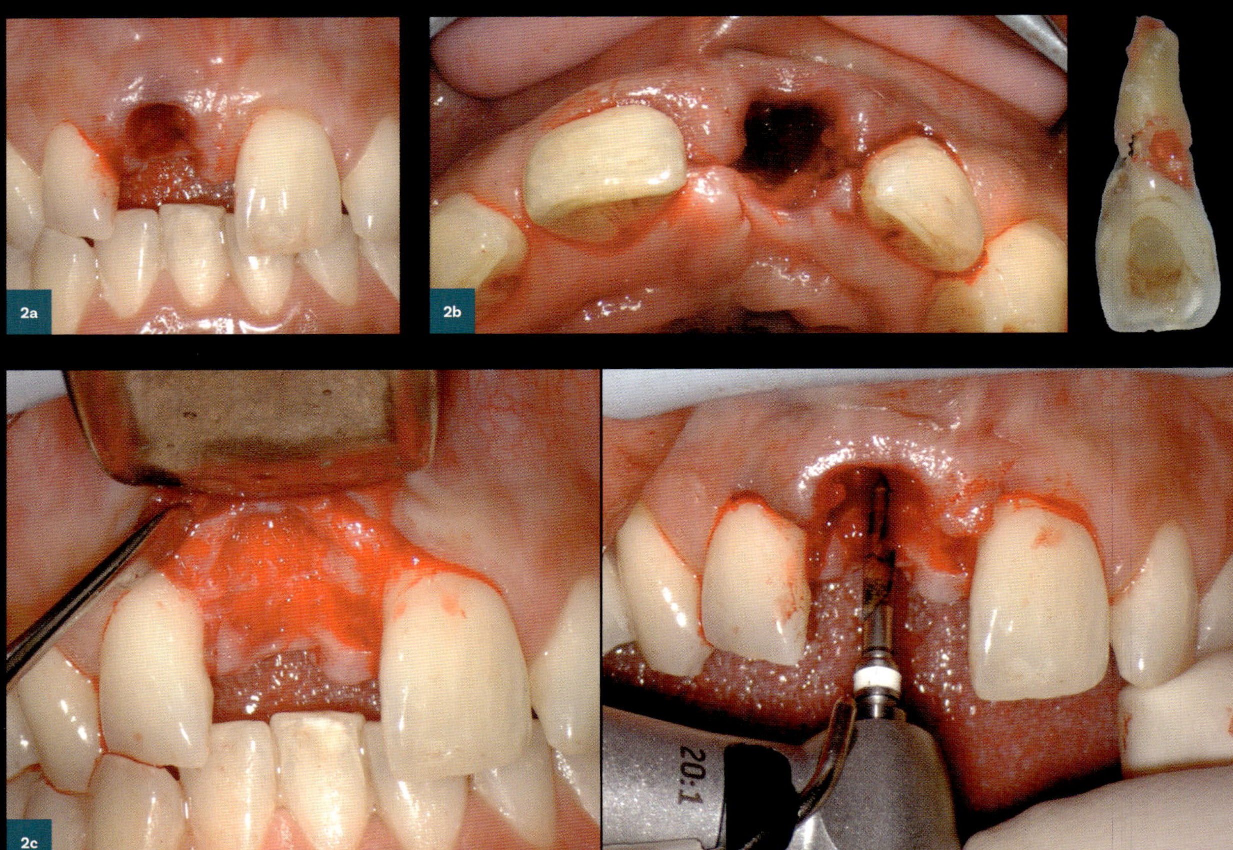

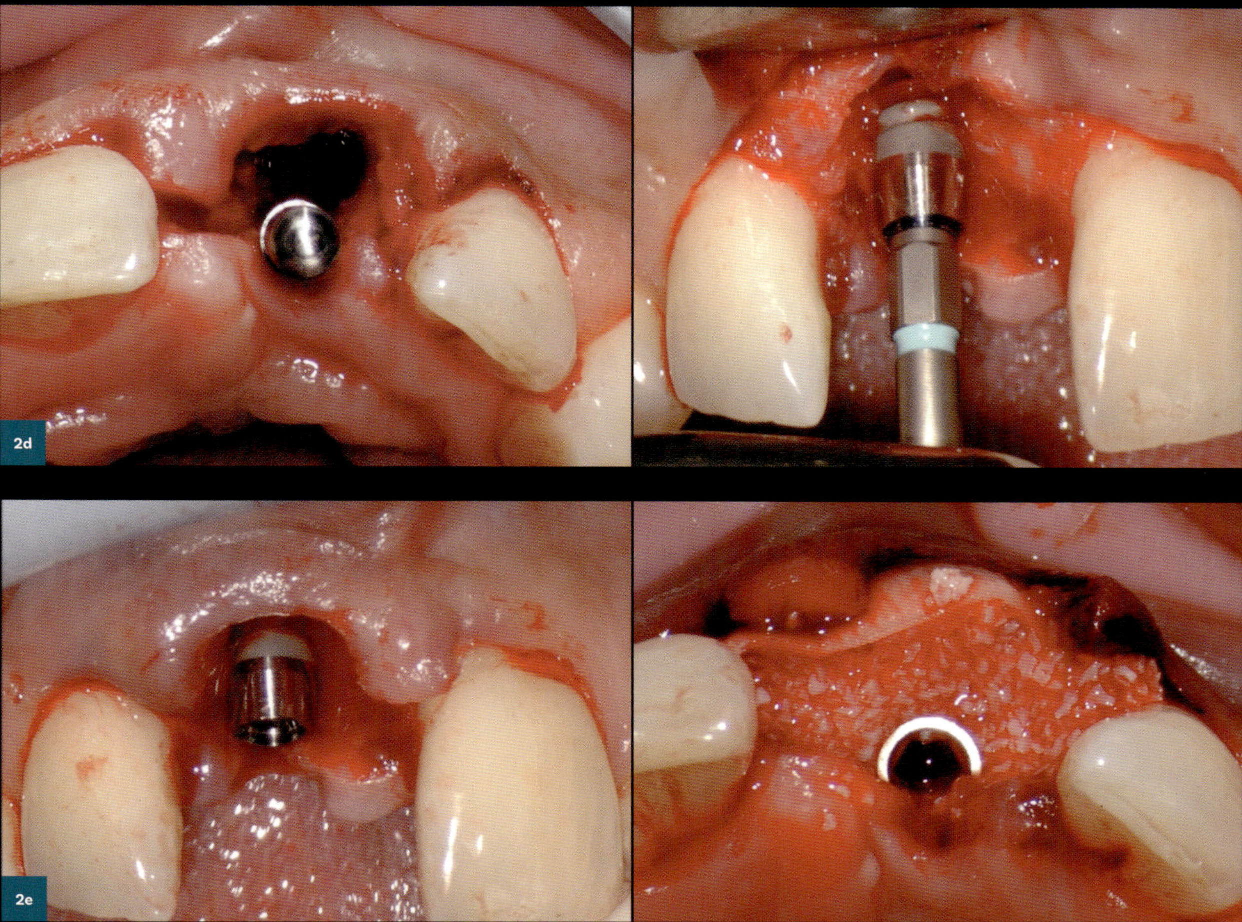

Figs. 2a-e ■ Intraoperative phases, from extraction to implant placement and successive tissue regeneration.

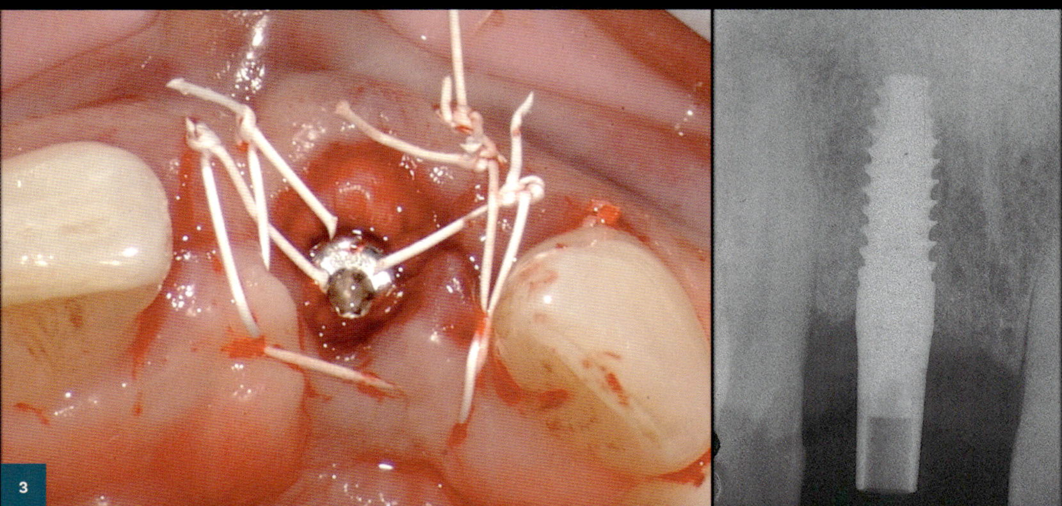

Fig. 3 ■ Post-operative radiograph and sutures. It should be noticed how regenerative techniques tend to maintain and increase the peri-implant tissue.

CONT'D >

> CONT'D

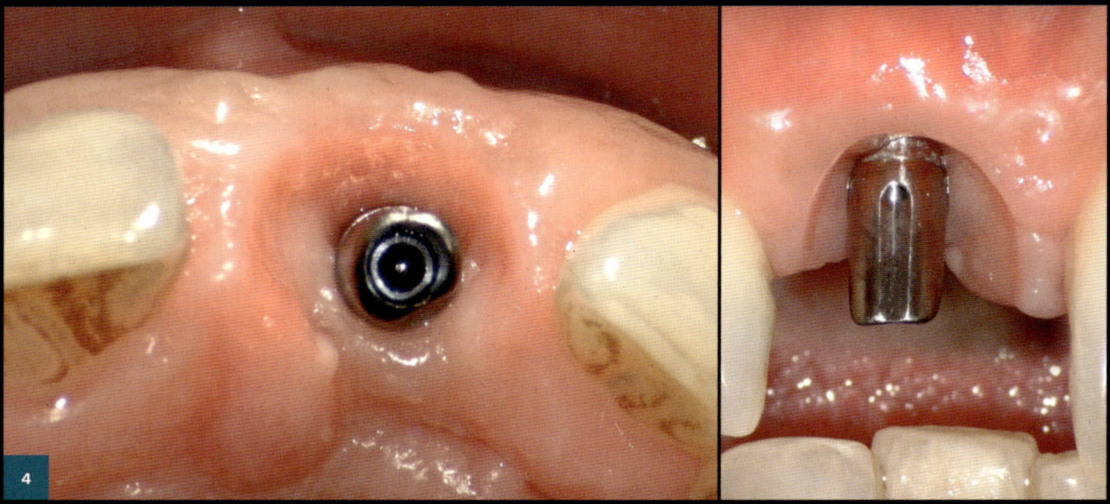

Fig. 4 ■ The healing phases of the peri-implant tissue demonstrate a perfect adaptation around the implant's collar. The strategic placement of a series of temporary crowns guided the gingival margin to the desired position around the implant's abutment.

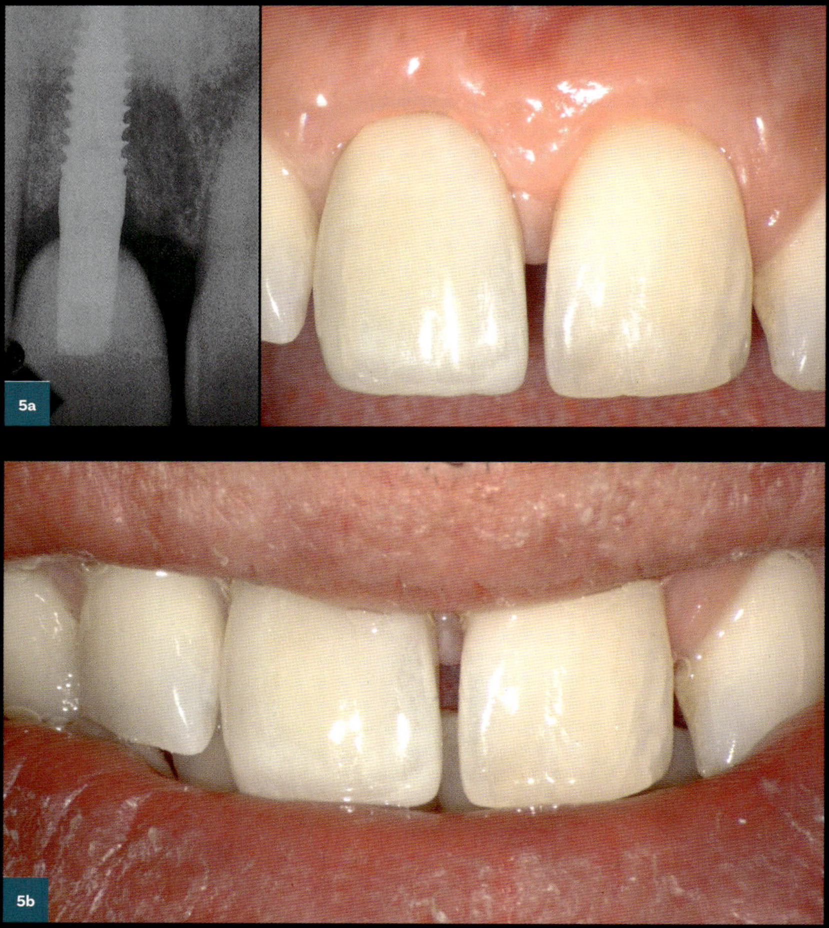

Figs. 5a,b ■ Final restoration and follow-up. Soft tissue management has enabled an adequate aesthetic rehabilitation with restoration of function of the treated area.

Bibliography

1. Pinheiro LHM, Guimarães LS, Antunes LS, Küchler EC, Kirschneck C, Antunes LAA. Genetic variation involved in the risk to external apical root resorption in orthodontic patients: a systematic review. *Clin Oral Investig.* 2021;25(10):5613-5627.
2. Andreasen JO. Luxation of permanent teeth due to trauma. A clinical and radiographic follow-up study of 189 injured teeth. *Scand J Dent Res.* 1970;78(3):273-286.
3. Trope M. Root Resorption due to Dental Trauma. *Endodontic Topics.* 2002;1(1):79-100.
4. Tronstad L. Root resorption aetiology, terminology and clinical manifestations. *Endod Dent Traumatol.* 1988;4(6):241-252.
5. Heithersay GS. Management of tooth resorption. *Aust Dent J.* 2007;52(Suppl 1):S105-S121.
6. Patel S, Kanagasingam S, Pitt Ford T. External cervical resorption: a review. *J Endod.* 2009;35(5):616-625.
7. Aidos H, Diogo P, Santos JM. Root Resorption Classifications: A Narrative Review and a Clinical Aid Proposal for Routine Assessment. *Eur Endod J.* 2018;3(3):134-145.
8. Patel S, Saberi N. The ins and outs of root resorption. *Br Dent J.* 2018;224(9):691-699.
9. Andreasen FM, Kahler B. Pulpal response after acute dental injury in the permanent dentition: clinical implications-a review. *J Endod.* 2015;41(3):299-308.
10. Tindol JE. Internal resorption: a case presentation with bruxism as the possible etiology. *Tex Dent J.* 1992;109(10):13-15.
11. Silveira FF, Nunes E, Soares JA, et al. Double "pink tooth" associated with extensive internal root resorption after orthodontic treatment: a case report. *Dent Traumatol.* 2009;25(3):e43-e47.
12. Kanter J. Idiopathic internal resorption. Report of a case. *J Am Acad Gold Foil Oper.* 1973;16(2):43-47.
13. Ne RF, Witherspoon DE, Gutmann JL. Tooth resorption. *Quintessence Int.* 1999;30(1):9-25.
14. Patel S, Durack C, Ricucci D. Root resorption. In: Hargreaves KM, Berman LH (eds.). Pathways of the pulp. 11th ed. St Louis, Elsevier;2016:660-683.
15. Malmgren B, Malmgren O, Andreasen JO. Alveolar bone development after decoronation of ankylosed teeth. *Endod Topics.* 2006;14(1):35-40.
16. Cohenca N, Stabholz A. Decoronation - a conservative method to treat ankylosed teeth for preservation of alveolar ridge before permanent prosthetic reconstruction: literature review and case presentation. *Dent Traumatol.* 2007;23(2):87-94.
17. Heithersay GS. Invasive cervical resorption: an analysis of potential predisposing factors. *Quintessence Int.* 1999;30(2):83-95.
18. Patel K, Schirru E, Niazi S, Mitchell P, Mannocci F. Multiple apical radiolucencies and external cervical resorption associated with varicella zoster virus: a case report. *J Endod.* 2016;42(6):978-983.
19. Neely AL, Gordon SC. A familial pattern of multiple idiopathic cervical root resorption in a father and son: a 22-year follow-up. *J Periodontol.* 2007;78(2):367-371.
20. Chu EY, Deeb JG, Foster BL, et al. Multiple Idiopathic Cervical Root Resorption: A Challenge for a Transdisciplinary Medical-Dental Team. *Front Dent Med.* 2021;2:1-9.
21. Gorrel C, Larsson A. Feline odontoclastic resorptive lesions: unveiling the early lesion. *J Small Anim Pract.* 2002;43(11):482-488.
22. Heithersay GS. Clinical, radiologic and histopathologic features of invasive cervical resorption. *Quintessence Int.* 1999;30(1):27-37.
23. Patel S, Foschi F, Mannocci F, Patel K. External cervical resorption: a three-dimensional classification. *Int Endod J.* 2017;51(2):206-214.
24. Gunraj MN. Dental root resorption. *Oral Surg Oral Med Oral Pathol Oral Radiol Endod.* 1999;88(6):647-653.
25. Andreasen FM. Transient apical breakdown and its relation to colour and sensibility changes after luxation injuries to teeth. *Endod Dent Traumatol.* 1986;2(1):9-19.

PART III

The replacement of a severely compromised tooth with an immediate implant

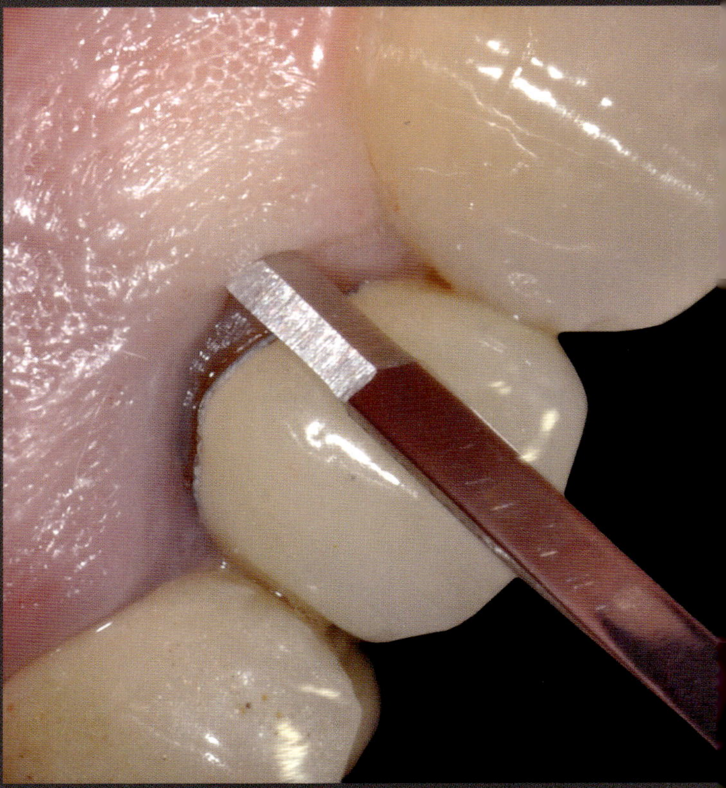

Matteo Antonio **Deflorian**

Fabio **Galli**

Fabio **Gorni**

Pierfrancesco **Zuffetti**

Andrea **Pittaluga**

Riccardo **Scaini**

Tiziano **Testori**

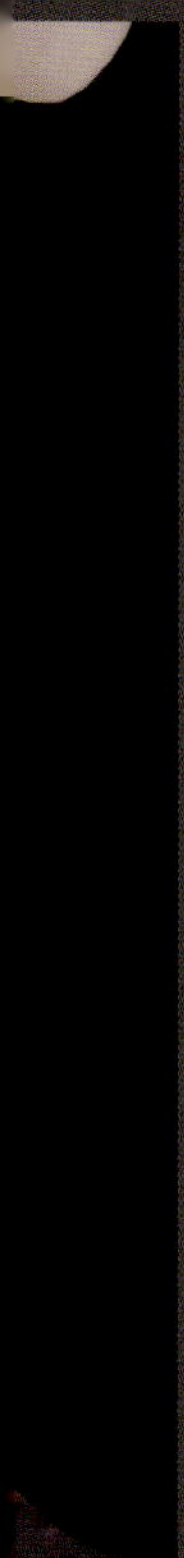

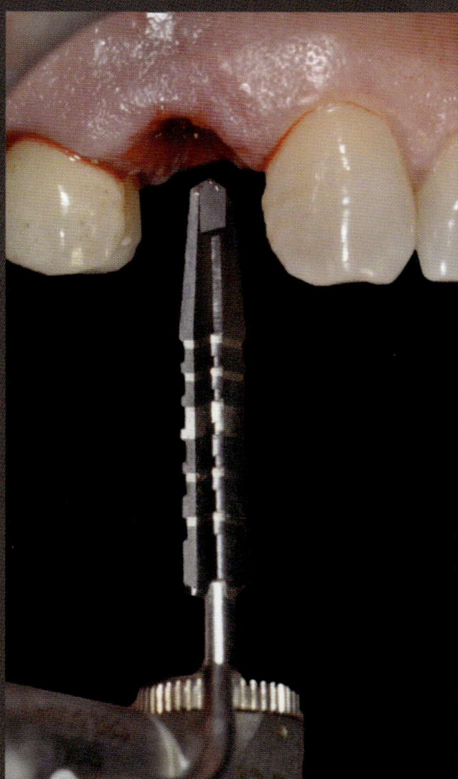

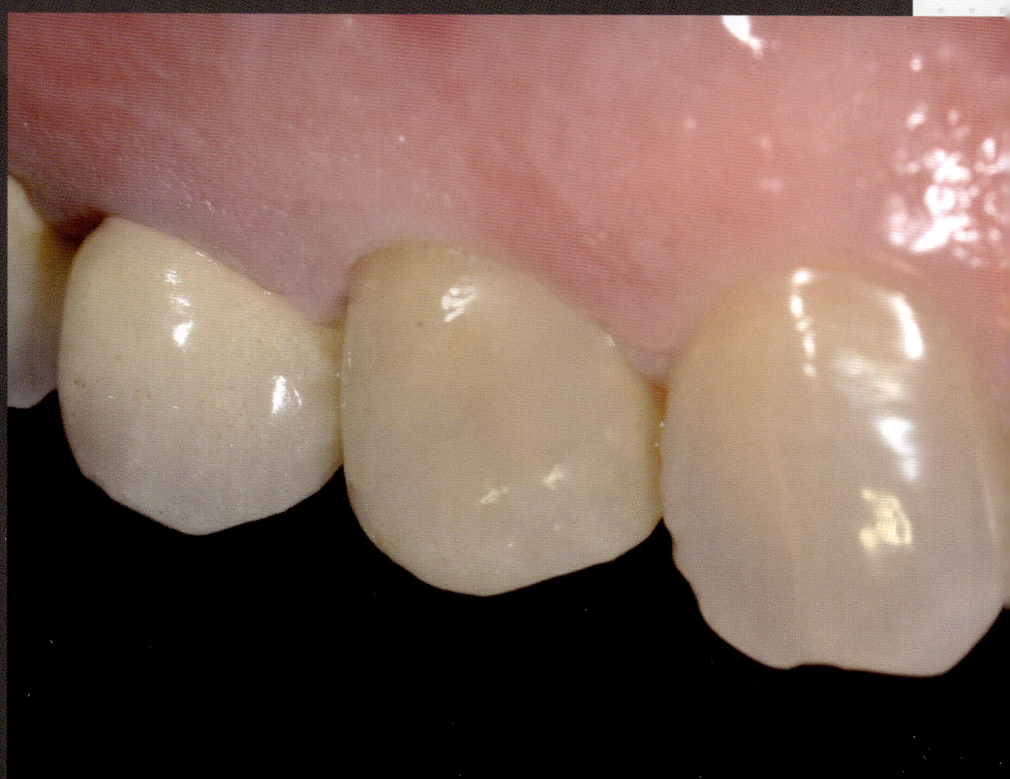

Introduction

Implant treatment for tooth replacement is often a last resort or an alternative when other techniques like restorative, periodontal, and endodontic techniques are not effective to preserve the tooth. Therefore, developing a scientifically supported and ethically oriented treatment plan relies on evaluating the prognosis of each tooth, which is not universally agreed upon due to cultural backgrounds and varying professional experiences, resulting in opposing judgments in some cases.[1-3] Nevertheless, certain essential aspects in the diagnostic phase hold universally recognized value and importance in the restorative/prosthetic, periodontal, and endodontic fields.

The clinician's difficult decision-making process of choosing between repeating root canal therapy or opting for more invasive therapies like implants requires multiple areas of expertise, often necessitating a multidisciplinary approach.[4,5]

Even before evaluating the endodontic aspect, considering the prosthetic/conservative and periodontal perspectives is crucial. In fact, ensuring adequate residual dental structure for reconstruction is essential even if the tooth is recoverable through endodontic treatment.[4,6,7] Previously devitalized teeth often have definitive restorations like crowns or inlays, which may require evaluation if recurrent caries necessitates replacement. The compromised gingival margin may require periodontal (clinical crown lengthening),[6,7] surgical (surgical extrusion in single-rooted cases)[8-10] or orthodontic (orthodontic extrusion)[10,11] interventions. It is also important to account for the possibility of a radiological underestimation of carious lesions present in the analogical detection, which is more relevant in digital detection (phosphorous) when making treatment decisions. If none of these options are feasible, extraction and implant rehabilitation should be considered after balancing the cost-benefit ratio of such interventions.[12] Additionally, it is essential to rule out the possibility of a vertical fracture, which often presents symptoms and manifests as a punctiform probing of the affected area.

Before selecting an endodontic approach, accurate periodontal probing should be performed.[13,14] In cases of diagnosed vertical fractures, extraction therapy becomes inevitable to avoid treatment failure. It is also important to note that this type of probing could arise from the fistulous tract of an endodontic lesion.[15,16] A previously endodontically treated tooth may or may not have a chronic apical lesion, which can be symptomatic or asymptomatic. If there is no apical lesion and no symptoms, and prosthetic tooth restoration is necessary, the clinician should consider if the previous treatment can be improved. If the previous therapy is deemed correct, retreatment (except for the loss of its coronal seal) may be dangerous and counterproductive, possibly leading to the decision not to retreat the tooth.[17]

However, if the clinician is confident in improving the previous therapy, a new endodontic approach is recommended. If a tooth has acceptable and asymptomatic root canal therapy with no signs of apical distress, it is neither acceptable nor unethical to cause iatrogenic damage.[4,5] Conversely, if the tooth has a chronic lesion or is symptomatic, and conservative, prosthetic and periodontal maintenance is possible, retreatment is indicated. The retreatment complexity can vary from simple to extremely complex cases, often directly proportional to the amount of iatrogenic damage present and anatomical complexity of the tooth, often requiring specific instruments like an operating microscope, lasso extractor, root canal post removal devices or dedicated ultrasonic tips.[4,5] A thorough radiographic analysis is essential for a correct approach to retreatment.[4] By utilizing it, we can proactively identify various treatment challenges, such as:

- marginal congruity of the pre-existing restoration
- underfilling/overfilling
- intracanal posts
- false paths/perforations
- broken files
- important apical dimensions.

One of the clinician's initial decisions revolves around retaining the pre-existing restorations. If marginal seal loss is absent, they may decide to preserve the restoration. However, it is crucial to acknowledge that this choice complicates the treatment further, necessitating meticulous cavity access due to potential discrepancies between the prosthetic restoration's inclination and the original one. Consequently, perforation of the coronal third becomes more frequent in such cases. Several factors contraindicate access through the restoration, including the possibility of having damaged internal tissue (which compromises the long-term therapy success), sub-optimal adhesion between the adhesive restoration and the old restoration, and challenges posed by metallic elements inside the old crown, making electronic apex locators difficult to use. The key to endodontic success lies in the three-dimensional sealing of the root canal system, as treatment failure can result from filling the canal short of the apex or leaving voids.[4,18] A careful analysis of the number of untreated/obturated canals, the quality of the previous treatment (considering taper, shaping and three-dimensional filling), as well as radiological visibility of the canal lumen and previous treatment, thereby form the basis for formulating an appropriate endodontic treatment plan.

In fact, if the previous therapy presented a correct shape (albeit "short") and the canal was invisible beyond that point, the retreatment of the element is strongly discouraged, thereby favouring a surgical approach (apical surgery) as the first choice.[4] In cases with overfilling, the decision to retain the tooth may require a surgical approach based on the amount of extruded material and the operator's skills.[19] Root canal posts, prevalent before and after the advent of adhesive reconstructive techniques, frequently pose challenges in retreatment dentistry, necessitating particular extraction techniques. Therefore, identifying them in advance allows proper preparation before starting therapy.[20,21] False pathways and perforations, among the most common iatrogenic errors, may not be identifiable through simple two-dimensional imaging alone. If there is any suspicion, it should prompt the use of three-dimensional imaging with a Cone-Beam CT scan for early identification and localization. The position and size of the perforations may require different obturation techniques and operating strategies. Therefore, it is useful to identify them in advance to allow formulation of a more accurate tooth prognosis.[22] Another significant obstacle yet common iatrogenic error is the presence of fractured root canal instrument fragments inside the canal lumen. Depending on the instrument type, the fragment length and its position within the canal, the clinician may decide to bypass or remove it, necessitating the use of an operating microscope during fragment removal.[23,24]

Chronic apical lesions can remodel the apex, considerably increasing its calibre and reducing its taper, which complicates obturation. The advanced identification of this clinical situation helps the operator plan retreatment effectively, prepare instruments for possible closure with a silicate-based apical plug, and communicate with the patient more effectively.[25] As we have seen, evaluating a previously endodontically treated tooth requires multidisciplinary skills. Furthermore, a correct diagnosis, as in all areas of medicine, is essential for treatment success. This shares the same importance as the early identification of retreatment dentistry-related problems, which is fundamentally important for therapy preparation and proper ergonomics. In a small but substantial percentage of cases, particularly when developing complex treatment plans, it is crucial to consider a well-established orthodontic treatment concept known as "strategic extraction for implant placement".

In summary, as clinicians and as authors, we find it essential to evaluate the possibility of extracting teeth that could be preserved, following the above criterion, in cases where their maintenance would result in more complex and invasive treatment carrying a greater risk of developing complications. (**Figs. 1.1a-d, 1.2**).

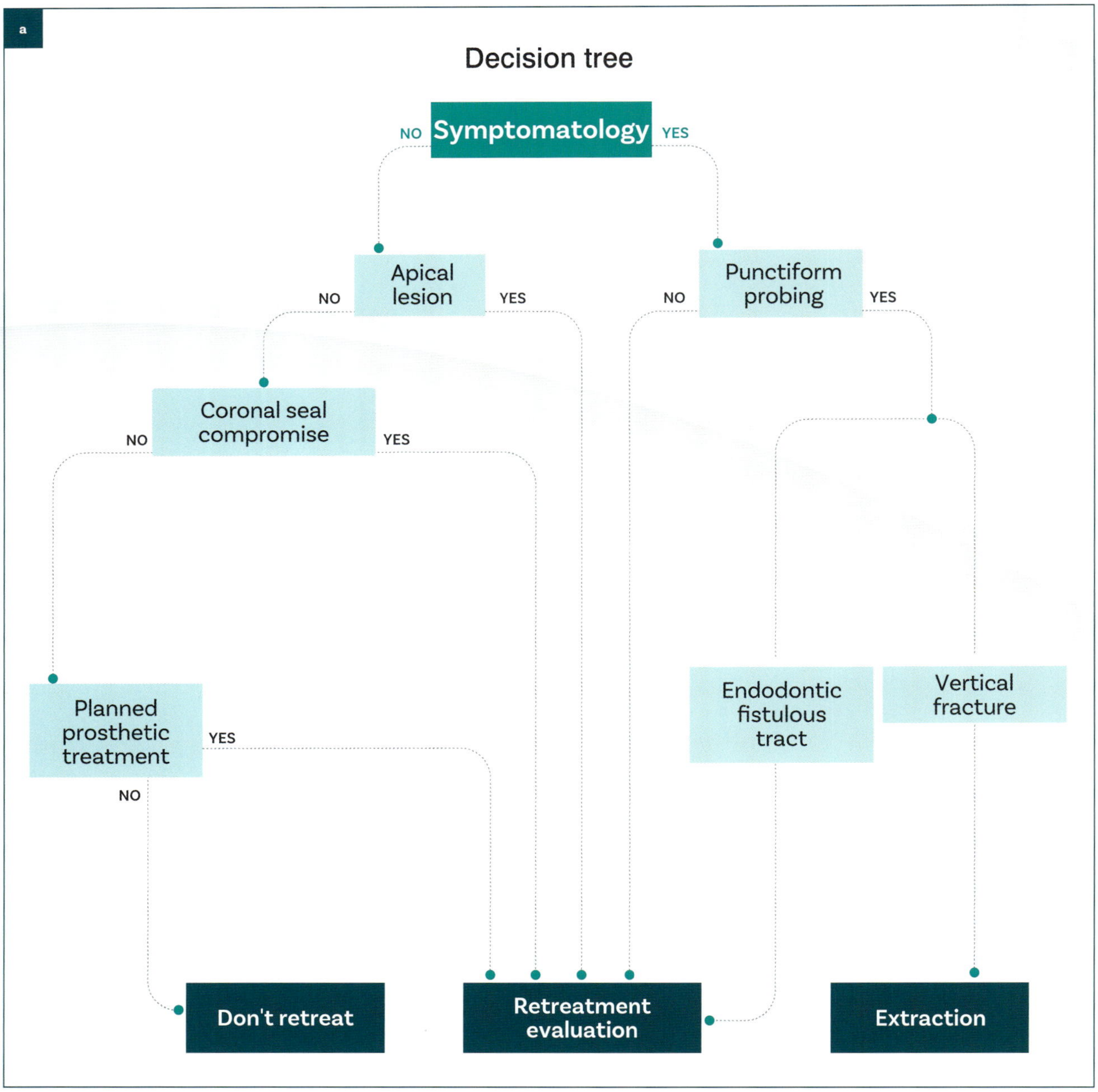

Figs. 1.1a-d ■ The decision tree presents the structural and periodontal analyses required in case of retreatment.

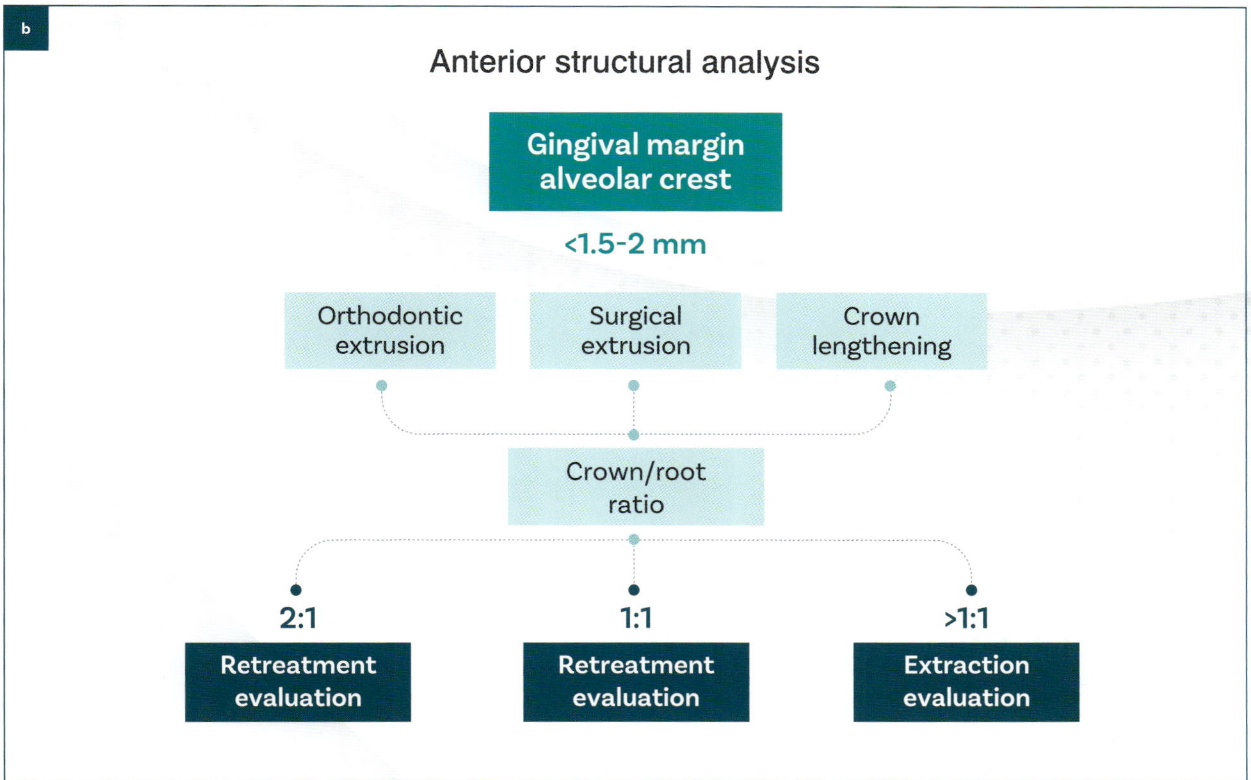
b
Anterior structural analysis
Gingival margin alveolar crest
<1.5-2 mm
Orthodontic extrusion
Surgical extrusion
Crown lengthening
Crown/root ratio
2:1
1:1
>1:1
Retreatment evaluation
Retreatment evaluation
Extraction evaluation

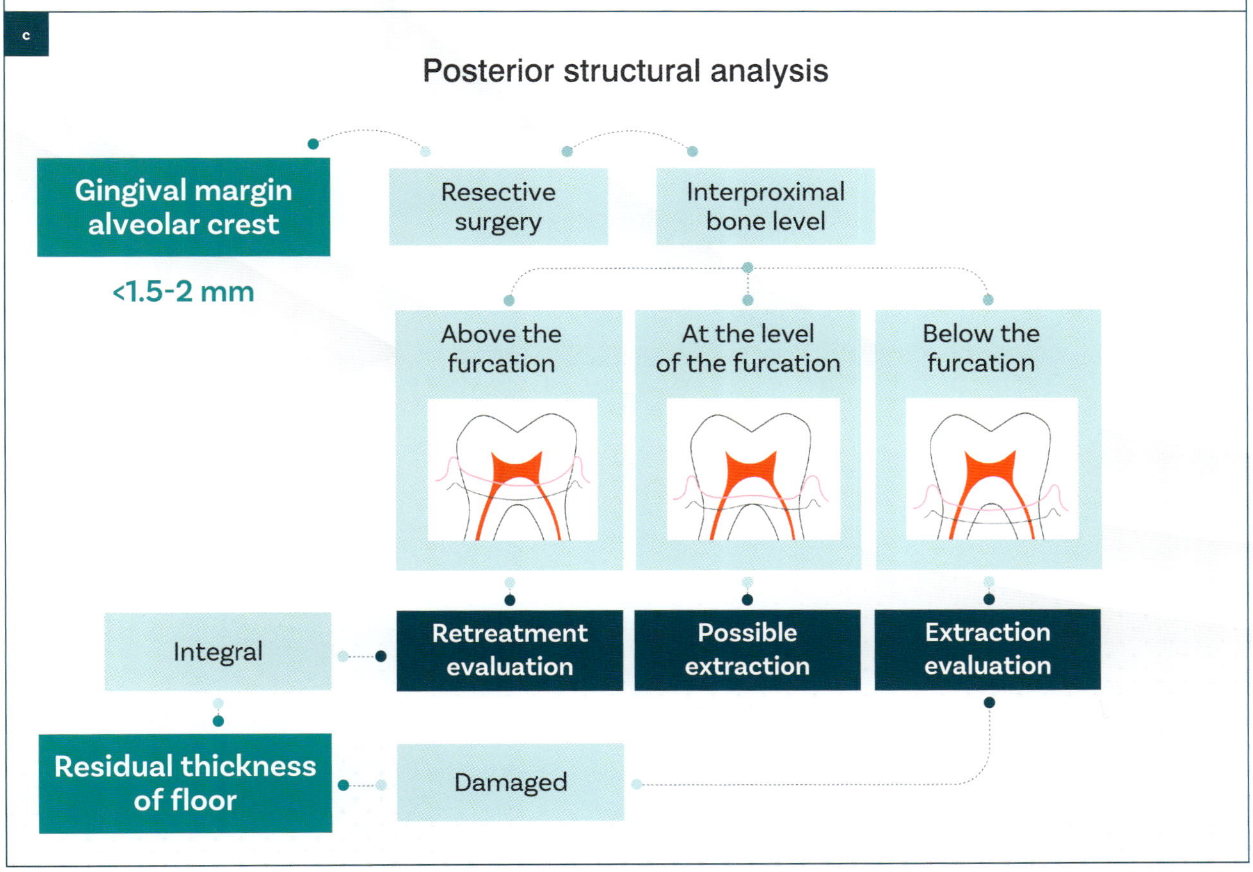
c
Posterior structural analysis
Gingival margin alveolar crest
<1.5-2 mm
Resective surgery
Interproximal bone level
Above the furcation
At the level of the furcation
Below the furcation
Integral
Retreatment evaluation
Possible extraction
Extraction evaluation
Residual thickness of floor
Damaged

CONT'D >

> CONT'D

d

Periodontal analysis

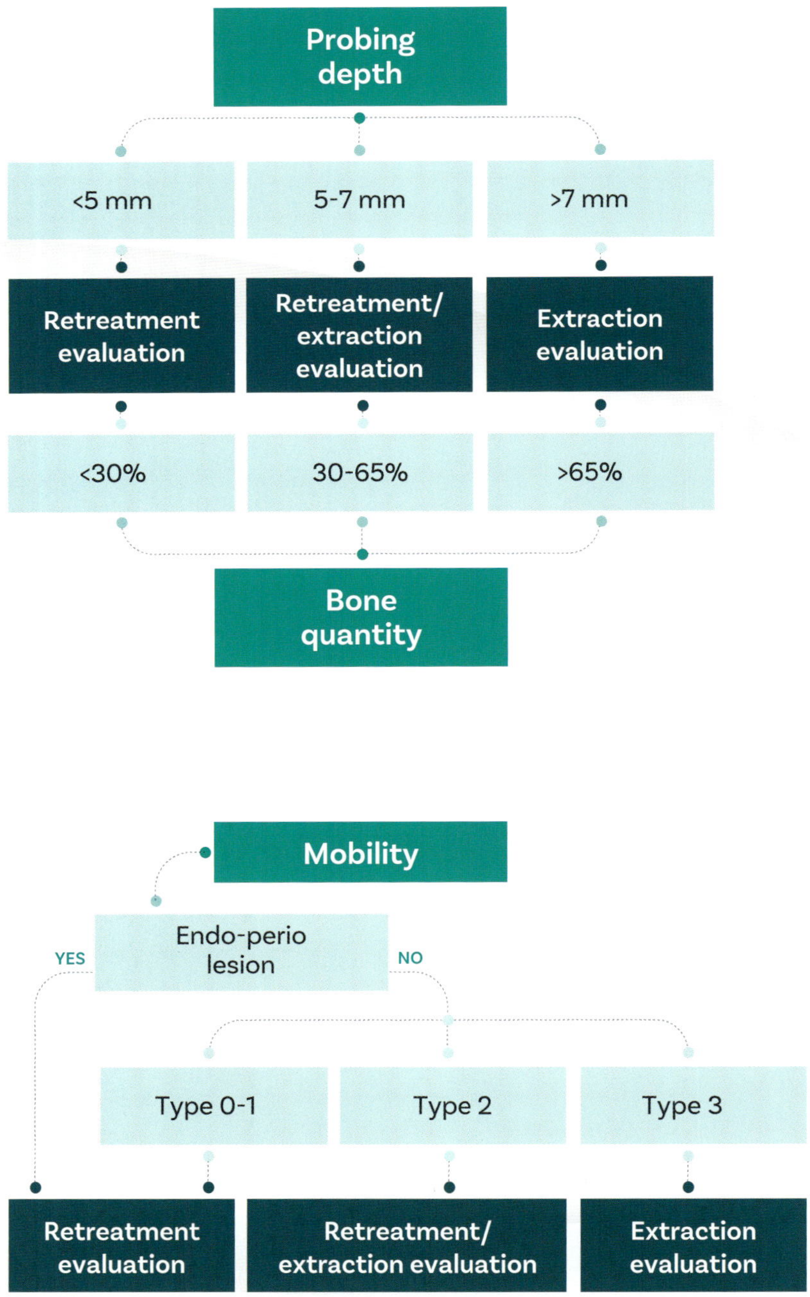

Difficulty level

UNDERFILLING	1	2	3	4	5
Inadequate taper and 3D obturation, visible apical endodontium	X				
Inadequate taper and 3D obturation, no visible apical endodontium			X		
Adequate taper and 3D obturation, visible apical endodontium				X	
Adequate taper and 3D obturation, no visible apical endodontium					X*
OVERFILLING					
Inadequate taper and 3D obturation, canal space visible laterally			X		
Adequate taper and 3D obturation, canal space completely obturated					X*

APICAL DIAMETER	1	2	3	4	5
25-40	X				
40-70			X		
>70					X
Resorption or altered anatomy					X*

FIBRE POST	1	2	3	4	5
coronal 1/3		X			
middle 1/3				X	
apical 1/3					X*
"DENTATUS" POST					
coronal 1/3	X				
middle 1/3		X			
apical 1/3				X	
CAST POST					
coronal 1/3		X			
middle 1/3			X		
apical *1/3					X

* Retreatment is contraindicated: apical surgery or extraction is indicated.

CONT'D >

Fig. 1.2 ■ Evaluation of the case difficulty.

> *CONT'D*

Difficulty level

BROKEN FILE	1	2	3	4	5
coronal 1/3		X			
middle 1/3					X
apical 1/3					X
PERFORATION: POSITION					
Floor/crown			X		
Furcation/stripping					X
apical 1/3					X
PERFORATION: DIMENSION					
<1.5 mm			X		
1.5-3 mm				X	
>3 mm					X*

* Retreatment is contraindicated: apical surgery or extraction is indicated.

Add the score indicated according to the tooth to be examined

TOOTH POSITION	
Single-rooted	0
Multi-rooted	+5

The presence of a tooth scoring 5 categorizes the case as a "**complex retreatment**".

If there are multiple teeth scoring 5, retreatment may be contraindicated. Careful evaluation is required regarding the patient's willingness to maintain them, their importance as prosthetic abutments, and the availability of appropriate instrumentation.

0-9 | 9-15 | 16-21 | >21

0-9 SIMPLE RETREATMENT:
It can be performed with basic instruments, and the use of a magnification system is necessary.

9-15 MODERATE RETREATMENT:
It may require specific instrumentation, and the use of an operating microscope is advisable.

16-21 COMPLEX RETREATMENT:
It requires specific instrumentation, with the use of an operating microscope being essential.

>21 UNFAVOURABLE COST/BENEFIT RATIO
It is important to carefully assess the patient's willingness to maintain the tooth as a prosthetic abutment. Additionally, the availability of instruments must be considered. If these factors pose challenges, extraction should be considered.

Bibliography

1. Azarpazhooh A, Dao T, Figueiredo R, Krahn M, Friedman S. A survey of dentists' preferences for the treatment of teeth with apical periodontitis. *J Endod.* 2013;39(10):1226-1233.
2. Azarpazhooh A, Dao T, Figueiredo R, Krahn M, Friedman S. A survey of patients' preferences for the treatment of teeth with apical periodontitis. *J Endod.* 2013;39(12):1534-1541.
3. Censi R, De Micheli L, Borgonovo AE, Vavassori V, Re D. Treatment of seriously compromised teeth: decision-making criteria and treatment options. *Minerva Stomatol.* 2013;62(9):321-333.
4. Gagliani MM, Gorni FG, Martignoni M. Ritrattamenti. Soluzioni per patologie periapicali di origine endodontica. Capitolo I: "Gli insuccessi in endodonzia. Un'analisi clinica ed epidemiologica". Edra 2018.
5. Gorni FG, Gagliani MM. The outcome of endodontic retreatment: a 2-yr follow-up. *J Endod.* 2004;30(1):1-4.
6. Ghezzi C, Brambilla G, Conti A, Dosoli R, Ceroni F, Ferrantino L. Cervical margin relocation: case series and new classification system. *Int J Esthet Dent.* 2019;14(3):272-284.
7. Veneziani M. Adhesive restorations in the posterior area with subgingival cervical margins: new classification and differentiated treatment approach. *Eur J Esthet Dent.* 2010;5(1):50-76.
8. Plotino G, Abella Sans F, Duggal MS, et al. Clinical procedures and outcome of surgical extrusion, intentional replantation and tooth autotransplantation - a narrative review. *Int Endod J.* 2020;53(12):1636-1652.
9. Angerame D, De Biasi M, Kalaj B, Maglione M. Surgical extrusion: A dental technique. *J Prosthet Dent.* 2021;125(1):23-28.
10. Cordaro M, Staderini E, Torsello F, Grande NM, Turchi M, Cordaro M. Orthodontic Extrusion vs. Surgical Extrusion to Rehabilitate Severely Damaged Teeth: A Literature Review. *Int J Environ Res Public Health.* 2021;18(18):9530.
11. Paolone MG, Kaitsas R. Orthodontic-periodontal interactions: Orthodontic extrusion in interdisciplinary regenerative treatments. *Int Orthod.* 2018;16(2):217-245.
12. Li G, Qu XM, Chen Y, Zhang J, Zhang ZY, Ma XC. Diagnostic accuracy of proximal caries by digital radiographs: an in vivo and in vitro comparative study. *Oral Surg Oral Med Oral Pathol Oral Radiol Endod.* 2010;109(3):463-467.
13. Khasnis SA, Kidiyoor KH, Patil AB, Kenganal SB. Vertical root fractures and their management. *J Conserv Dent.* 2014;17(2):103-110.
14. Walton RE. Vertical root fracture: Factors related to identification. *J Am Dent Assoc.* 2017;148(2):100-105.
15. Shenoy N, Shenoy A. Endo-perio lesions: diagnosis and clinical considerations. *Indian J Dent Res.* 2010;21(4):579-585.
16. Al-Fouzan KS. A new classification of endodontic-periodontal lesions. *Int J Dent.* 2014;2014:919173.
17. Del Fabbro M, Corbella S, Sequeira-Byron P, et al. Endodontic procedures for retreatment of periapical lesions. *Cochrane Database Syst Rev.* 2016;10(10):CD005511.
18. Muliyar S, Shameem KA, Thankachan RP, Francis PG, Jayapalan CS, Hafiz KA. Microleakage in endodontics. *J Int Oral Health.* 2014;6(6):99-104.
19. Li BY, Gong QM. [Research progress in clinical prognosis of apical overfilling of root canal obturation]. *Zhonghua Kou Qiang Yi Xue Za Zhi.* 2021;56(2):210-215.
20. Dickie J, McCrosson J. Post removal techniques part 1. *Dent Update.* 2014;41(6):490-492, 495-498.
21. Foroughi K, Sedaghat-Zandi A, Friedman S. Post removal techniques used in nonsurgical endodontic retreatment. *N Y State Dent J.* 1999;65(5):28-29.
22. Gorni FG, Andreano A, Ambrogi F, Brambilla E, Gagliani M. Patient and Clinical Characteristics Associated with Primary Healing of Iatrogenic Perforations after Root Canal Treatment: Results of a Long-term Italian Study. *J Endod.* 2016;42(2):211-215.
23. Heydari A, Rahmani M, Heydari M. Removal of a Broken Instrument from a Tooth with Apical Periodontitis Using a Novel Approach. *Iran Endod J.* 2016;11(3):237-240.
24. Fu M, Zhang Z, Hou B. Removal of broken files from root canals by using ultrasonic techniques combined with dental microscope: a retrospective analysis of treatment outcome. *J Endod.* 2011;37(5):619-622.
25. Torabinejad M, Nosrat A, Verma P, Udochukwu O. Regenerative Endodontic Treatment or Mineral Trioxide Aggregate Apical Plug in Teeth with Necrotic Pulps and Open Apices: A Systematic Review and Meta-analysis. *J Endod.* 2017;43(11):1806-1820.

9

Technique for atraumatic extraction and alveolar preservation

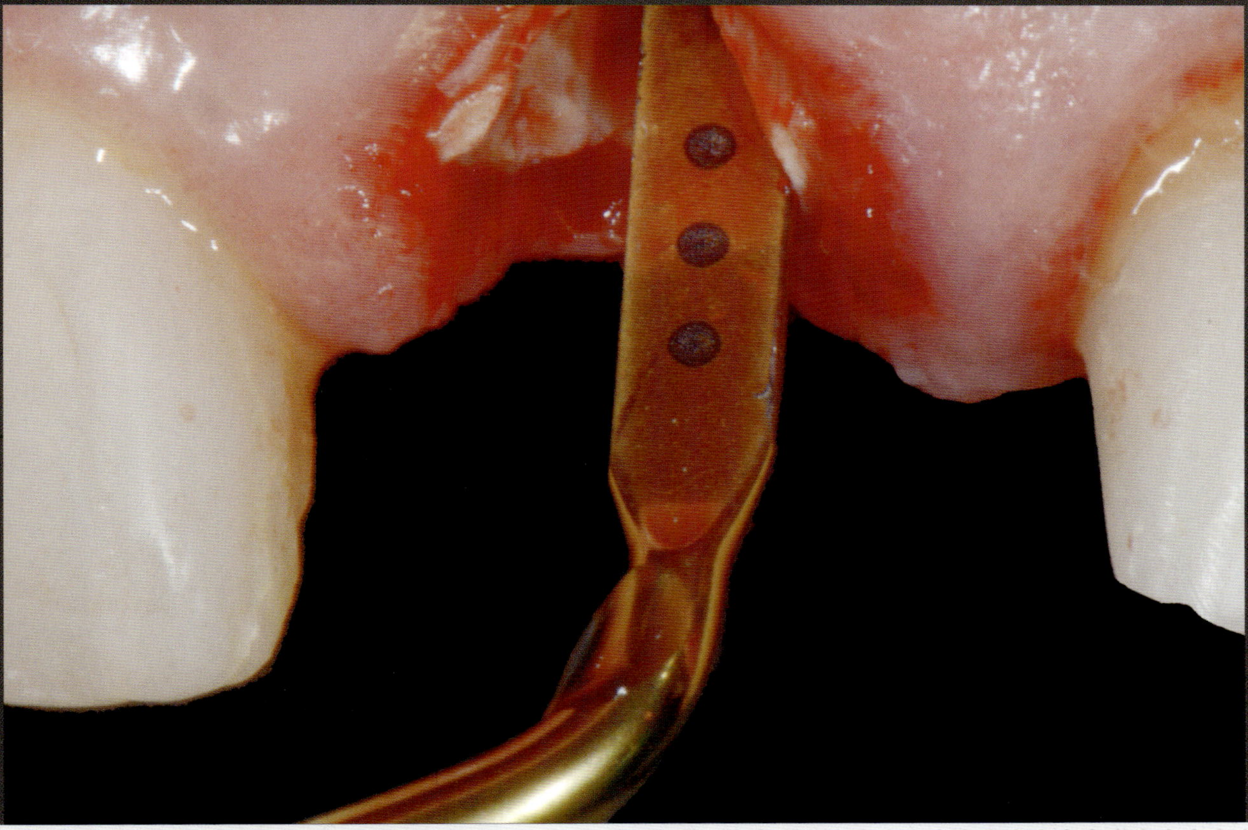

After tooth loss, alveolar bone resorption occurs, with greater resorption observed on the buccal side compared to the lingual and palatal sides. However, the horizontal component is predominant in this process.[1,2] Initial studies on the bone healing process post-tooth extraction were conducted on an animal model in 1952[3] and biopsies on humans in 1969.[4] Recently, morphological changes following dental extractions have been analysed using diagnostic models and measurements during implant insertion.[5] Within the first year, ~50% of the initial crestal thickness is reabsorbed, with two-thirds of this resorption occurring within the first three months. Numerous studies have examined post-extraction morphological alterations,[1,2] highlighting potential clinical limitations of immediate loading protocols in aesthetically important areas. The periodontal ligament fibres insert into the bundle bone, a crucial part of the alveolar bone structure. Araujo et al. demonstrated in an animal model that the bundle bone structure is crucial in influencing post-extraction morphological alterations.[6] The bundle bone receives its blood supply from the periodontal ligament and from the periosteum, while the endosteum is not present given the low bone thickness of the post-extraction socket in its coronal areas. Once the tooth is extracted, the bundle bone begins to undergo resorption as it loses vascular support from the periodontal ligament, and the periosteal vascularization alone is insufficient for complete bundle bone preservation. Especially in patients with a thin biotype, bundle bone may be the sole buccal mineralized structure with significant post-extraction horizontal resorption. Hence, a meticulous pre-operative diagnosis is necessary to allow the operator to determine appropriate cases for inserting immediately loaded post-extraction implants and identify at-risk cases where a delayed loading protocol associated with regenerative techniques is recommended. Various studies[7-10] have proposed the following surgical techniques for preserving the bone crest post-dental element extraction:

1. atraumatic extraction
2. positioning of a membrane
3. positioning of an intra-alveolar graft.

Atraumatic extraction aims to minimize vascular damage in the extraction area. This involves designing access flaps with reduced mesio-distal extensions and limited detachment of mucosal tissue from the bone plane in the apical-coronal direction. Large detachment leads to lower vascular supply with increased post-extraction bone resorption. Atraumatic extraction also involves preserving the alveolar bone structure and, therefore, performing dental avulsions by using delicate movements primarily in the mesio-distal direction or rotating along the dental axis for single-rooted teeth. Contrastingly, root resections are necessary for multi-rooted teeth to facilitate the avulsion of individual roots. Instruments like periotomes, piezoelectric handpiece inserts, and co-axial mono-radicular extractors can be used to reduce trauma to surrounding structures.

To minimize bone crest resorption after extraction, the possibility of placing a resorbable or non-resorbable membrane to protect the extraction site was evaluated. Both types of membranes guaranteed less alveolar crest reabsorption with comparable outcomes. After six months, re-entry into the treated area revealed 1.31 mm of reabsorption in sites with the membrane compared to 4.56 mm in the control sites. These values were statistically significant and offered a clinical alternative to complex regenerative surgical techniques. The use of grafts within socket sites has been proposed to reduce bone resorption, although concerns have been raised regarding the interference with normal healing processes caused by the presence of a graft inside the socket.[11] Studies on human models demonstrated that autologous demineralized bone grafts or different alloplastic grafts showed the graft granules surrounded by connective tissue or immature bone 6-9 months after their insertion.[12-14] The use of deproteinized bovine bone has been analysed in post-extraction sites of dog mandibles, and the Authors have highlighted its osteoconductive function for new bone formation.[15] Artzi et al.[12] inserted deproteinized bovine bone grafts into 15 human extraction sockets and performed biopsies after nine months. The Authors concluded that this graft type can preserve the bone crest. These results contrast with those of Becker et al.,[11] who found graft granules after 3-7 months. Carmagnola et al.[14] report that only 40% of biomaterial particle circumference contacts immature bone, but successful implant placement is possible due to graft quality and quantity. Many variables make study comparisons difficult, including defect type and size, flap closure, graft type, and the absence of landmarks. Few studies[5,7,8,13] tried adopting a reproducible method to evaluate socket healing based on material type. The use of deproteinized bovine bone was analysed[10] using CT scans before and at 30- and 90-days post-operative to assess buccal bone resorption. The Authors found a minor bone reduction (20%) compared to sites without grafting material (79%).

Surgical technique for pocket preservation

During the surgical phase, after appropriate anaesthesia, one initially proceeds with a periotomy to reach the bone crest. This can be achieved using 15c blades or all-around type microsurgical blades for thin periodontal biotypes. An envelope flap may be done, if necessary, without involving the interdental papillae, using the previously reported papilla preservation techniques. If a flap is chosen, minimal tissue detachment is recommended, focussing on the most coronal 2 mm of the bone crest. For multirooted teeth, it is mandatory to do root resection for removal. To facilitate root separation, a partial coronectomy is performed beforehand to improve visibility during the root separation procedure. Surgical drill mounted on a straight blue ring handpiece (rather than on a red ring contra-angle or surgical turbine) or a piezoelectric instrument is recommended, depending on the clinician's preference.

Once the roots are separated, extraction elevators are used for normal luxating movements. Instead, extraction forceps are preferred for single-rooted elements. After extraction, the integrity of the alveolar walls must be evaluated, followed by surgical revision of the post-extraction alveolus to completely remove any granulation tissues and/or sinus tracts. Once this phase is concluded, abundant irrigation of the site with sterile physiological solution is recommended. Prior to graft positioning, socket isolation with a sterile gauze dam is useful, similar to the lateral approach used when performing sinus grafts. The socket must be filled up to the level of the bone crest to protect the graft. For this phase, various principles have been proposed. We discourage primary intention closure through flap passivation as it contradicts the biological principles of minimizing vascular trauma associated with the periosteum contribution.

The various alternatives involve the use of:

1. A type 1 collagen sponge with secondary intention healing.
2. A resorbable membrane with secondary intention healing.
3. A socket seal using a palatal connective tissue graft with primary intention healing.
4. A socket seal using a collagen matrix.

All these techniques have demonstrated positive outcomes in mitigating post-extraction volumetric reabsorption. A recent systematic literature review indicates a wide heterogeneity in treatments used, evaluated variables, and observation periods, making it impossible to recommend specific techniques and/or materials for better outcomes. However, limited data suggest that the use of a membrane yields better results.[16]

Bibliography

1. Cardaropoli G, Araujo M, Lindhe J. Dynamics of bone tissue formation in tooth extraction sites. An experimental study in dogs. *J Clin Periodontol.* 2003;30(9):809-818.
2. Araujo M, Lindhe J. Dimensional ridge alterations following tooth extraction. An experimental study in the dog. *J Clin Periodontol.* 2005;32(2):212-218.
3. Huebsch RF, Caleman RD, Frandsen AM, Becks H. The healing process following molar extraction. I. Normal male rats (long-evans strain). *Oral Surg.* 1952;5(2):864-876.
4. Amler MH. The time sequence of tissue regeneration in human extraction wounds. *Oral Surg Oral Med Oral Pathol.* 1969;27(3):309-318.
5. Schropp L, Wenzel A, Kostopolulos L, Karring T. Bone healing and soft tissue contour changes following single-tooth extraction: a clinical and radiographic 12-month prospective study. *Int J Period Rest Dent.* 2003;23(4):313-323.
6. Araujo M, Wennström JL, Lindhe J. Modeling of the buccal and lingual bone walls of fresh extraction sites following implant installation. *Clin Oral Implants Res.* 2006;17(6):606-614.
7. Lekovic V, Kenney EB, Weinlaeder M, et al. A bone regenerative approach to alveolar ridge maintenance following tooth extraction. Report of 10 cases. *J Periodontol.* 1997;68(6):563-570.
8. Lekovic V, Camargo PM, Klokkevold PR, et al. Preservation of alveolar bone in extraction sockets using bioabsorbable membranes. *J Periodontol.* 1998;69(9):1044-1049.
9. Hämmerle CH, Chen ST, Wilson Jr TG. Consensus statements and recommended clinical procedures regarding the placement of implants in extraction sockets. *Int J Oral Maxillofac Impl.* 2004;19 Suppl:26-28.
10. Nevins M, Camelo M, De Paoli S, et al. A study of the fate of the buccal wall of extraction sockets of teeth with prominent roots. *Int J Period Rest Dent.* 2006;26(1):19-29.
11. Becker W, Cameron S, Sennerby L, Urist MR, Becker BE. Histologic findings after implantation and evaluation of different grafting materials and titanium micro screws into extraction sockets: case reports. *J Periodontol.* 1998;69(4):414-421.
12. Artzi Z, Tal H, Davan D. Porous bovine bone mineral in healing of human extraction sockets. Part 1: histomorphometric evaluations at 9 months. *J Periodontol.* 2000;71(6):1015-1023.
13. Froum S, Cho SC, Rosemberg F, Rohrer M, Tarnow D. Histological comparison of healing extraction sockets implanted with bioactive glass or demineralized freeze-dried bone allograft. *J Periodontol.* 2002;73(1):94-102.
14. Carmagnola D, Adriaensens P, Berglundh T. Healing of human extraction sockets filled with Bio-Oss. *Clin Oral Impl Res.* 2003;14(2):137-143.
15. Berglundh T, Lindhe J. Healing around implants placed in bone defects treated with Bio-Oss. An experimental study in the dog. *Clin Oral Impl Res.* 1997;8(2):117-124.
16. Faria-Almeida R, Astramskaite-Januseviciene I, Puisys A, Correia F. Extraction Socket Preservation With or Without Membranes, Soft Tissue Influence on Post Extraction Alveolar Ridge Preservation: *A Systematic Review. J Oral Maxillofac Res.* 2019;10(3):e5.

PART III - Chapter 10

10

Immediate post-extraction implantology

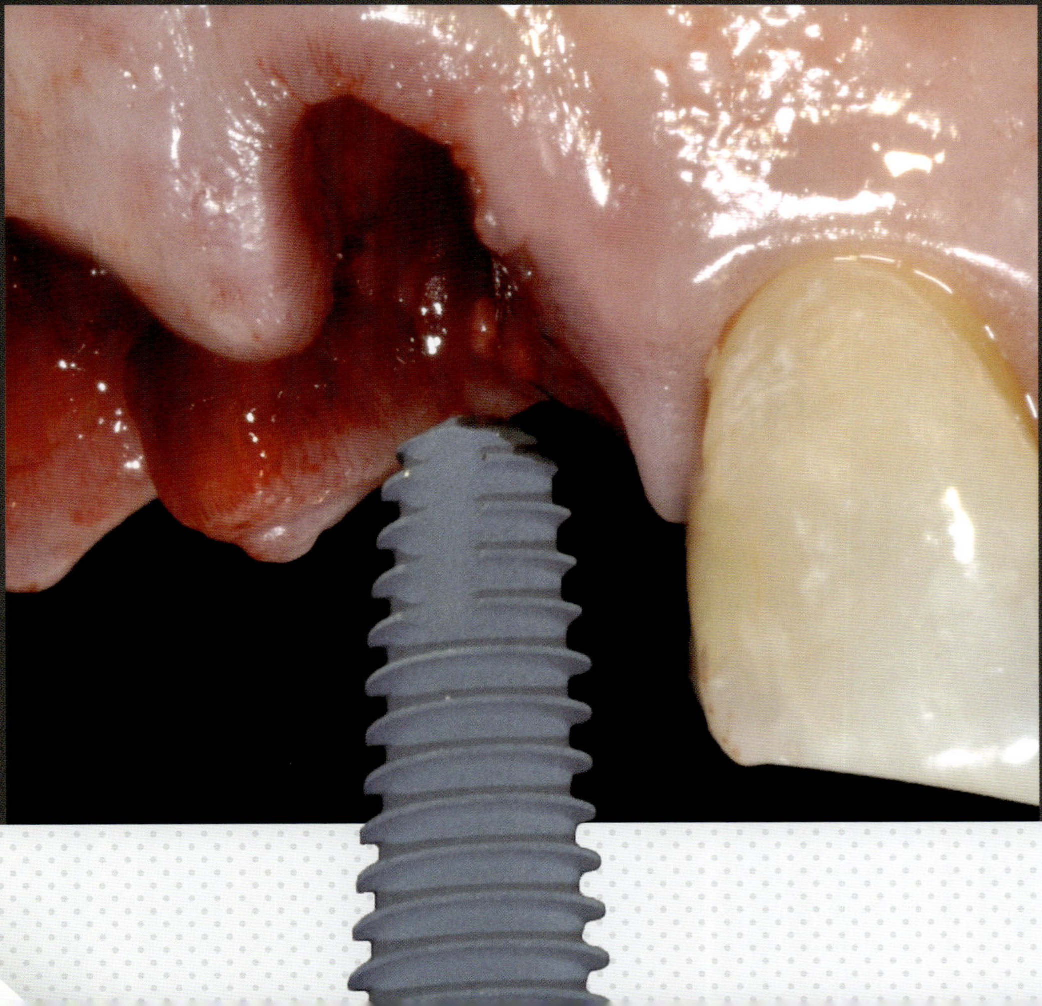

The insertion of post-extraction implants has been highly successful among clinicians, offering indisputable advantages: reducing surgical sessions and treatment times, while allowing utilization of a wider bone crest.[1] Although there is literary consensus regarding the high reliability of these protocols, an immediate post-extraction approach cannot be universally considered the treatment of choice for every clinical situation. The technique classification proposed by Hämmerle et al. in 2004 as to the timing of implant insertion to which we will refer was and is divided into four protocols:[1]

- **TYPE 1**: Immediate post-extraction implant placement (at the time of extraction).
- **TYPE 2**: Early post-extraction implants (within 4-8 weeks after extraction).
- **TYPE 3**: Delayed implant placement (between 12 and 16 weeks after extraction, in the healed bone).
- **TYPE 4**: Delayed implant placement (16 weeks after extraction, in the healed bone).

Post-extraction implants serve different purposes depending on the prosthetic timing:

- Implant placement with immediate temporary crown application.
- Implant placement with healing abutment positioning (one-stage).
- Implant placement with submerged coverage (two-stage).

To ensure perfect osseointegration, the implant loading times are not crucial, but it is important to control micro-movements at the bone-implant interface.

The tolerance threshold for micro-movements depends on the macro- and micro-geometrical design of the implant.[2]

Primary stability in a post-extraction site at the anterior portion of the jaw requires consideration of the anatomical characteristics of the site to be treated and its alignment with the prosthetically guided implant positioning. The following key anatomical characteristics are:

1. Alignment between the long axis of the tooth and the alveolar process, considering parallelism or dis-parallelism.
2. Presence or absence of a bone portion of at least 4 mm apical to the root apex of the extracted tooth.
3. Amount of palatal bone in the post-extraction socket.[3]
4. Extent of the vestibular concavity of the pre-maxilla between the canine teeth, assessed radiologically and clinically (through palpatory examination).

Based on these points, we can expect to obtain primary stability when:

1. The implant can be anchored apically/palatally in the post-extraction alveolus by at least 4 mm.
2. Surgical techniques involve under-preparation of the osteotomy site.
3. Implants with conical morphology and sharp threads are used instead of cylindrical implants.
4. In the absence of adequate palatal/apical bone volumes, larger diameter implants are used, seeking stability in the mesio-distal portions of the alveolus. In such cases, maintaining an adequate distance[3] between the implant shoulder and the buccal bone housing,[4] as well as between the implant shoulder and the root of the adjacent teeth,[5] is necessary.

Surgical technique

The elevation of a mucoperiosteal flap, as previously mentioned, impairs periosteal vascularization, causing a vascular deficit in the underlying bone.[6]
Consequently, bone crest resorption occurs, resulting in a soft tissue recession, especially in thin gingival biotypes. To minimize these negative outcomes, some authors[7] recommend avoiding mucoperiosteal flap elevation. However, implant insertion without mucoperiosteal flap elevation presents surgical challenges. Therefore, the operator must adhere to the following operating guidelines:

- Perform atraumatic extractions (**Fig. 10.1a-c**).
- Use a surgical guide to compensate for reduced visibility.
- Verify the buccal cortical bone integrity during implant site preparation by sounding the buccal bone wall.
- Avoid using the same alveolar angulation and opt for a diverging axis with the palatal wall as a guide.
- The implant position in the frontal group of teeth must refer to the cingulum of the adjacent teeth.

As previously emphasised, implant position significantly impacts aesthetic outcomes. In the buccal-lingual direction, the implant must have three-dimensional references that must be placed in the palatal portion of the socket, aligning with the cingulum of the adjacent teeth. The apical-coronal position of the implant platform should maintain a 3-4 mm distance from the most apical buccal gingival margin of adjacent teeth.
For post-extraction implants in the latero-posterior regions, the implant position should be centred within the socket. Evaluating the bucco-lingual dimension of the residual socket is critical. If this dimension becomes excessive, the implant must be positioned more buccally. This bucco-lingual position of the implant must be 2 mm more lingual than the tangent of the adjacent teeth to facilitate the design of a correct emergence profile. This approach is more feasible in the molar areas, whereas in the premolars, particularly the first upper premolar, it may cause fenestration of the buccal cortex due to the natural bone undercut. To avoid this intraoperative complication, the implant axis can be tilted buccally, while maintaining a centred-implant position in the socket.

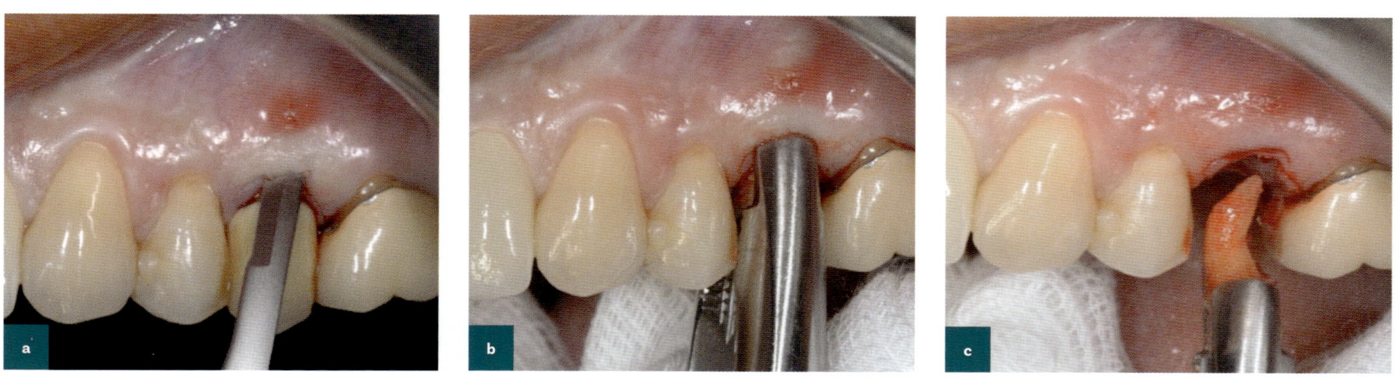

Figs. 10.1a-c ■ Step by step atraumatic extraction of an unsalvageable tooth.

Long-term follow-up

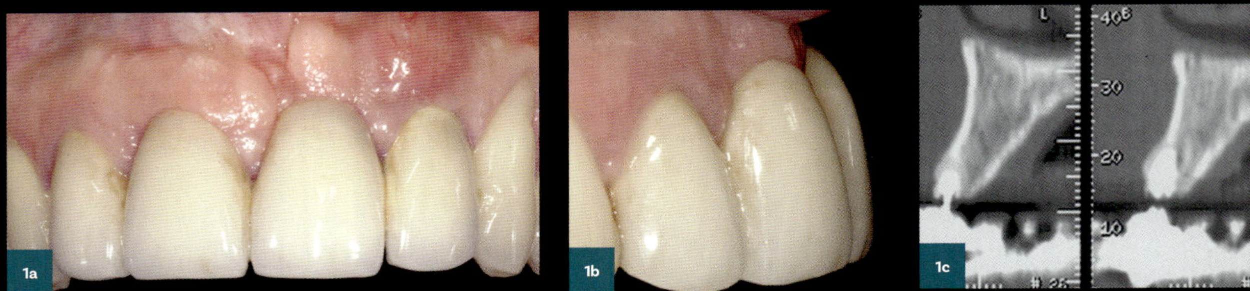

Figs. 1a-c ■ A 43-year-old male patient presented for a consultation, complained about both functional and aesthetic problems with the traditional prosthetic rehabilitation of the upper frontal sector, specifically with post abutments in teeth 12 and 22. Radiographic examination revealed that these teeth cannot be kept. The patient inquired about the possibility of receiving single crowns instead.

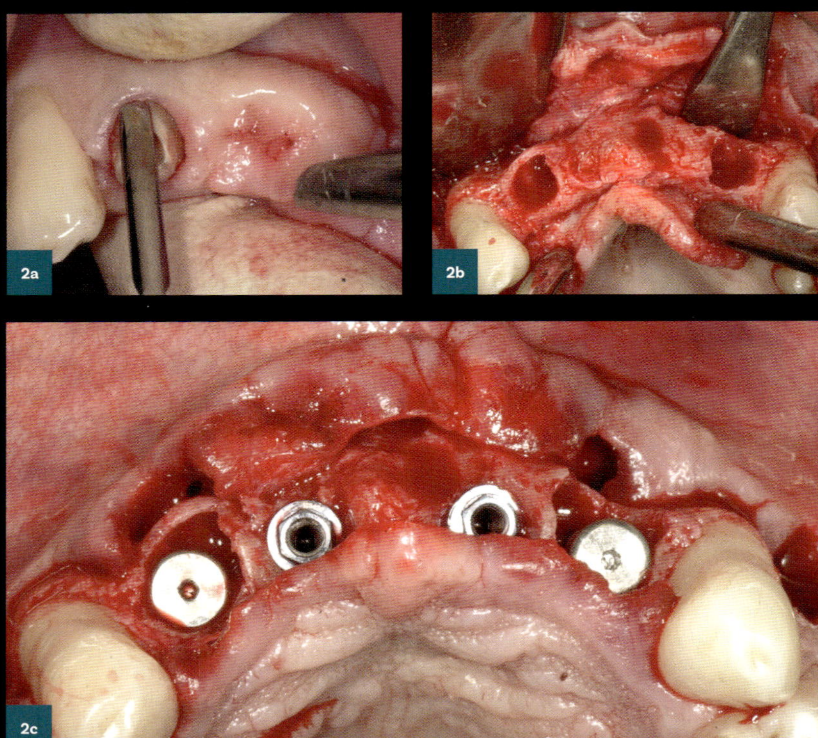

Figs. 2a-c ■ Insertion of 4 implants in the 12-11-21-22 area: Implants inserted in the 12-22 area are post-extraction, while the implants in 11-21 were inserted into the alveolar bone. Consequently, due to the high aesthetic importance of this area, a decision was made to immediately load only the latter two implants. The implants in 12-22 were submerged and loaded subsequently after achieving osseointegration. In this case, all 4 implants were successfully placed while maintaining proper inter-implant distances. Temporary sutures were applied, and two impression copings were placed for taking an intraoperative impression using sterile and radiopaque material.

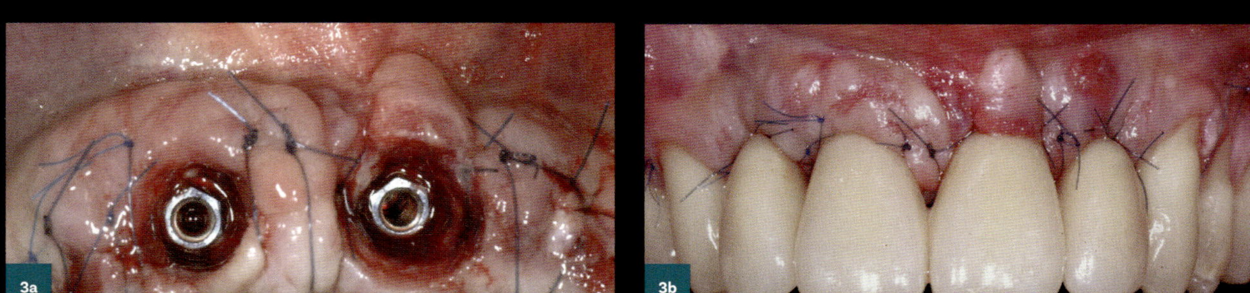

Figs. 3a,b ■ Occlusal view of the completed procedure, following connection of the screw-retained provisional prosthesis.

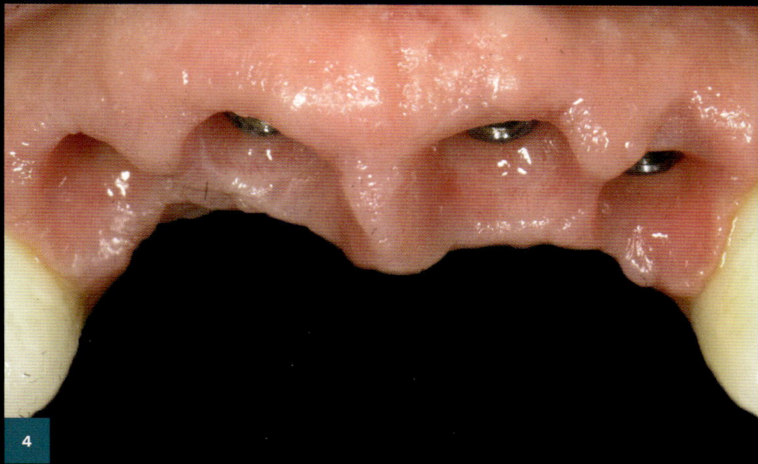

4

Fig. 4 ■ Soft tissue appearance 6 months post-surgery.

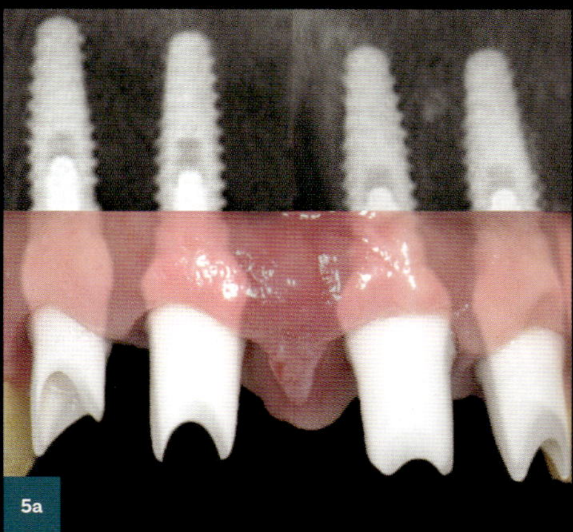

5a

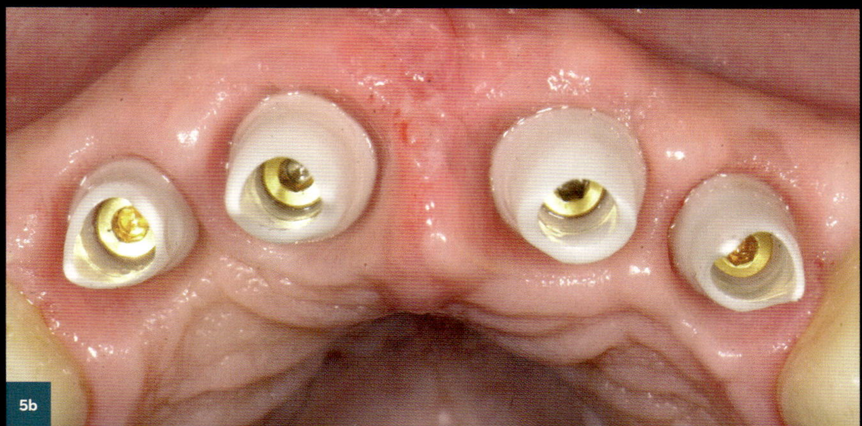

5b

Figs. 5a-c ■ Clinical and radiographic images of the final rehabilitation with 4 ceramic zirconium single crowns cemented on zirconium implant abutments.

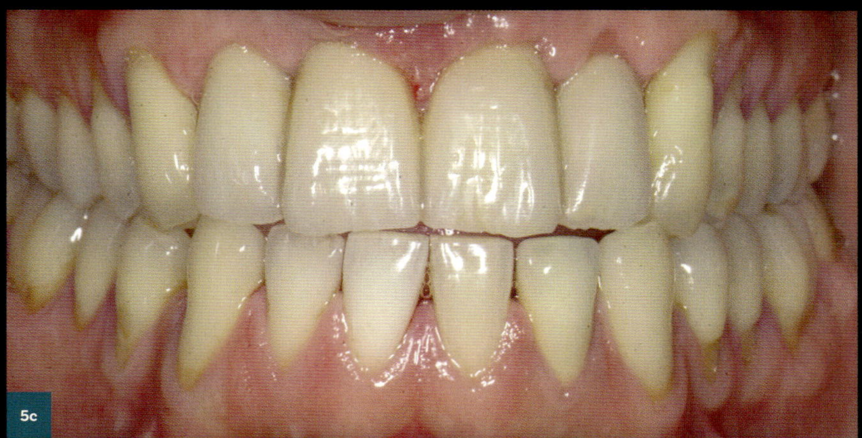

5c

CONT'D

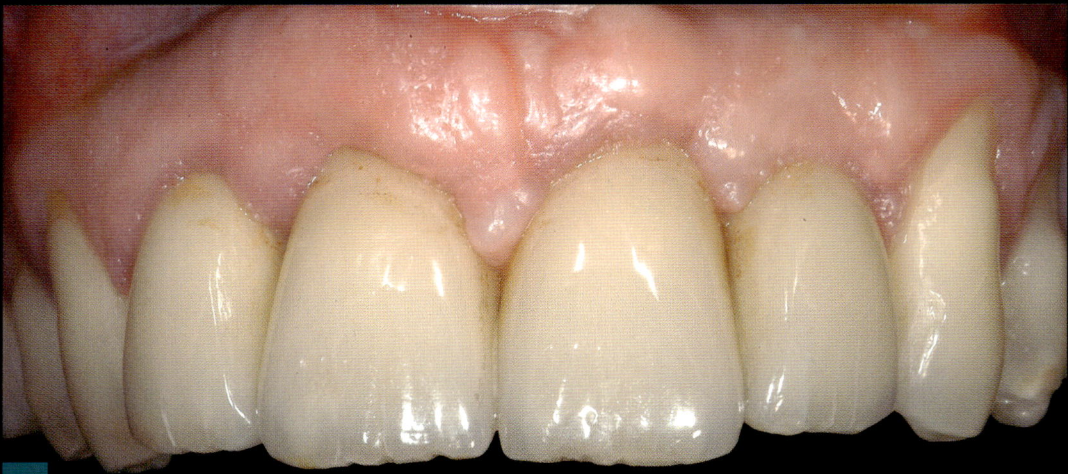

6a

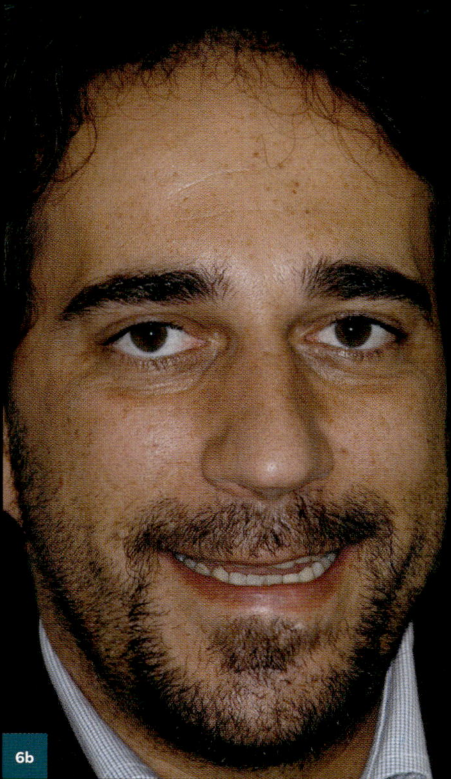

6b

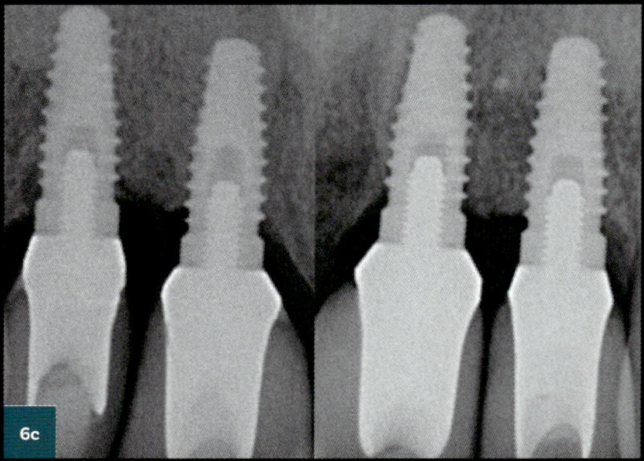

6c

Figs. 6a-c ■ Clinical and radiographic images depicting the 18-year of treatment follow-up.

Teeth are often extracted due to an irreversible infectious process. In the past, any ongoing infections were considered contraindications for implant placement as they could hinder healing and osseointegration, and cause implant failure.

Subsequent investigations, however, demonstrated that thorough socket debridement prior to implant placement could allow its successful osseointegration. Studies show that the survival rate of implants placed in uninfected or healed sockets does not differ significantly.[8-16] A recent retrospective study of 369 patients and 527 implants placed in infected and uninfected sites, followed up for an average of 54 months, found no statistical difference in implant survival rates.[17] Regardless of implant survival, the presence of endodontic and/or periodontal lesions results in morphological alterations of the post-extraction site that should be considered for proper treatment planning.

The variables to consider for this purpose include:

- Predictability of obtaining adequate primary stability.
- Presence/absence of vestibular bone housing.
- Periodontal biotype.
- Presence/absence of recessions.

Excluding the predictability of obtaining primary stability as previously described, the above points form the basis of diagnostic algorithms illustrated in **Figure 10.2**.

Presence/absence of the buccal bone housing

Previous literature demonstrated that intact buccal bone housing is essential for the stability of the buccal soft tissues at the treatment site.[18] When there is a bone defect buccal to the tooth to be extracted, the careful analysis of the defect morphology becomes critical in determining the correct therapeutic approach. A study on immediate post-extraction implants revealed that defects limited to the facial component of the buccal bone resulted in a gingival recession rate >1.5 mm in 8.3% of cases. Conversely, defects involving the mesial and distal components of the tooth to be extracted or even those of the adjacent teeth led to a recession rate >1.5 mm of 42.8% and 100% of cases treated, respectively.[19] Therefore, evaluating the absence of buccal bone housing is crucial when considering an immediate post-extraction approach, taking the periodontal biotype into account as well.

An innovative technique, known as the "socket-shield technique," has recently been introduced to preserve the thin and prone-to-fracture buccal bone crest during root extraction. Hülzeler et al. were the first to describe this technique in an experiment involving Beagle dogs, where a premolar was hemi-sectioned, and a portion (referred to as the "shield") at the buccal zone, 1 mm coronal to the buccal bone crest, was preserved. The implant was then positioned immediately close to the "shield" at the palatal/lingual level but without direct contact. No complications were found, and subsequent histology subsequently revealed cementum formation between the implant surface and the remaining portion of the root.[20]

Schwimer provided further histological confirmations of this technique in 2018,[21] and although various authors have made modifications, underlying biological principles remain unchanged.[22-24] The promising results currently encourage continuous efforts to improve and enhance the predictability of this technique.[25] The possibility of leaving this portion of the root, which often originates from an endodontically pathological tooth, is due to the fact that the remaining portion consists mainly of external root cement. In this area, the dentinal tubules, which can serve as potential bacterial micro niches, can be cleaned and treated intra-surgically with low surface tension products and EDTA, followed by bactericidal treatment with 0.2% chlorhexidine.

Socket shield

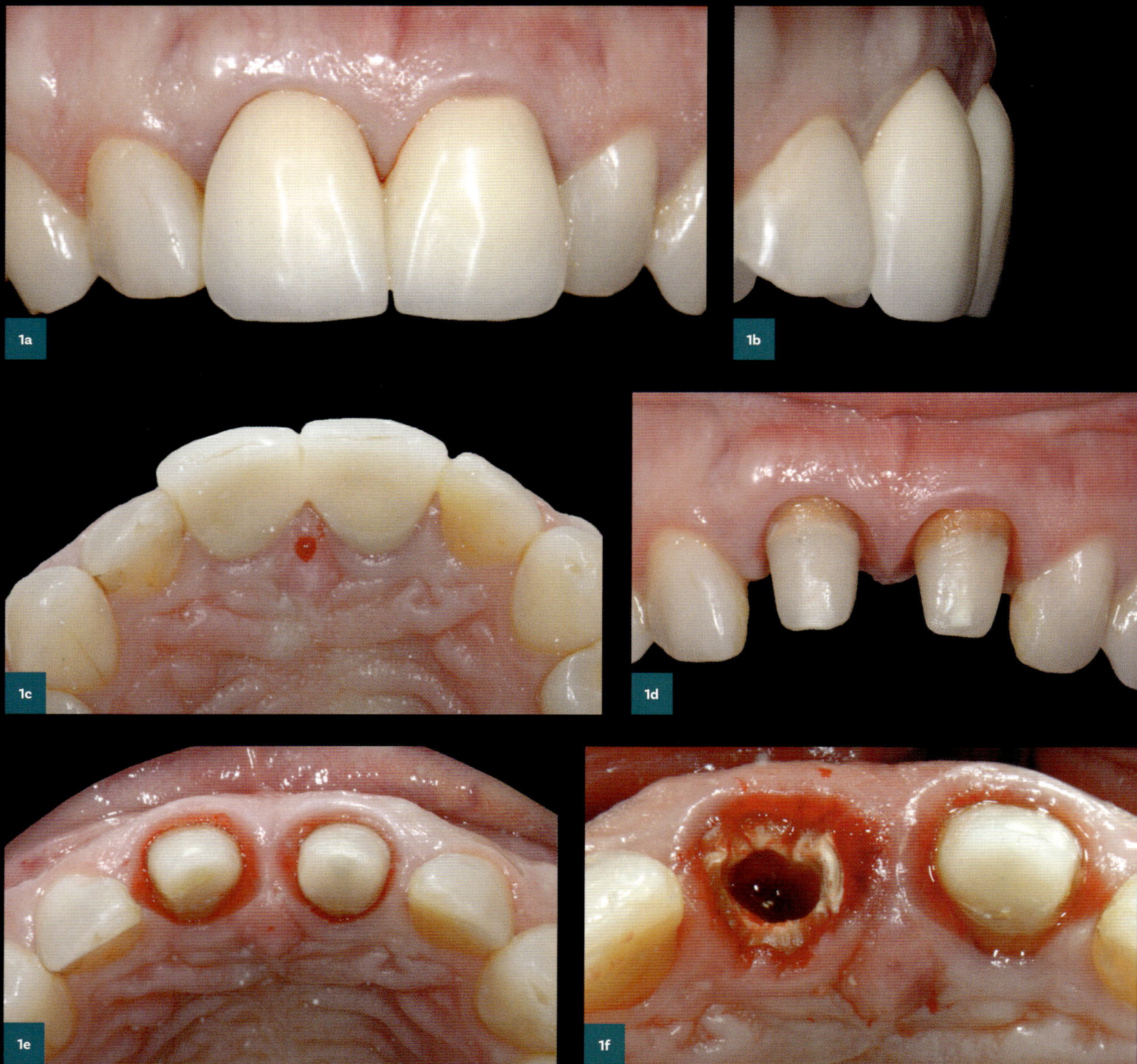

Figs. 1a-f ■ A female patient presented with prosthetic crown mobility of tooth 11 during a consultation. After removing the crown, the root showed root canal overpreparation and recurrent intracanal caries. Since the root had no ferrule, the tooth was deemed unsavable.

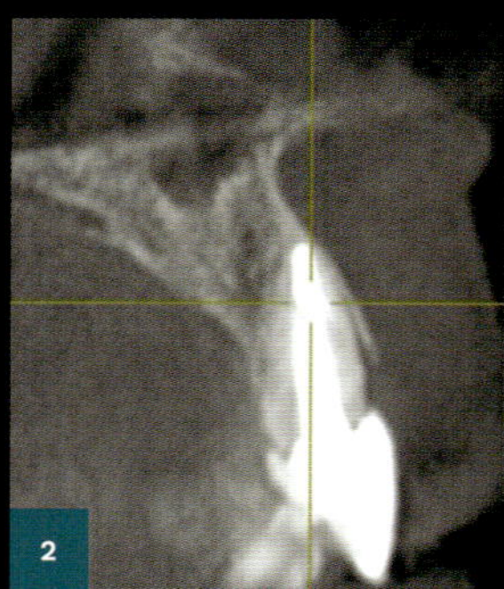

Fig. 2 ■ It was decided to integrate the diagnostic phase with a CBCT examination and proceed with an implant-prosthetic rehabilitation using the socket shield technique.

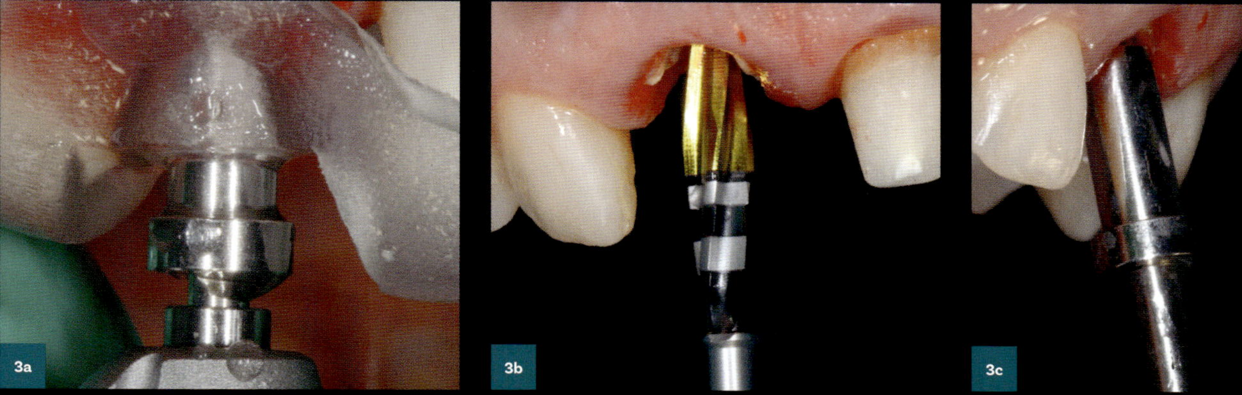

Figs. 3a-c ■ Following the removal of the coronal reconstruction and the endodontic material, computer-guided root shaving was performed. It is crucial to assess the root shaving's preparation axis and the implant site preparation at each step.

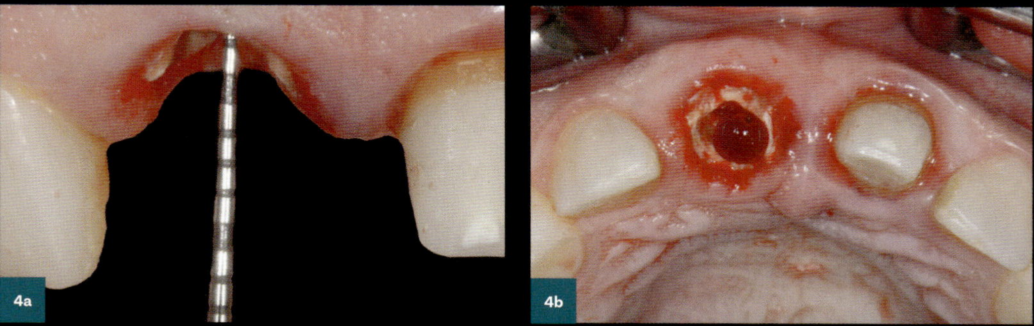

Figs. 4a,b ■ Once the root remnant's internal shaving has been completed, buccal mapping was conducted to determine the relationship between the root margin and the marginal soft tissues

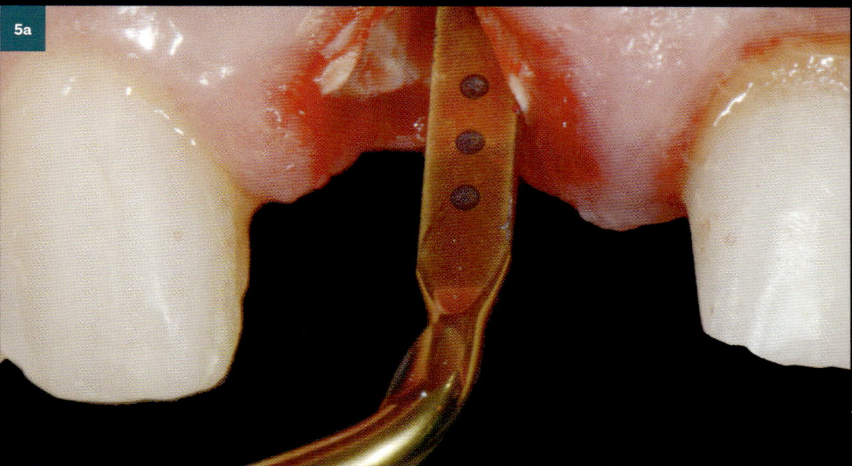

Figs. 5a-d ■ At this point, the palatal portion of the root was extracted using piezoelectric instruments.

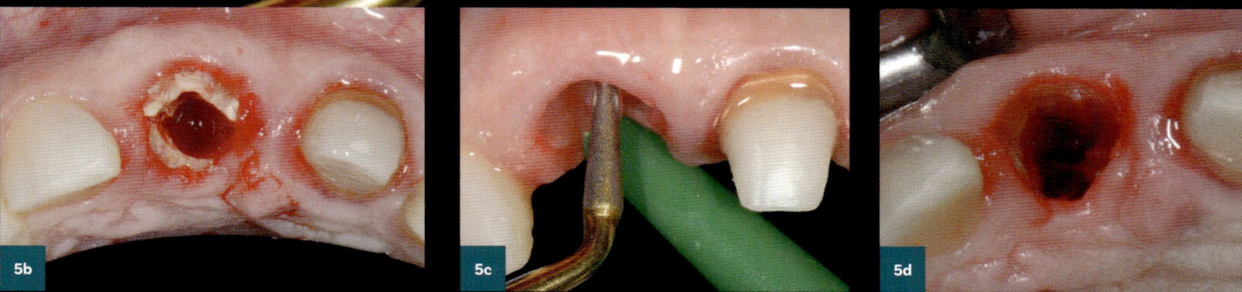

CONT'D >

> CONT'D

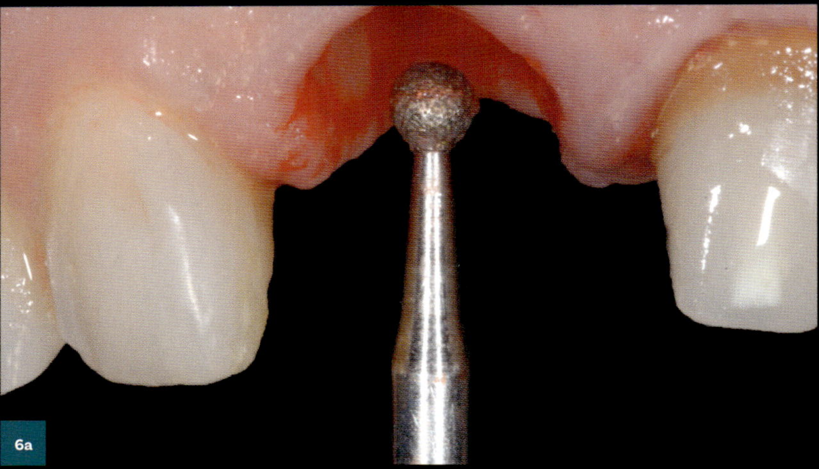

6a

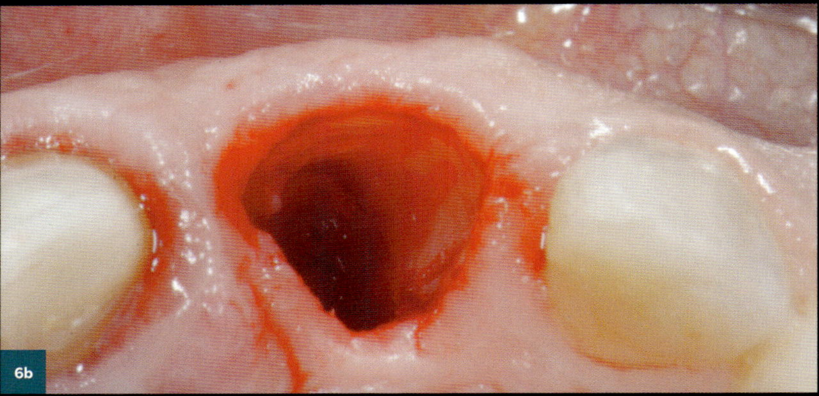

6b

Figs. 6a,b ■ After extraction of the palatal portion of the root, the vestibular shield was shaped using a diamond ball bur.

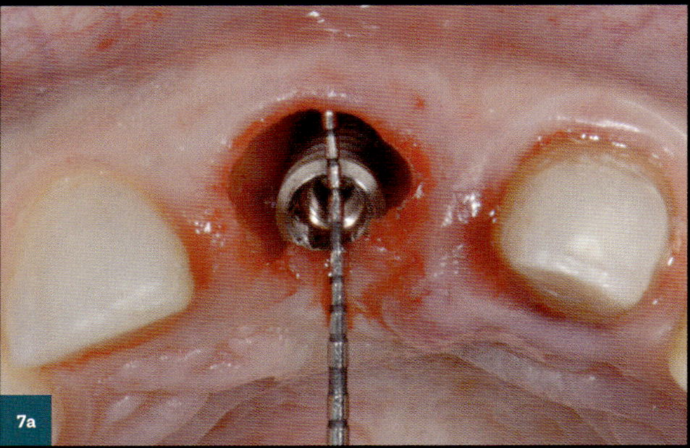

7a

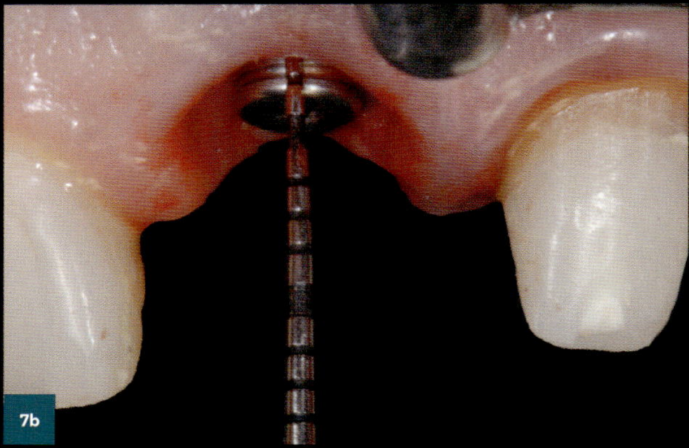

7b

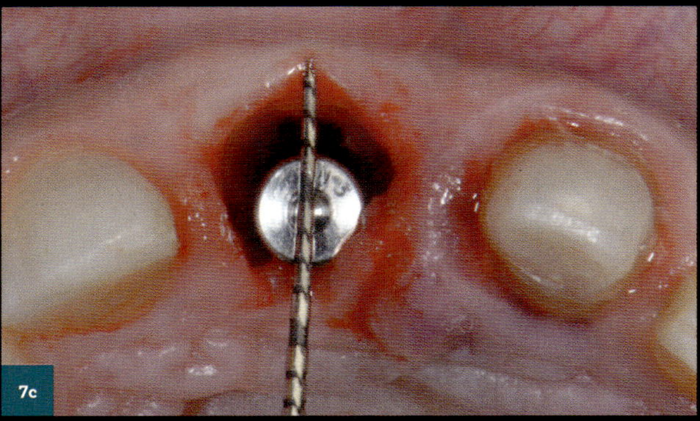

7c

Figs. 7a-c ■ The implant was then inserted, and its accurate positioning in the three spatial planes was carefully evaluated.

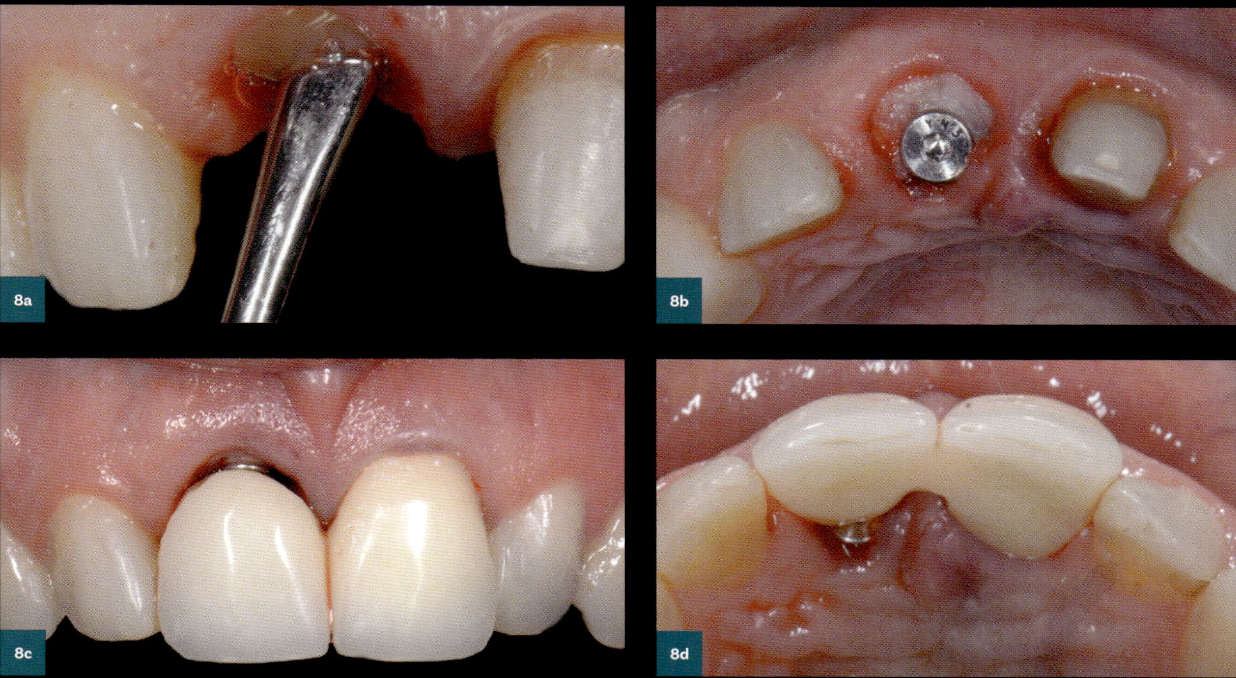

Figs. 8a-d ■ At the end of the surgery, the healing abutment and PRF membrane were placed. The provisional phase involved resin rehabilitation of tooth 21 with extension to 11 to avoid immediate loading of the implant.

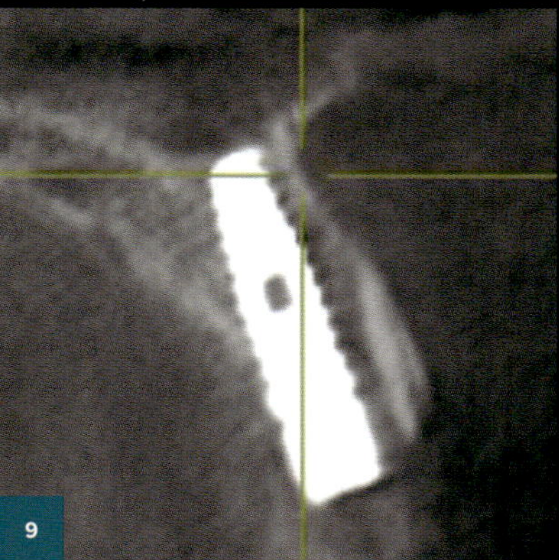

Fig. 9 ■ Tomographic evaluation confirmed the correct implant position.

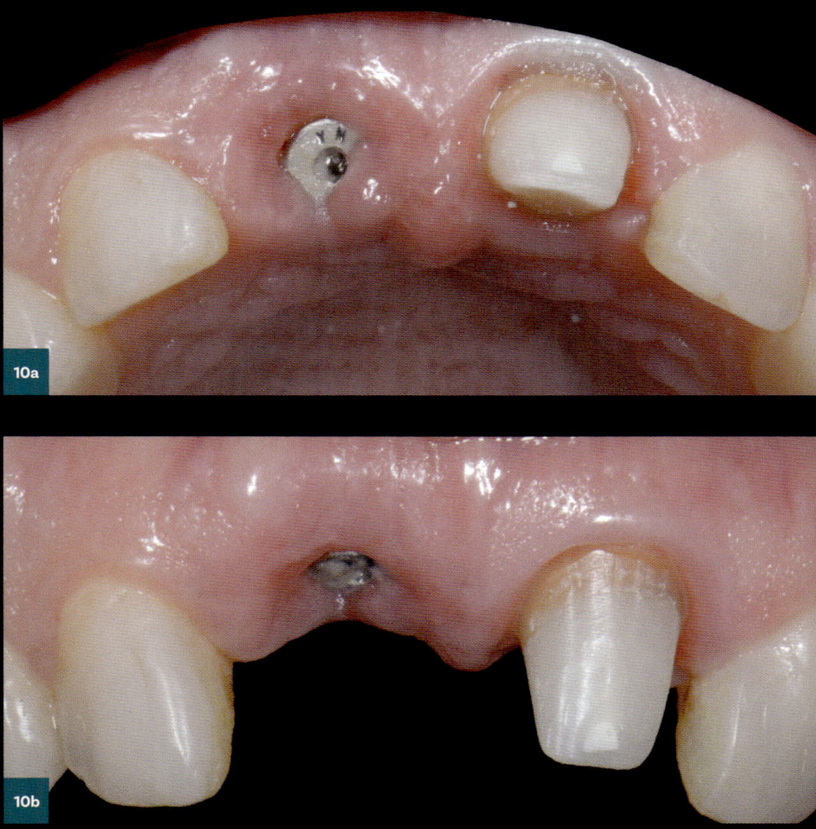

Figs. 10a,b ■ Soft tissue condition after 6 months of healing.

> CONT'D

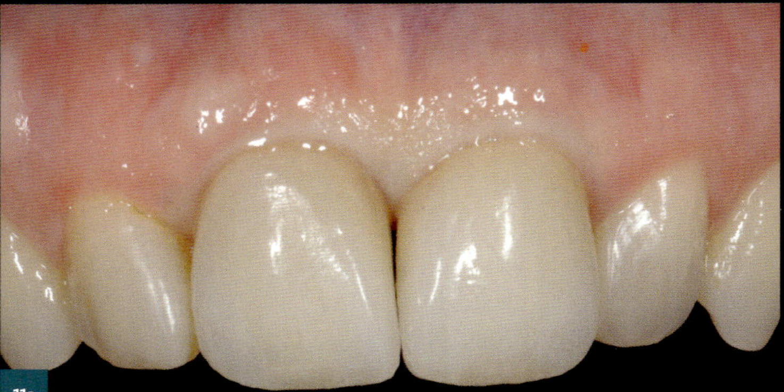

11a

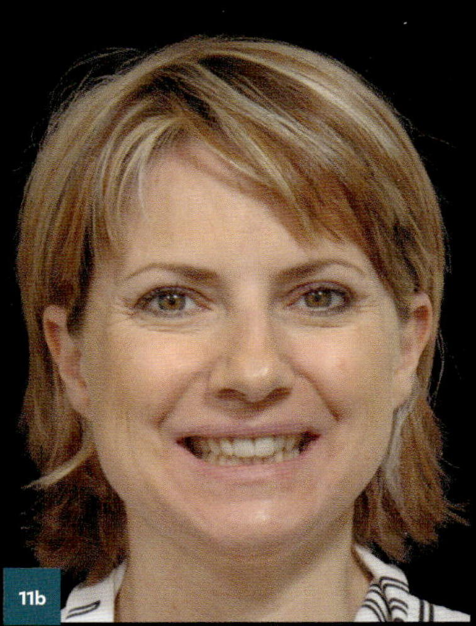

11b

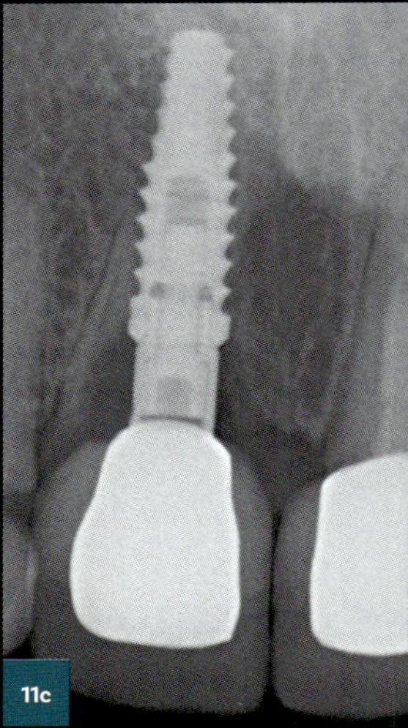

11c

Figs. 11a-c ■ Clinical and radiographic images of the definitive rehabilitation.

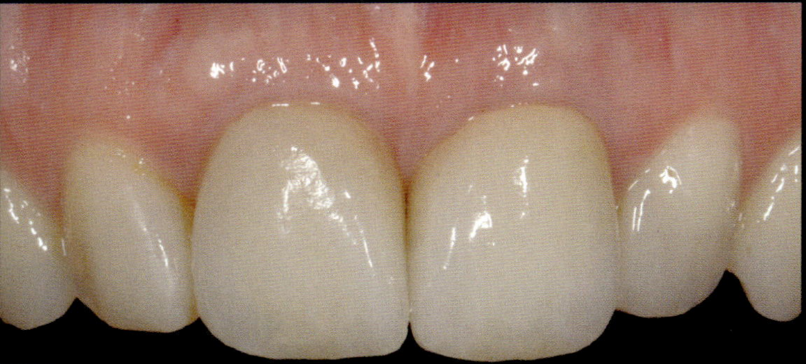

12a

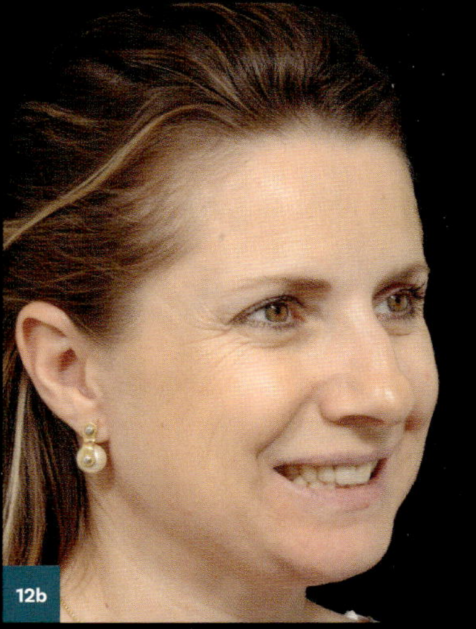

12b

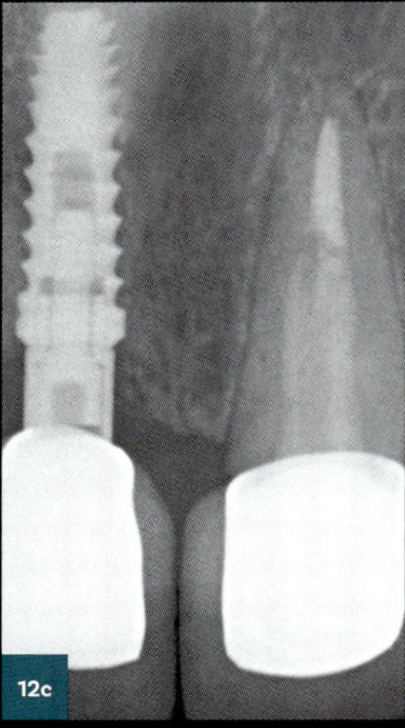

12c

Figs. 12a-c ■ Clinical and radiographic images taken 1 year after delivery.

Periodontal biotype

Over the years, efforts have been made to classify the population based on a series of morphological characteristics of gingival tissues. These characteristics are influenced by genetic traits and local factors like the shape, size and position of the teeth. Existing literature has characterized gingival phenotypes associated with varying soft tissue thicknesses.[26,27] Correlations have been found between gingival biotype and buccal bone thickness of the alveolar process, determined intraoperatively and via CBCT exams.[28] Different periodontal biotypes have also been found to have an important clinical relevance.[29] Specifically, in implantology, patients with a reduced thickness (<1 mm) show increased vestibular recession over a medium period evaluation of the vestibular cortex of the sites treated with immediate post-extraction implants.[30,31] Therefore, thin periodontal biotype was found to be associated with buccal recession in immediate post-extraction implants performed with both flapless[32] and flap procedures.[33] Although thin periodontal biotypes present a challenging clinical trend that distinguishes the post-extraction implant treatment of thin periodontal biotypes, the prognosis of the onset of buccal/labial recession can be improved by performing buccal/labial connective tissue grafts at the treated site, thereby modifying the soft tissue thickness.[34]

Absence/presence of recession

Gingival recession refers to the pathological displacement of the gingival tissues apically, exposing the root surface.[34] The presence of a recession in dental diagnostics is diagnostically important for treatment planning due to the anatomical alterations. The first crucial aspect is that the recession is characterized by loss of clinical attachment, resulting in the loss of a significant portion of the buccal bone housing. Furthermore, gingival recession involves the loss of keratinized tissue. Therefore, extracting a dental element with gingival recession poses various unfavourable aesthetic prognostic factors, particularly when considering an immediate post-extraction approach.[18] In such cases, a deferred approach may prove more effective compared to immediate post-extraction procedures.[35]

Predictability of primary stability

Anatomy	*Class I, II, III**	*Class IV**
Implant morphology	*Conical implant*	*Cylindric implant*
Surgical technique	*Under preparation*	*Normal/over-preparation*

*according to Kan 2011

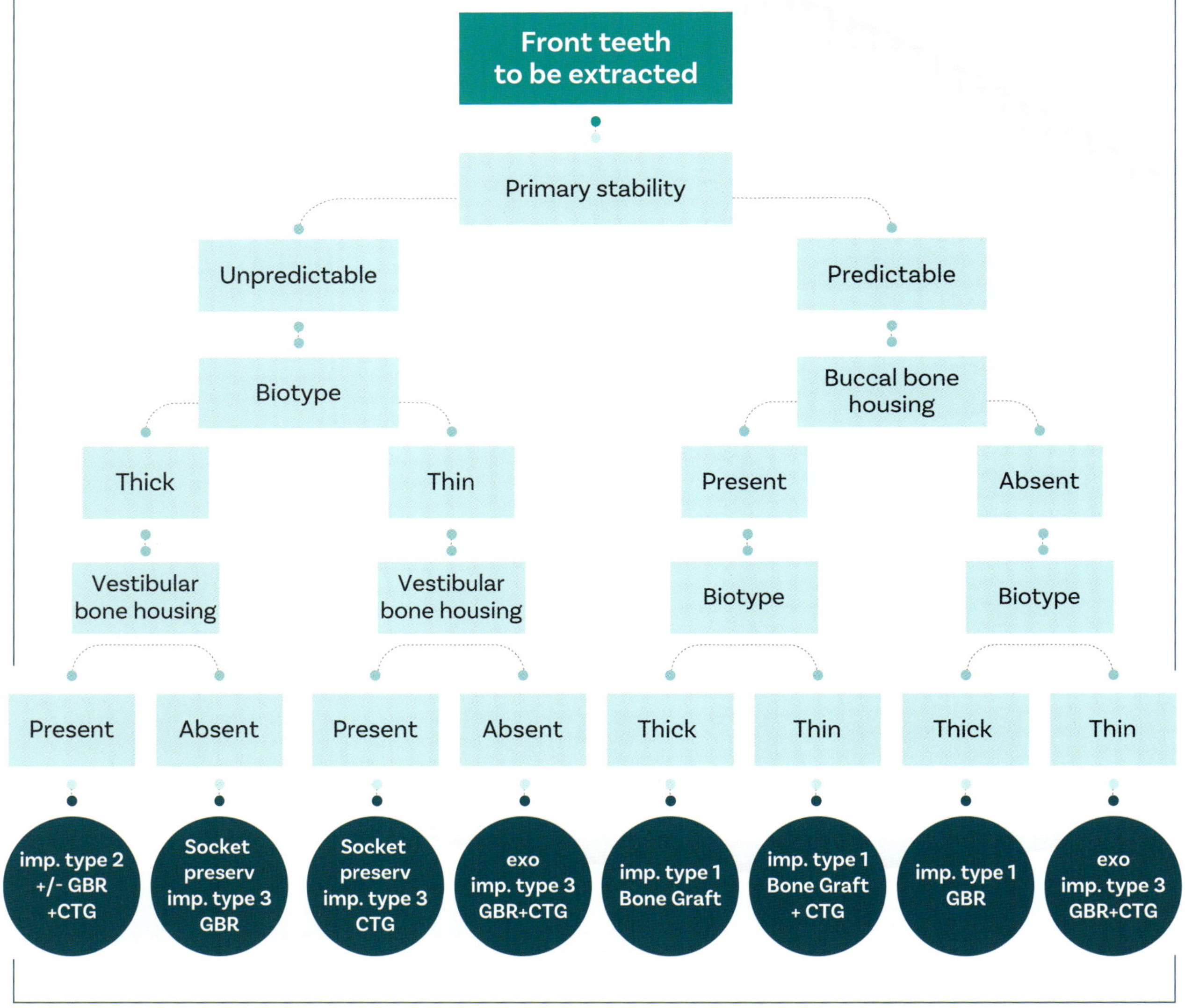

Fig. 10.2 ■ Decision-making diagnostic algorithm for immediate implant placement in aesthetic sectors.

Bibliography

1. Hämmerle CH, Chen ST, Wilson TG Jr. Consensus statements and recommended clinical procedures regarding the placement of implants in extraction sockets. *Int J Oral Maxillofac Implants. 2004*;19 Suppl:26-28.
2. Brunski JB. Biomechanical factors affecting the bone-dental implant surface. *Clin Mater*. 1992;10(3):153-201.
3. Kan JYK, Roe P, Rungcharassaeng K, et al. Classification of Sagittal Root Position in Relation to the Anterior Maxillary Osseous Housing for Immediate Implant Placement: A Cone Beam Computed Tomography Study. *Int J Oral Maxillofac Implants*. 2011;26(4):873-876.
4. Capelli M, Testori T, Galli F, et al. Implant-buccal plate distance as diagnostic parameter: a prospective cohort study on implant placement in fresh extraction sockets. *J Periodontol*. 2013;84(12):1768-1774.
5. Tarnow DP, Magner AW, Fletcher P. The effect of the distance from the contact point to the crest of bone on the presence or absence of the interproximal dental papilla. *J Periodontol*. 1992;63(12):995-996.
6. Bragger U, Hafeli U, Huber B, Hämmerle CH, Lang NP. Evaluation of postsurgical crestal bone levels adjacent to non-submerged dental implants. *Clin Oral Implants Res*. 1998;9(4):218-224.
7. Esposito M, Grusovin M, Maghaireh H, Maghaireh H, Coulthard P, Worthington HV. Interventions for replacing missing teeth: management of soft tissues for dental implants. *Cochrane Database Syst. Rev*. 2007;3:CD006697.
8. Fugazzotto P. A retrospective analysis of immediately placed implants in 418 sites exhibiting periapical pathology: results and clinical considerations. *Int J Oral Maxillofac Implants*. 2012;27(1):194-202.
9. Fugazzotto PA. A retrospective analysis of implants immediately placed in sites with and without periapical pathology in sixty-four patients. *J Periodontol*. 2012;83(2):182-186
10. Bell CL, Diehl D, Bell BM, Bell RE. The immediate placement of dental implants into extraction sites with periapical lesions: a retrospective chart review. *J Oral Maxillofac Surg*. 2011;69(6):1623-1627.
11. Lindeboom JA, Tjiook Y, Kroon FH. Immediate placement of implants in periapical infected sites: a prospective randomized study in 50 patients. *Oral Surg Oral Med Oral Pathol Oral Radiol Endod*. 2006;101(6):705-710.
12. Siegenthaler DW, Jung RE, Holderegger C, Roos M, Hämmerle CH. Replacement of teeth exhibiting periapical pathology by immediate implants: a prospective, controlled clinical trial. *Clin Oral Implants Res*. 2007;18(6):727-737.
13. Chang SW, Shin SY, Hong JR, et al. Immediate implant placement into infected and noninfected extraction sockets: a pilot study. *Oral Surg Oral Med Oral Pathol Oral Radiol Endod*. 2009;107(2):197-203.
14. Crespi R, Capparè P, Gherlone E. Fresh-socket implants in periapical infected sites in humans. *J Periodontol*. 2010;81(3):378-383.
15. Crespi R, Capparè P, Gherlone E. Immediate loading of dental implants placed in periodontally infected and noninfected sites: a 4-year follow-up clinical study. *J Periodontol*. 2010;81(8):1140-1146.
16. Truninger TC, Philipp AO, Siegenthaler DW, Roos M, Hämmerle CH, Jung RE. A prospective, controlled clinical trial evaluating the clinical and radiological outcome after 3 years of immediately placed implants in sockets exhibiting periapical pathology. *Clin Oral Implants Res*. 2011;22(1):20-27.
17. Zuffetti F, Capelli M, Galli F, Del Fabbro M, Testori T. Post-extraction implant placement into infected versus non-infected sites: a multicenter retrospective clinical study. *Clin Implant Dent Relat Res*. 2017;19(5):833-840.
18. Kois JC, Kan JYK. Predictable peri-implant gingival esthetics: surgical and prosthodontic rationales. *Pract Proced Aesthet Dent. 2001;13(9):711-715.*
19. Kan JYK, Rungcharassaeng K, Sclar A, Lozada J. Effects of the facial osseous defect morphology on gingival dynamics after immediate tooth replacement and guided bone regeneration: 1-year results. *J Oral Maxillofac Surg*. 2007;65(Suppl 1):13-19.
20. Hürzeler MB, Zuhr O, Schupbach P, Rebele SF, Emmanouilidis N, Fickl S. The socket-shield technique: A proof-of-principle report. *J Clin Periodontol*. 2010;37(9):855-862.
21. Schwimer C, Pette GA, Gluckman H, Salama M, Du Toit J. Human Histologic Evidence of New Bone Formation and Osseointegration Between Root Dentin (Unplanned Socket-Shield) and Dental Implant: Case Report. *Int J Oral Maxillofac Implants*. 2018;33(1):e19-e23.
22. Kan JY, Rungcharassaeng K. Proximal socket shield for interimplant papilla preservation in the esthetic zone. *Int J Periodontics Restorative Dent*. 2013;33(1):e24-e31.
23. Gluckman H, Salama M, Du Toit J. Partial Extraction Therapies (PET) Part 1: Maintaining Alveolar Ridge Contour at Pontic and Immediate Implant Sites. *Int J Periodontics Restorative Dent*. 2016;36(5):681-687.
24. Gluckman H, Salama M, Du Toit J. Partial Extraction Therapies (PET) Part 2: Procedures and Technical Aspects. *Int J Periodontics Restorative Dent*. 2017;37(3):377-385.
25. Gharpure AS, Bhatavadekar NB. Current evidence on the socket shield technique: a systematic review. *J Oral Implantol*. 2017;43(5):395-403.
26. Müller HP, Heinecke A, Schaller N, Eger T. Masticatory mucosa in subjects with different periodontal phenotypes. *J Clin Periodontol*. 2000;27(9):621-626.
27. Rasperini G, Acunzo R, Cannalire P, Farronato G. Influence of Periodontal Biotype on Root Surface Exposure During Orthodontic Treatment: A Preliminary Study. *Int J Periodontics Restorative Dent*. 2015;35(5):665-675.
28. Fu JH, Yeh CY, Chan HL, Tatarakis N, Leong DJ, Wang HL. Tissue Biotype and Its Relation to the Underlying Bone Morphology. *J. Periodontol*. 2010;81(4):569-574.

29. Chen ST, Darby IB, Reynolds EC. A prospective clinical study of non-submerged immediate implants: clinical outcomes and esthetic results. *Clin Oral Implants Res.* 2007;18(5):552-562.

30. Ferrus J, Cecchinato D, Pjetursson EB, Lang NP, Sanz M, Lindhe J. Factors influencing ridge alterations following immediate implant placement into extraction sockets. *Clin Oral Implants Res.* 2010;21(1):22-29.

31. Chen ST. Immediate implant placement postextraction without flap elevation. *J Periodontol.* 2009;80(1):163-172.

32. Evans CD, Chen ST. Esthetic outcomes of immediate implant placements. *Clin Oral Implants Res.* 2008;19(1):73-80.

33. Kan JY, Rungcharassaeng K, Morimoto T, Lozada J. Facial gingival tissue stability after connective tissue graft with single immediate tooth replacement in the esthetic zone: consecutive case report. *J Oral Maxillofac Surg.* 2009;67 (11 Suppl):40-48.

34. Zucchelli G. Eziologia delle recessioni gengivali. In: Zucchelli G (ed.). Chirurgia estetica mucogengivale. Milano, *Quintessenza Edizioni* 2012; pp. 13-60.

35. Buser D, Chen ST, Weber HP, Belser UC. Early implant placement following single-tooth extraction in the esthetic zone: biologic rationale and surgical procedures. *Int J Periodontics Restorative Dent.* 2008;28(5):441-451.

PART III - Chapter 11

11

Immediate loading

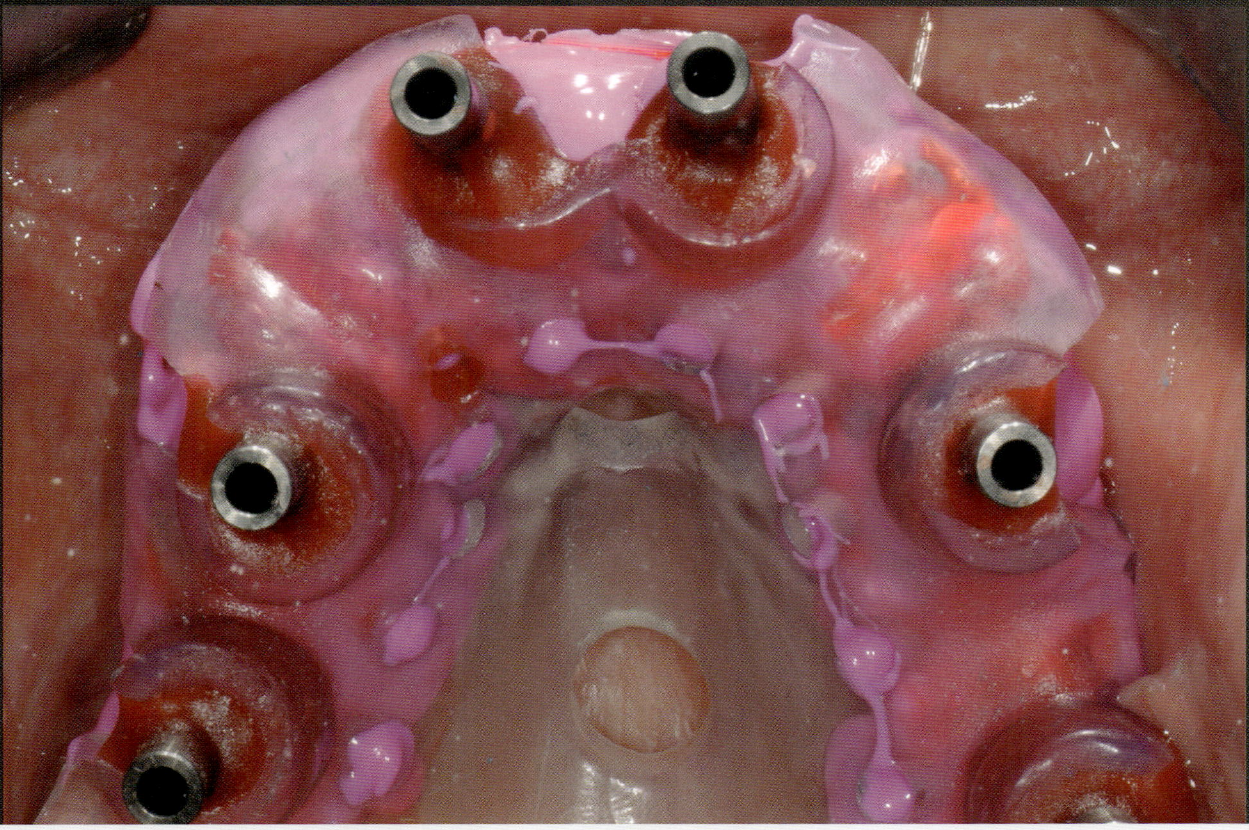

Among the significant advances in implant dentistry, immediate loading stands out as an innovative procedure with routine clinical applications.[1] Immediate loading is defined as the "application of functional or non-functional loading to an implant at the time of surgical placement or shortly after; generally considered to be loading within 48 hours of implant placement".[2] "Immediate functional loading" involves immediate occlusal loading of the implant prosthesis, whereas "non-functional loading" keeps the prosthesis out of direct occlusal contact. Here, loading occurs from lip and tongue pressure and food contact, but not from contact with the opposing teeth. The ultimate goal of an immediate loading protocol is to minimize surgeries and shorten the time between surgery and prosthesis delivery without compromising success rates. These protocols will ultimately reduce patient reservations, enhancing patient acceptance of implant therapy. Over the years, the uses of immediate loading in various indications have been well-documented, including implant placement in completely edentulous mandible and maxilla and their use in conjunction with immediate post-extraction implants.[3]

The bone healing process following implant placement resembles the primary healing of stabilized fractures.[4] Surgical trauma during the osteotomy procedure initiates bone healing following implant placement,[5] regardless of whether an implant is subsequently placed or not.

Optimal site preparation ensures primary stability through the bony walls of the implant bed. Immediately after implant placement, peri-implant bone resorption occurs naturally, creating biological space for new bone formation. Therefore, the bone remodelling process implies a reduction in the initial stability of the implant, with a certain time period necessary for the attainment of secondary stability, which is primarily due to the newly formed bone. The duration of this process varies based on peri-implant bone density and the implant's micrometry and macro-geometry.

Histological and biomechanical analyses suggest that immediate loading of implants results in rapid and intense peri-implant bone resorption between the second and fourth week of functional loading. Consequently, this reduces primary stability, potentially reaching a critical threshold. During this period, performing prosthetic procedures on the implants carries risks, as they could compromise implant stability and osseointegration, thereby causing early failure. Therefore, it is advisable to postpone the final phase of prosthetic rehabilitation for at least 2 or 3 months after implant placement. This delay allows the newly formed bone to provide sufficient secondary stability to the implant, enabling resistance to screwing and unscrewing procedures for prosthetic components.

Local bone density plays a crucial role in achieving and preserving primary implant stability during the healing process for optimal function. Studies indicate that reduced bone density leads to increased micro-mobility at the bone/implant interface under load-bearing conditions.[6,7] Therefore, the immediate loading of implants must be carefully planned in poor bone quality conditions. Hence, careful analysis of bone density using cone beam computed tomography (CBCT) is recommended.[8] If CBCT reveals very low values in the intended implant placement site, it is advisable to avoid the immediate loading protocol. Numerous histological and biomechanical studies on bone healing suggest that early or immediate mechanical stimulation, such as functional loading (unless it induces excessive micromovement at the bone-implant interface that compromises implant stability), can effectively stimulate osteoblast bioactivity (migration, proliferation, deposition of osteoid tissue) and osseointegration of the implant.[9] For instance, histological comparisons in monkeys revealed similar interfaces between osseointegrated implants in the posterior mandible under delayed loading and immediately functionalized implant samples.[10-12] Conversely, histological analysis showed that immediate loading promoted higher bone density in the interface near (but not in contact with) the implant surface compared to loading after a healing period.[10,13]

The pre-clinical results were confirmed by clinical trials involving consenting patients who underwent additional implants. These implants were immediately loaded and later retrieved for histological analysis without compromising their rehabilitation. Furthermore, another clinical study compared histological findings between loaded and unloaded implants.[14] Therefore, both biological rationale and histological evidence support the hypothesis that immediate implant loading can positively impact osseointegration.

From a clinical perspective, when considering the immediate prosthesis of a single post-extraction implant, we can make temporary crowns with retention that can either be cemented or screwed. The choice of prosthetic crown retention on implants depends on technical, mechanical, biological and surgical factors. This choice must already be made during the diagnostic phase, as it can influence the implant-prosthetic treatment plan formulation. Among technical factors, the main consideration is the space between the arches. Clinically measurable, but even better on study models, when this space measures <8 mm, it indicates a screw-retained prosthesis.[15] Biological/surgical aspects include the invasiveness of the implant positioning procedure, which can be influenced by factors such as patient age and their general health status. In cases where regenerative procedures may not be ideal for older patients or those with systemic pathologies, which would guarantee an ideal implant positioning, can be avoided by choosing a cemented-type prosthesis to correct the implant axis inclination.

The advent of digital systems enables sophisticated pre-operative programming through the CBCT elaboration. This technology allows predicting the implant's position and axis at the end of the surgery.

POST EXO + TRANS SINUS + IMMEDIATE LOADING

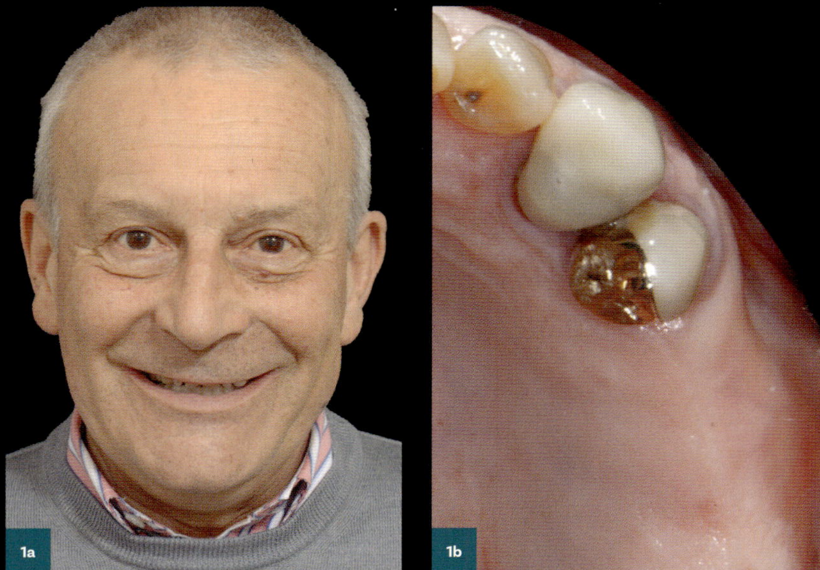

Figs. 1a,b ■ The patient attended for a consultation concerning rehabilitation of the second quadrant.

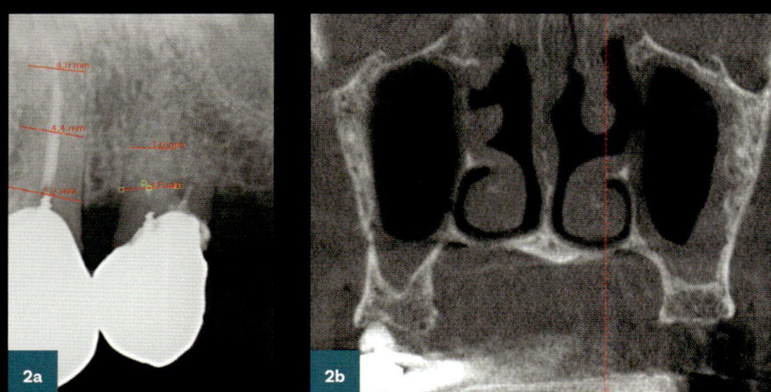

Figs. 2a,b ■ Intraoral radiographs taken during the clinical examination indicate that teeth 23 and 24 are unsalvageable due to the absence of a ferrule. The patient also reports that functional endoscopic surgery was performed on the maxillary sinus. Due to recurring polyposis, the ENT specialist said that a sinus lift was contraindicated. A minimally invasive sinus procedure could be accepted.

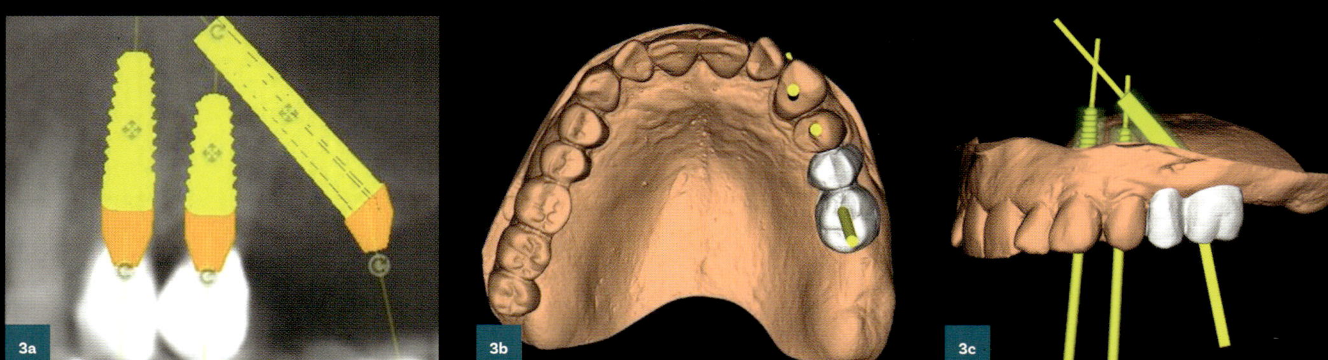

Figs. 3a-c ■ A digital planning was prepared for the rehabilitation using trans-sinus implants.

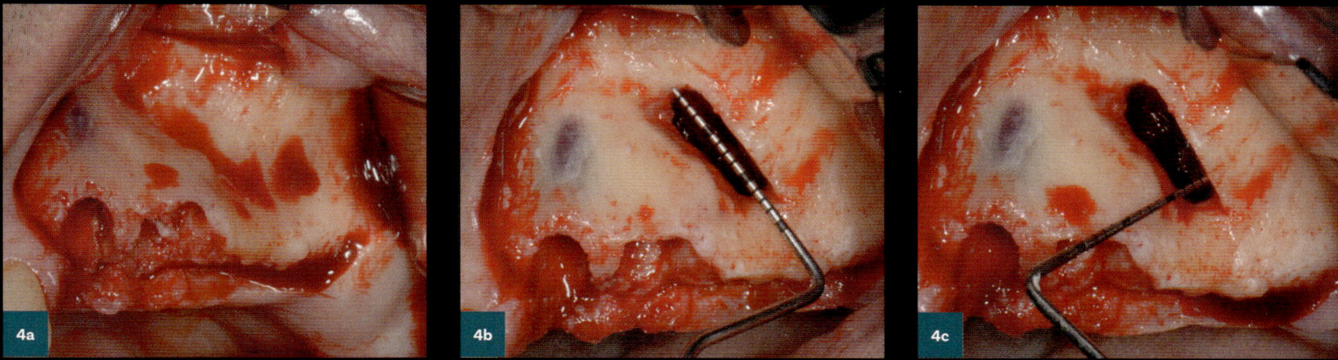

Figs. 4a-c ■ Preparation of the antrostomy and minimally invasive detachment of the sinus membrane to place the trans-sinus implant.

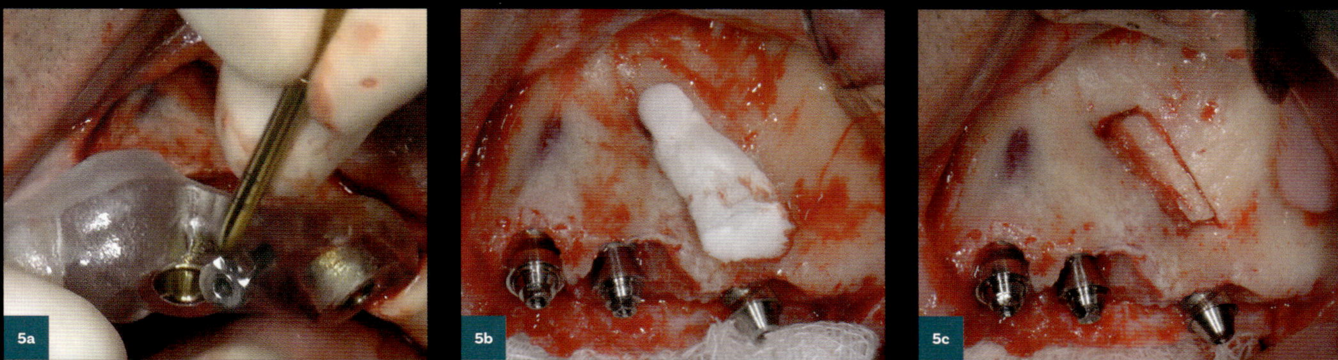

Figs. 5a-c ■ Due to the complexity of the case, implant positioning was performed using a computer-designed surgical guide. Post-extraction implants in teeth 23 and 24, as well as a trans-sinus implant in tooth 26. The cortical bone from the antrostomy is repositioned *in situ*.

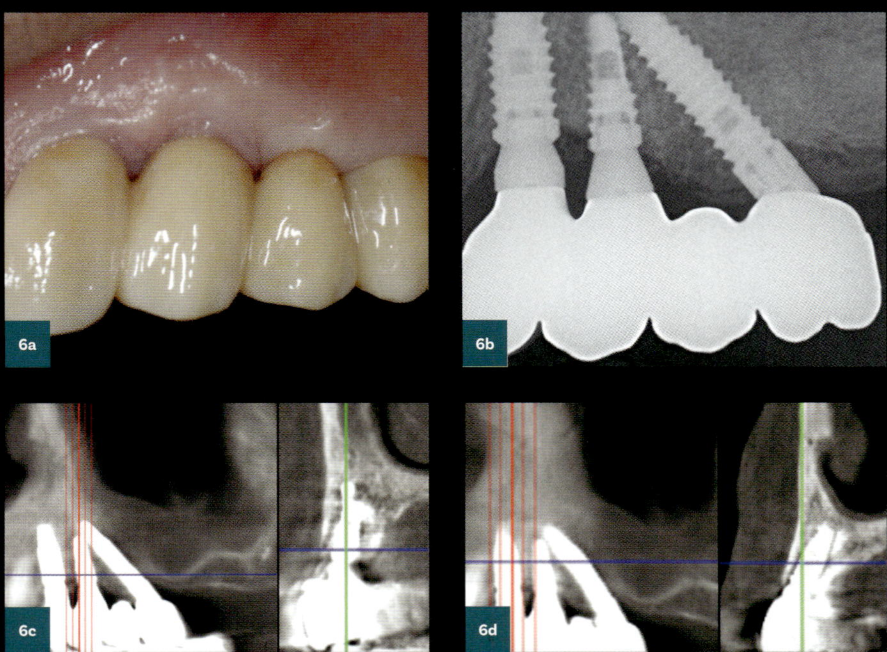

Figs. 6a-d ■ Definitive prosthetic rehabilitation, intraoral radiographs and CBCT check. (Prosthetics performed by Dr. A. Salici).

However, there are many scenarios that offer a choice between both solutions. Existing literature has extensively evaluated them under different aspects, with technological advancements significantly improving their outcomes. Pjetursson et al.[16] conducted a comparative analysis of implant survival studies published before and after 2000 and estimated a 5-year implant-prosthetic survival increase from 95.2% to 97.9% (cemented prosthesis) and from 77.6% to 96.8% (screwed prosthesis). A recent systematic review and meta-analysis of the screwed and cemented prosthesis focusing on bone resorption, showed that cemented type prosthesis had low bone resorption, thus presenting better survival and lower complications, with no statistically significant and clinically relevant differences. Currently, there is literary consensus regarding the screw-retained prosthesis as the first choice due to fewer biological complications and easier removal compared to the cemented prosthesis, despite the potential for higher complex surgery-associated biological costs and mechanical issues.[17] To address technical problems, especially related to screw-retained structural passivation, a mixed solution was proposed, wherein crowns with an occlusal access hole are cemented to titanium abutments directly in the laboratory with the adhesive technique. This approach ensures total structural passivity, eliminating any potential risks to patients associated with excessive cement in the peri-implant sulcus. Additionally, it provides the flexibility to adjust the emergence profile of the crown, both in the provisional phase and during the try-in, more apical or coronal according to aesthetic requirements. By adopting this method, we can leverage the benefits of both cemented and screwed prostheses while eliminating their disadvantages. Returning to the immediate loading phase, we currently consider the screw-retained temporary rehabilitation to be better performing from both biological and mechanical perspectives. In fact, a temporary cemented-type rehabilitation presents a greater risk of gingival inflammation at the abutment-cement-restoration interface, as well as the risk of cementation failure during the healing phases.[18]

As far as prosthetic procedures are concerned, accurate planning is a crucial start, which requires performing a diagnostic wax-up. Subsequently, the technical procedure basically pursues the following three paths:

1. Index technique
2. Intraoperative impression
3. Direct relining of a provisional with an access hole

Regarding the index technique, the procedure involves implant insertion using a modified or pre-prepared surgical guide as a template for transferring the implant position from the oral cavity to the laboratory. To accomplish this, a temporary abutment or impression transfer is connected to the implant for loading. The operating field is then isolated with a sterilized (cold technique) rubber dam, with prosthetic components attached to the guide using acrylic resin. This technique requires that the laboratory already possess models mounted in the articulator with the correct intermaxillary relationships. However, one limitation of this technique is the lack of information provided to the dental technician regarding soft tissues.

For intraoperative impressions, it is important to note that while this technique provides valuable information to the laboratory, it compromises the sterility of the operation. Therefore, if choosing this protocol, it is preferable to perform the impression phase before carrying out any bone regeneration procedures.

Direct relining of a perforated provisional requires more chairside operative time. However, thanks to the coordination with the laboratory, the open prosthetic crown can be connected to a temporary abutment using a flowable composite. This step should always be performed before any regenerative procedures, followed by unscrewing the abutment with the temporary crown fixed to it and delivery to the dental technician for finalizing the screw-retained temporary restoration.

GUIDED FLAPLESS SURGERY + USE OF PRE-EXISTING DEFINITIVE CROWN

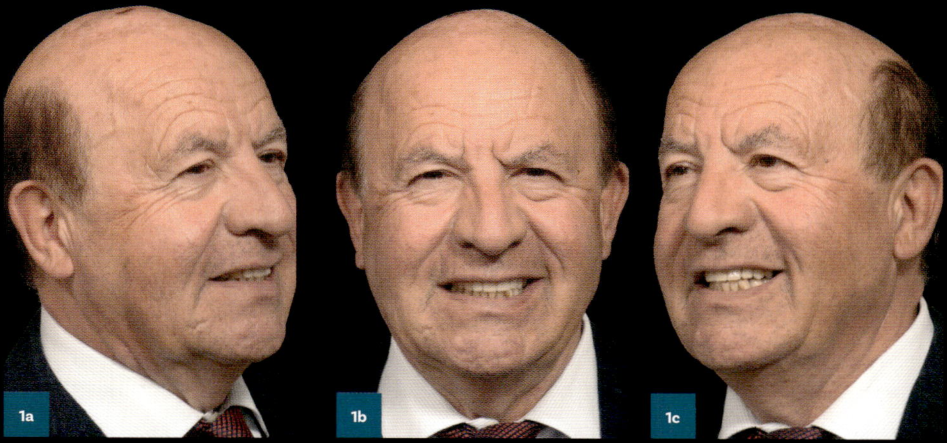

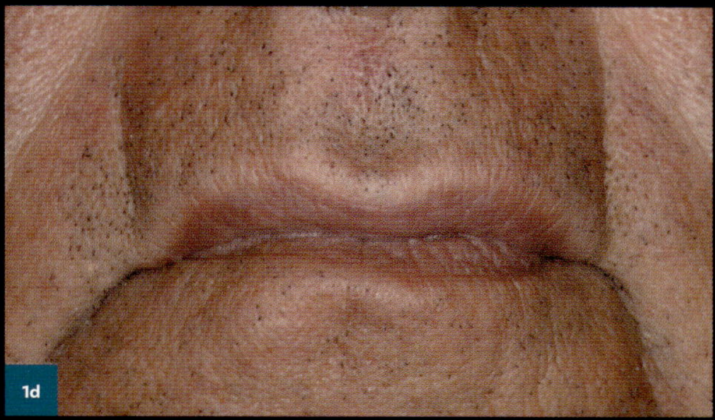

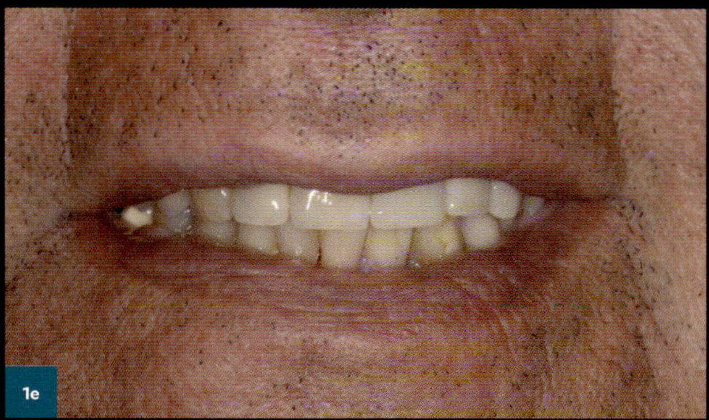

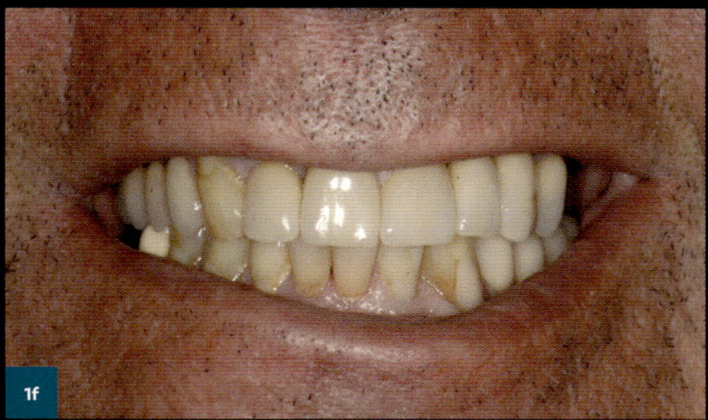

Figs. 1a-f ■ Extraoral images of the clinical case of a patient who presented for a consultation due to recurrent decementation of the prosthetic rehabilitation on tooth 12.

> CONT'D

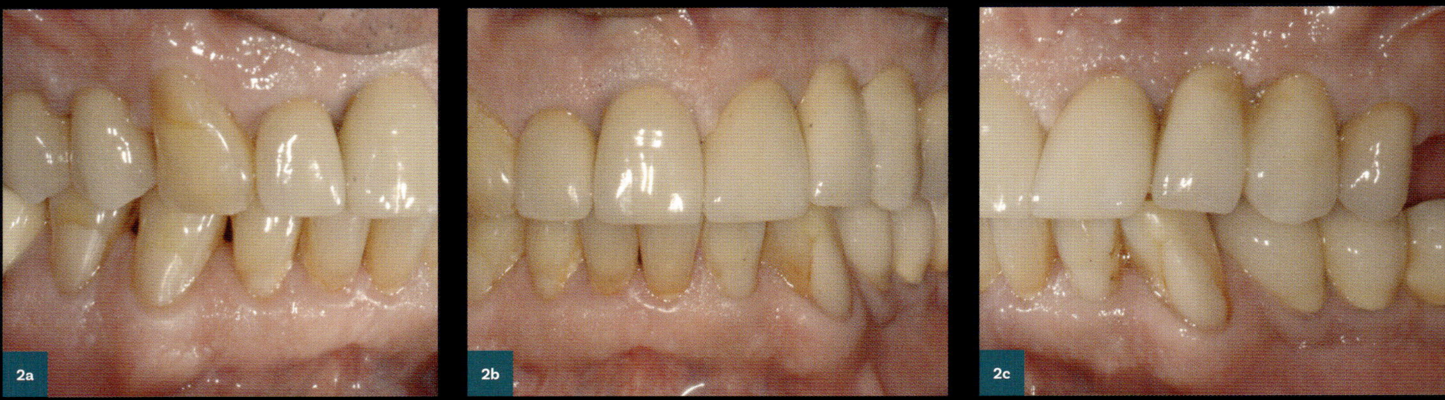

Figs. 2a-c ■ Intraoral images of the clinical case.

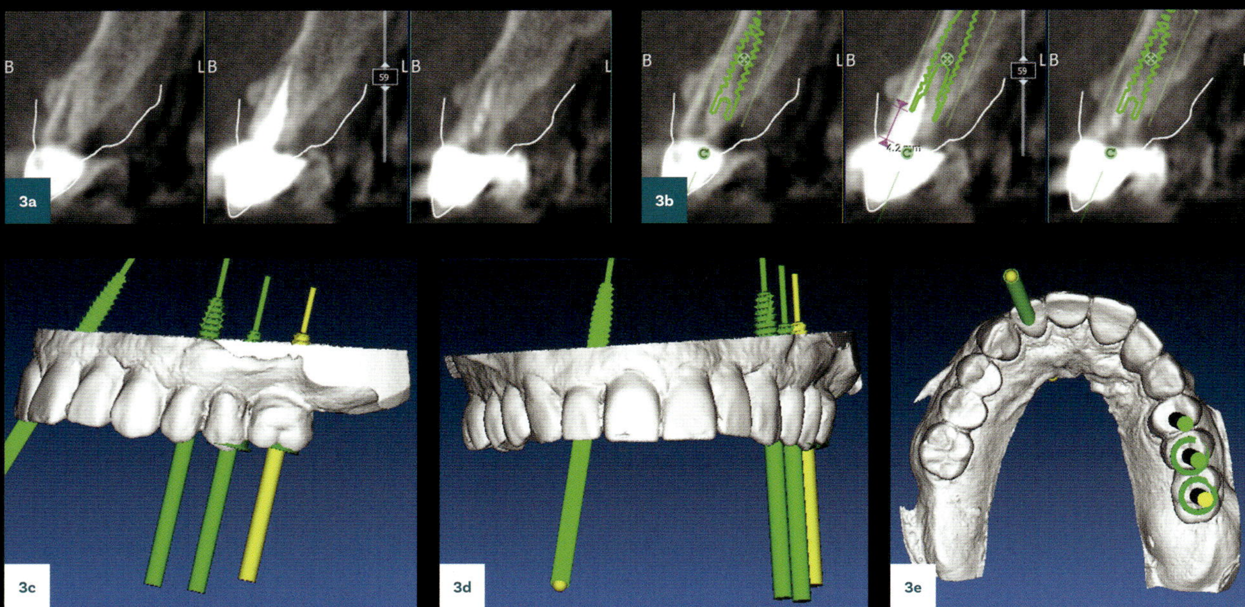

Figs. 3a-e ■ CBCT examination reveals root canal over-preparation in tooth 12, recurrent decementation of the prosthetic abutment reconstruction. Restoratively, tooth 12 is considered unsalvageable, prompting digital treatment planning for implant placement using a computer-guided template. The patient requests the possibility of having a fixed temporary rehabilitation.

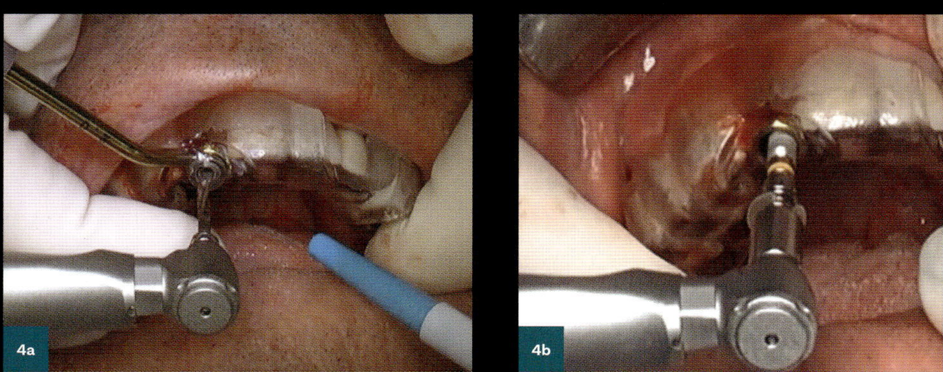

Figs. 4a,b ■ Surgical phases of computer-guided implant placement.

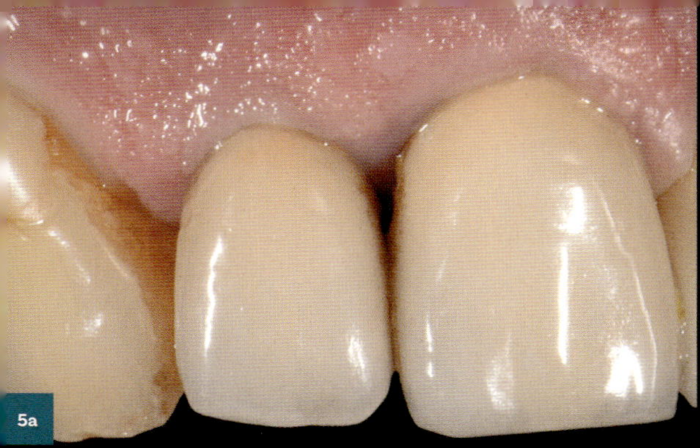

5a

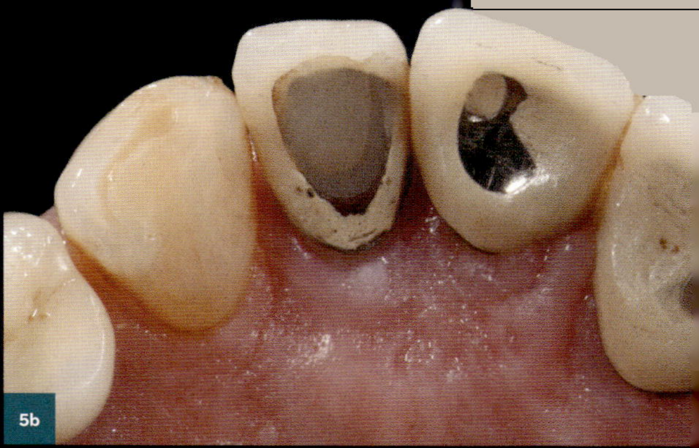

5b

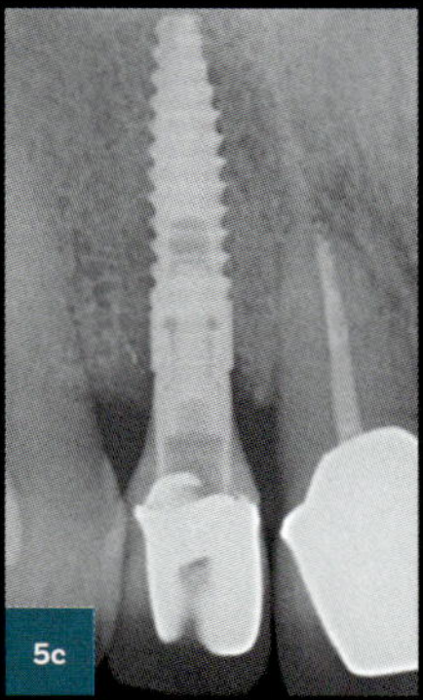

5c

Figs. 5a-c ■ Based on the high primary stability obtained immediate provisionalization was decided to be conducted using the pre-existing ceramic-metal prosthetic crown suitably modified for screw retention. Clinical and radiographic images are provided.

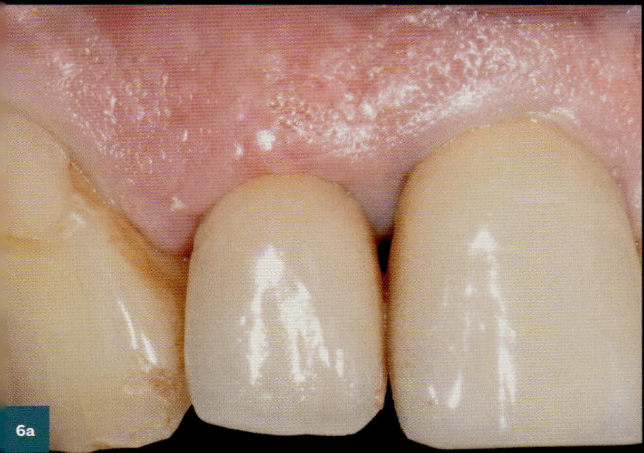

6a

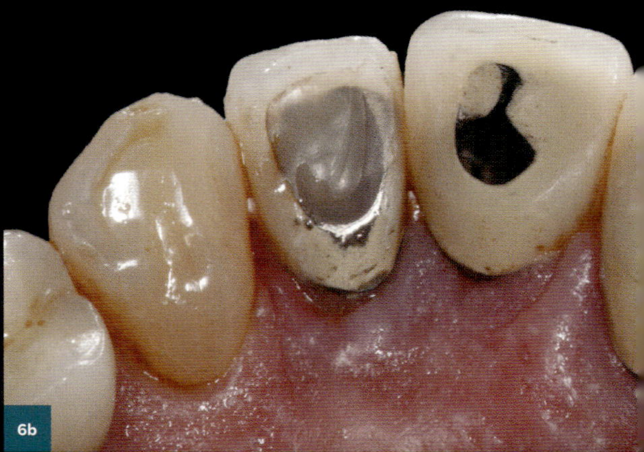

6b

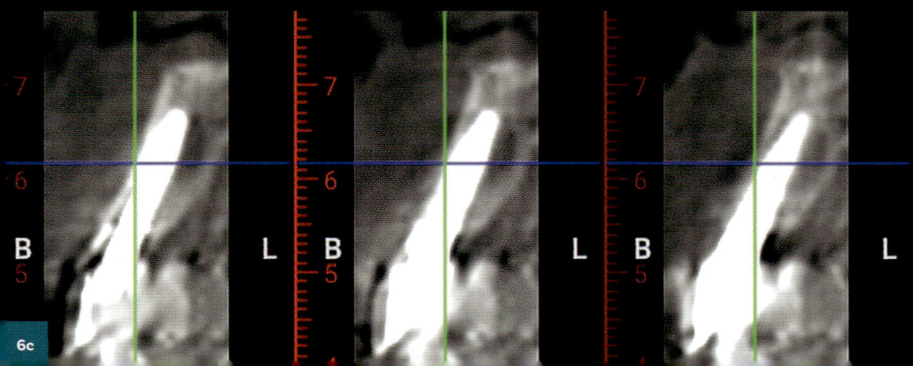

6c

Figs. 6a-c ■ Clinical and radiographic images taken 12 months post-loading.

FULL ARCH POST EXO

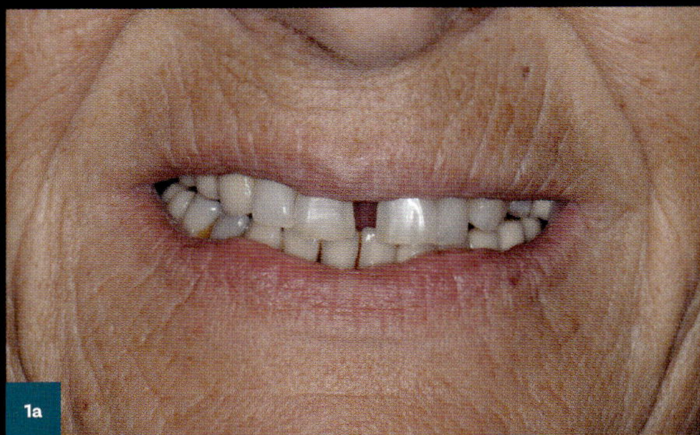

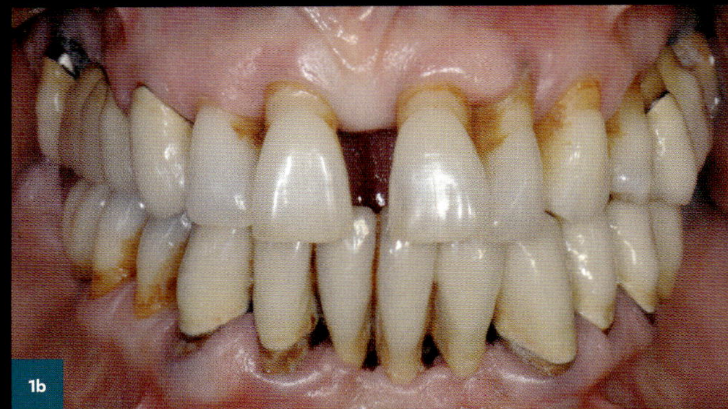

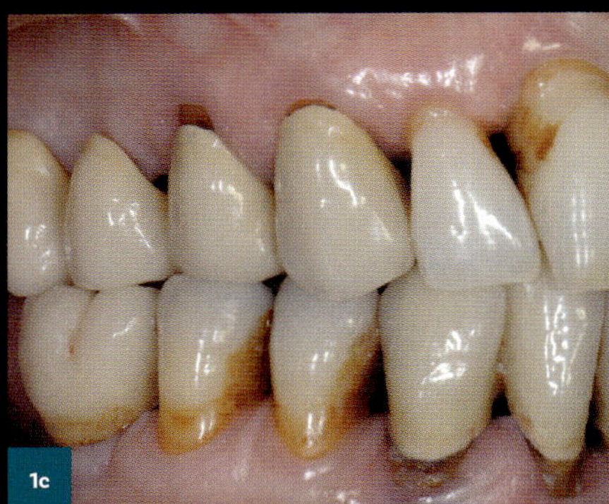

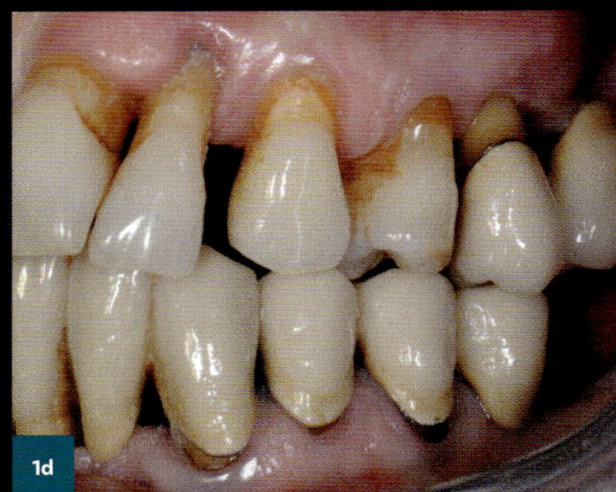

Figs. 1a-d ▪ Extraoral and intraoral images of the clinical case. The patient presents with complaints of masticatory difficulties and diffused mobility in the upper arch. Based on the clinical examination, an advanced periodontitis diagnosis was made. The teeth are deemed unsalvageable, and the patient was presented with the treatment plan for remediation and immediate loaded post-extraction implant-prosthetic rehabilitation.

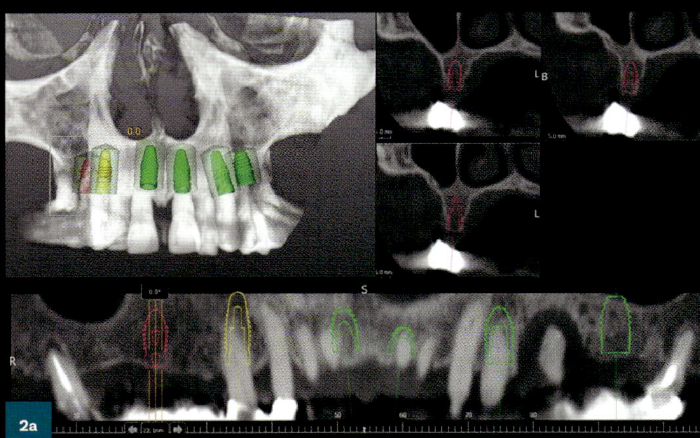

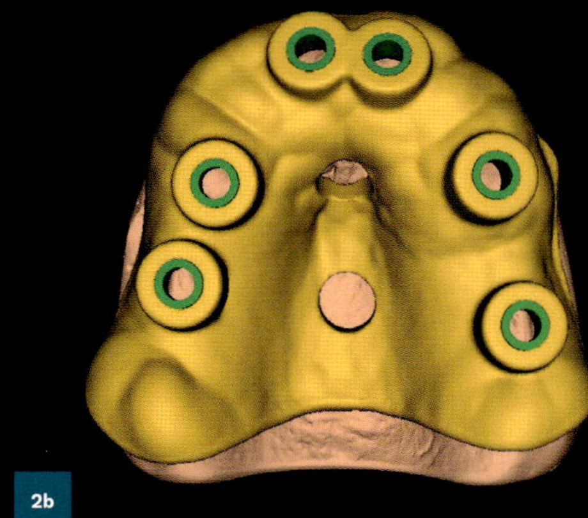

Figs. 2a,b ▪ Computerized planning of the surgical operation to create a computer-guided surgical template. The patient requests to maintain the diastema between teeth 11 and 21.

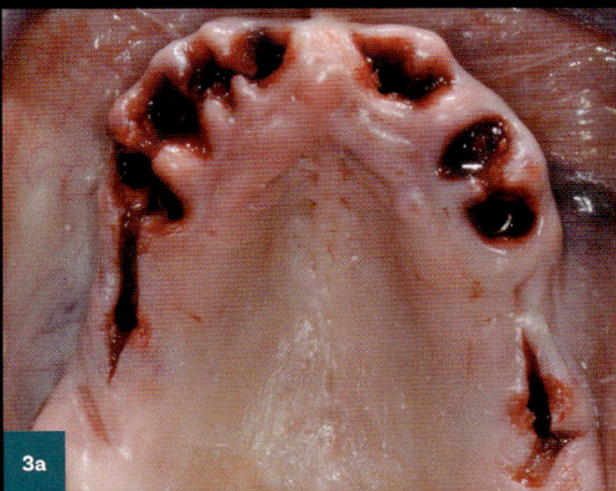

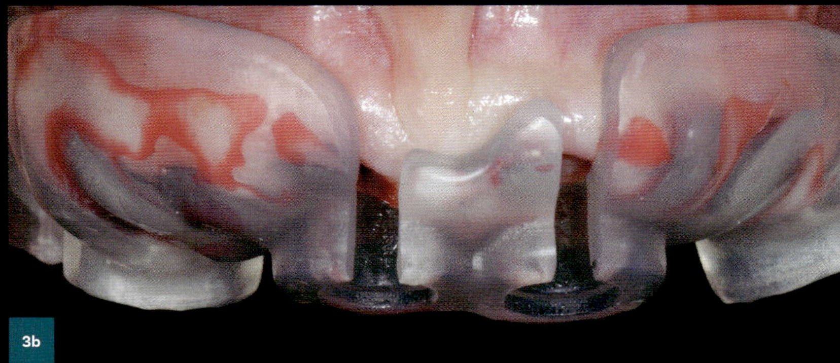

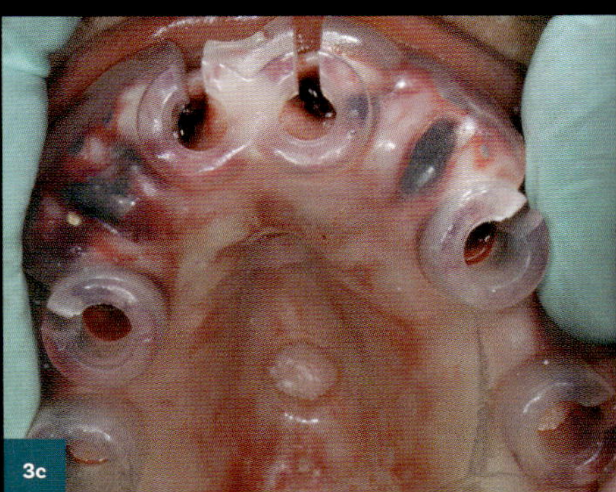

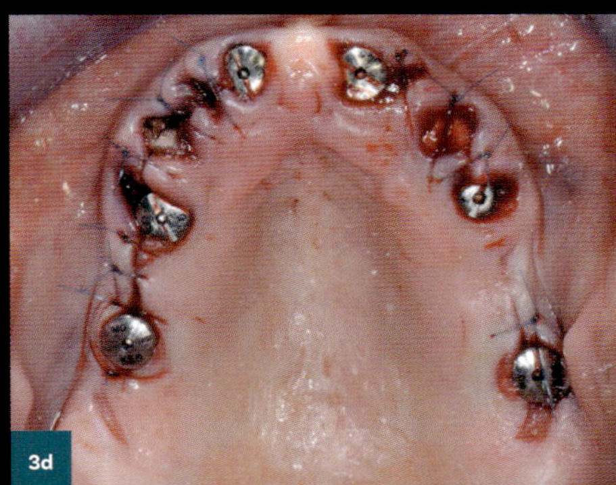

Figs. 3a-d ■ Surgical phases of teeth extraction and guided implant insertion.

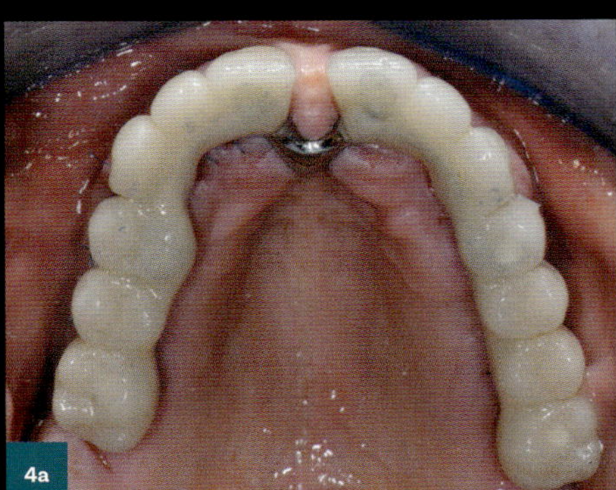

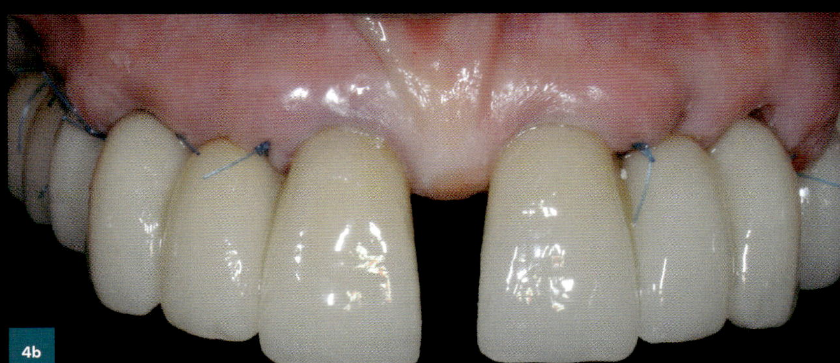

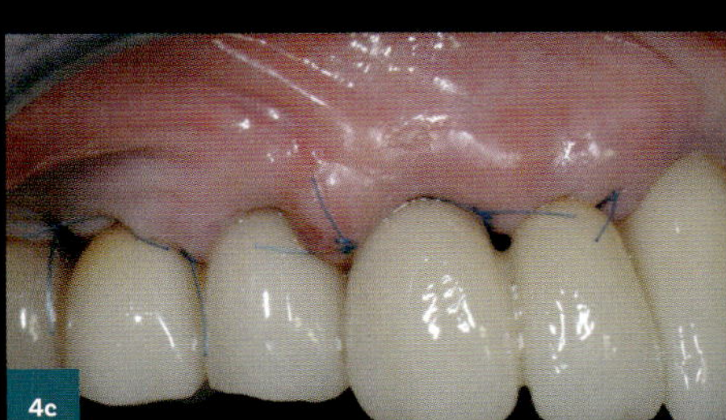

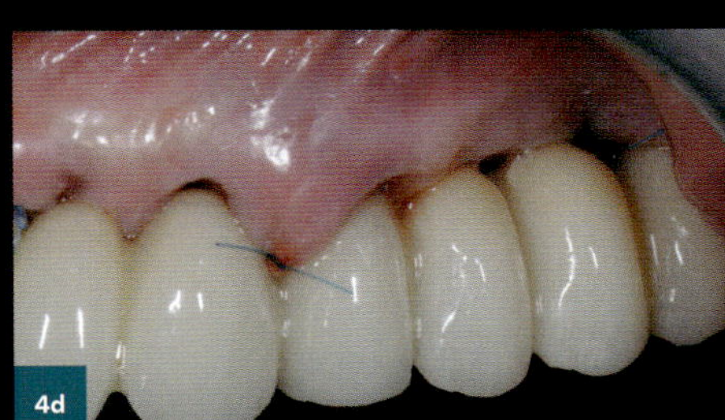

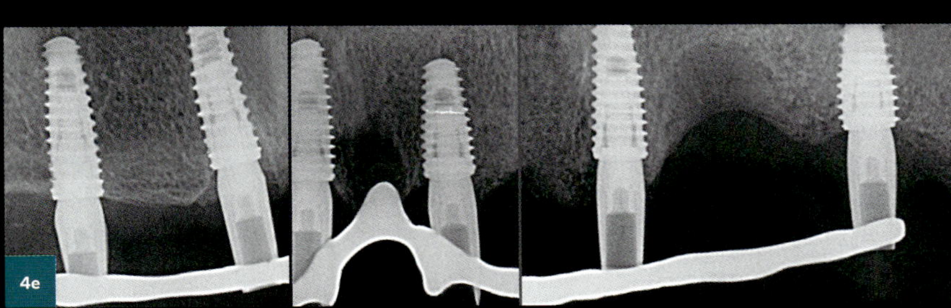

Figs. 4a-e ■ Connection of a immediately loaded screw-retained prosthesis. Clinical and radiographic images taken 24 hours after the surgical phase.

CONT'D ›

CONT'D

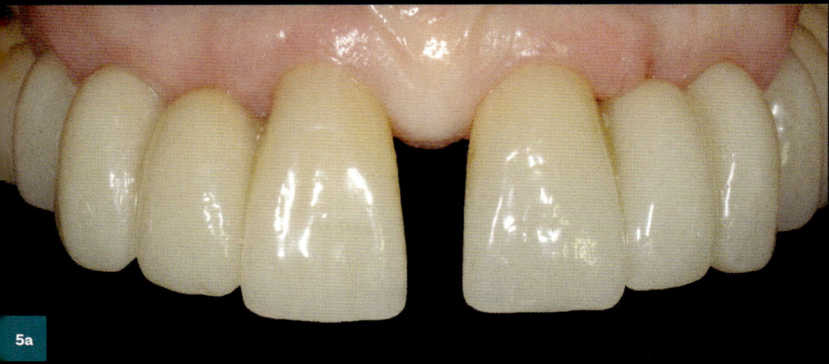

5a

Figs. 5a-c ■ Provisional rehabilitation observed 6 months after loading.

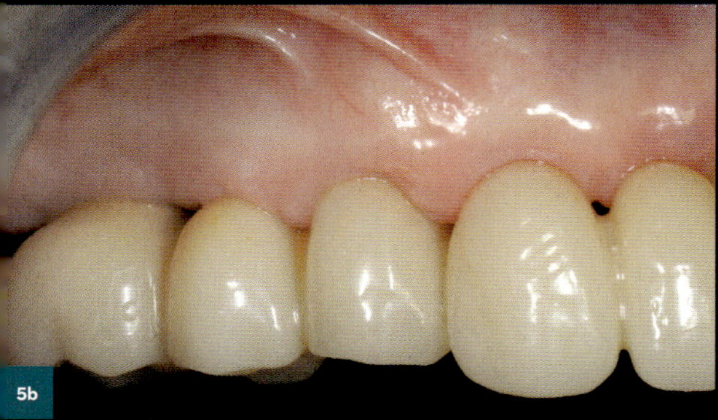

5b

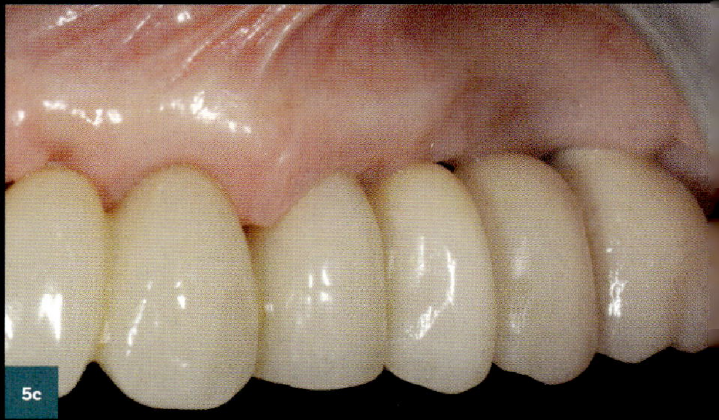

5c

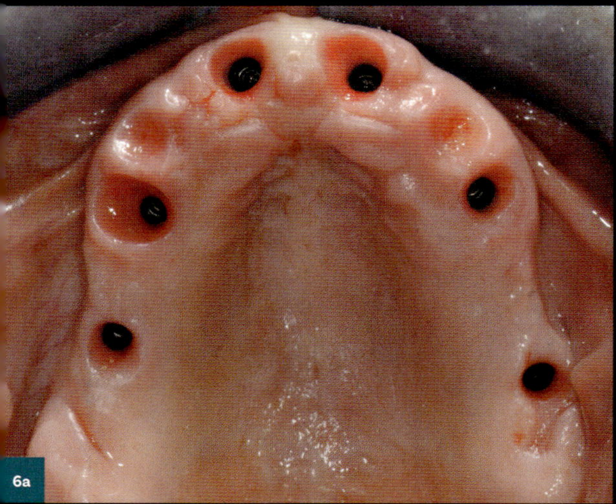

6a

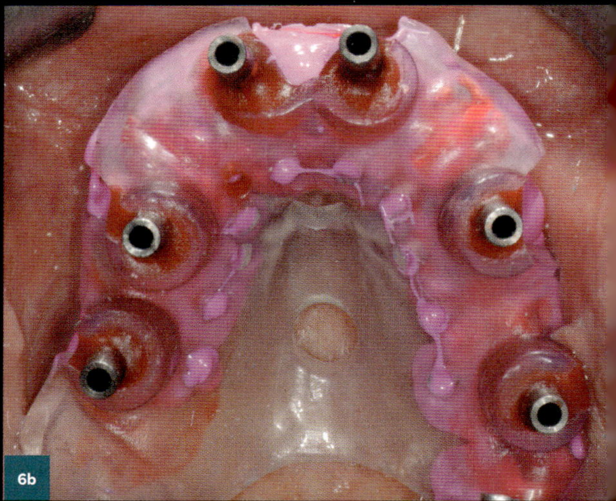

6b

Figs. 6a,b ■ Soft tissue condition prior to taking the final impression. The surgical guide is reused to transfer the implant positions and the soft tissue morphology to the dental technician. Titanium abutments are attached to the surgical guide by using self-curing resin. The soft tissue condition is recorded with the help of polyvinyl siloxane impression paste.

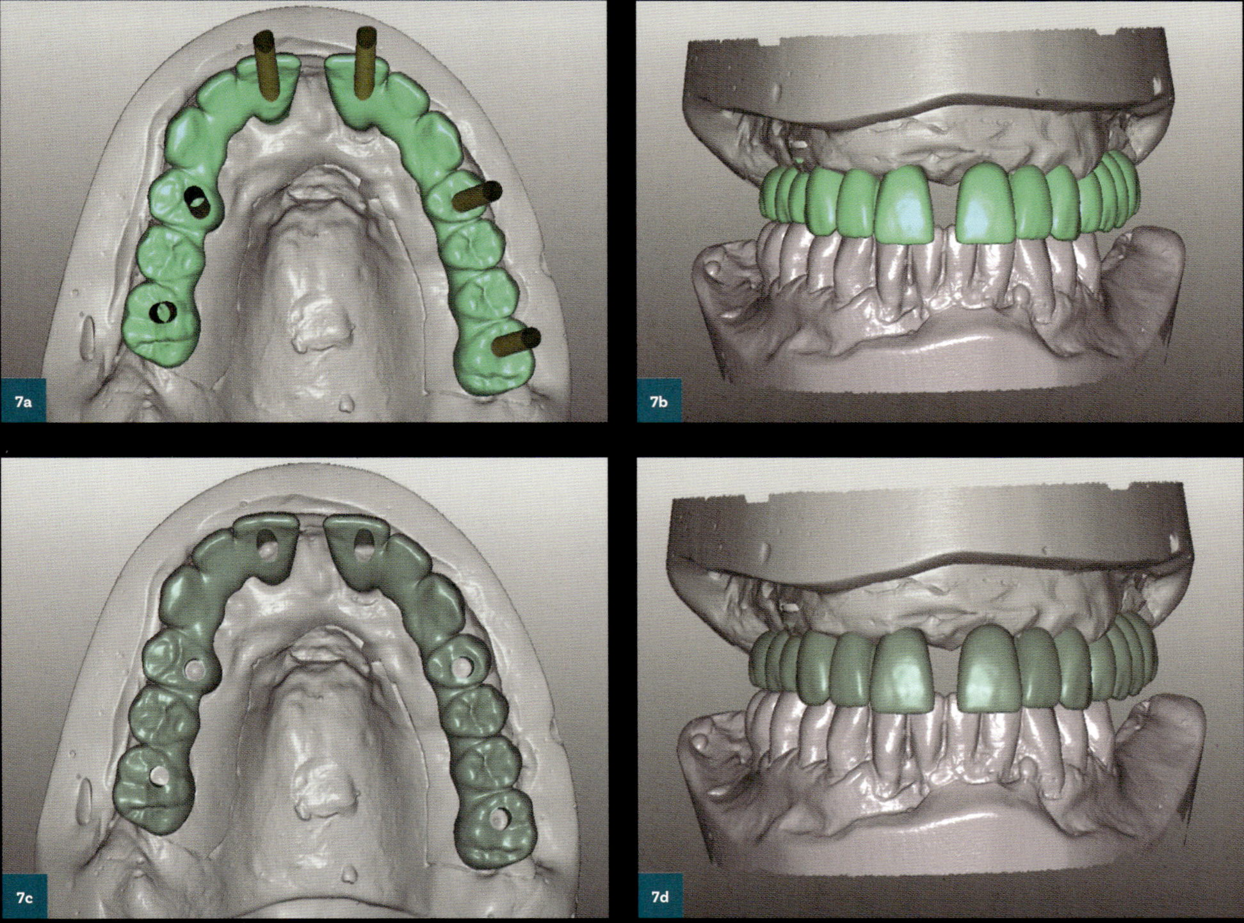

Figs. 7a-d ■ CAD phases of definitive rehabilitation.

> CONT'D

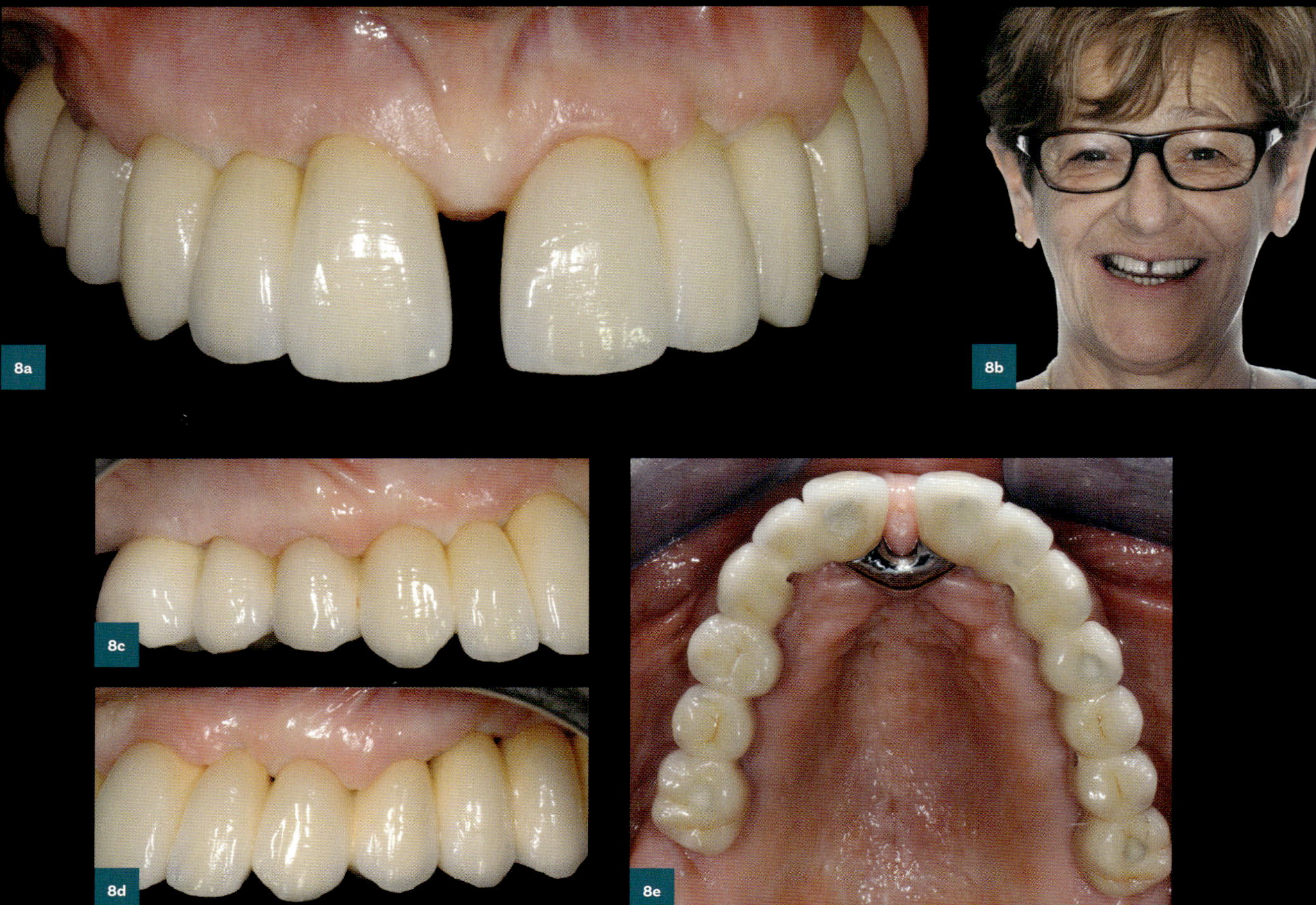

Figs. 8a-e ■ Clinical images of the definitive metal-ceramic screw-retained rehabilitation.

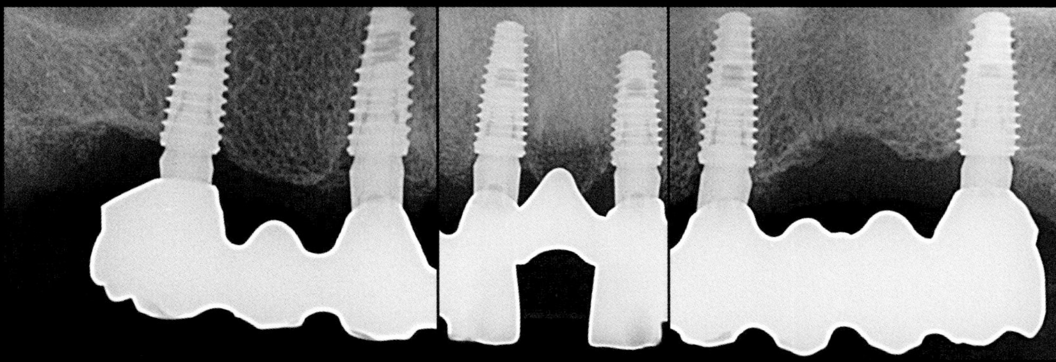

Fig. 9 ■ Intraoral radiographic images of the definitive rehabilitation.

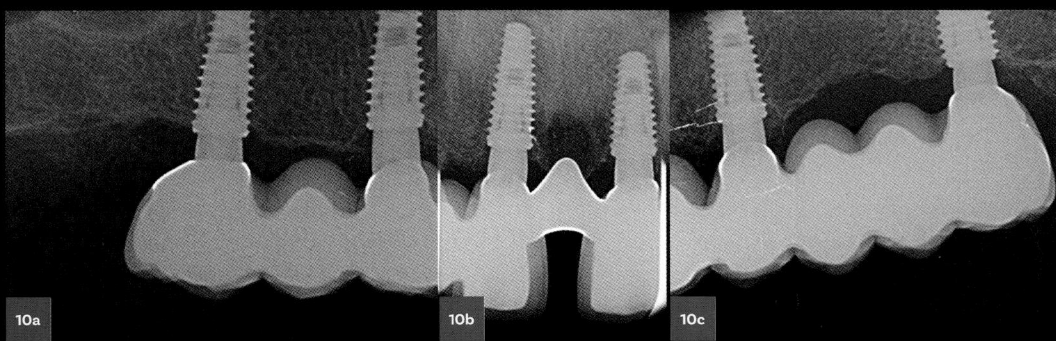

Figs. 10a-c ■ Radiographic and clinical follow-up at 3 years.

Bibliography

1. Misch CE, Hahn J, Judy KW, et al. Workshop guidelines on immediate loading in implant dentistry. *J Oral Implantol.* 2004;30(5):283-288.
2. Laney WR. Glossary of Oral and Maxillofacial Implants. *Int J Oral Maxillofac Implants.* 2017;32(4):1-200.
3. Nkenke E, Fenner M. Indications for immediate loading of implants and implant success. *Clin Oral Implants Res.* 2006;17(Suppl. 2):19-34.
4. Hobo S, Ichida E, Garcia LT. Osseointegration and Occlusal Rehabilitation. Tokyo, *Quintessence* 1990.
5. Schwartz Z, Lohmann CH, Cochran D, et al. Bone regulating mechanisms on implant surface. In: Lang NP, Karring T, Lindhe J (eds). Proceedings of the 3rd European Workshop on Periodontology: Implant Dentistry. Berlin, *Quintessence* 1999; pp. 41-54.
6. Engelke W, Decco OA, Rau MJ, Massoni MC, Schwarzwäller W. In vitro evaluation of horizontal implant micromovement in bone specimen with contact endoscopy. *Implant Dent.* 2004;13(1):88-94.
7. Trisi P, Perfetti G, Baldoni E, Berardi D, Colagiovanni M, Scogna G. Implant micromotion is related to peak insertion torque and bone density. *Clin Oral Implants Res.* 2009;20(5):467-471.
8. Todisco M, Trisi P. Bone mineral density and bone histomorphometry are statistically related. *Int J Oral Maxillofac Implants.* 2005;20(6):898-904.
9. Ko CC, Douglas WH, DeLong R, et al. Effects of implant healing time on crestal bone loss of a controlled-load dental implant. *J Dent Res.* 2003;82(8):585-591.
10. Romanos GE. Immediate loading of endosseous implants in the posterior area of the mandible. Animal and clinical studies. Berlin, *Quintessence* 2005.
11. Romanos G, Toh CG, Siar CH, et al. Peri-implant bone reactions to immediately loaded implants. An experimental study in monkeys. *J Periodontol.* 2001;72(4):506-511.
12. Romanos GE, Toh CG, Siar CH, Swaminathan D. Histologic and histomorphometric evaluation of peri-implant bone subjected to immediate loading: an experimental study with Macaca fascicularis. *Int J Oral Maxillofac Implants.* 2002;17(1):44-51.
13. Romanos GE, Toh CG, Siar CH, Wicht H, Yacoob H, Nentwig GH. Bone-implant interface around titanium implants under different loading conditions: a histomorphometrical analysis in the Macaca fascicularis monkey. *J Periodontol.* 2003;74(10):1483-1490.
14. Testori T, Szmukler-Moncler S, Francetti L, et al. Healing of Osseotite implants under submerged and immediate loading conditions in a single patient: A case report and interface analysis after 2 months. *Int J Periodontics Restorative Dent.* 2002;22(4):345-353.
15. Misch C. Priciples of fixed prosthodontics: cement-retained restorations. In: Dental Implant prosthetics. Elsevier, St Louis Missouri 2015; pp. 650-699.
16. Pjetursson B, Asgeirsson A, Zwahlen M, Sailer I. Improvements in Implant Dentistry over the Last Decade: Comparison of Survival and Complication Rates in Older and Newer Publications. *Int J Oral Maxillofac Implants.* 2014;29(Supplement):308-324.
17. Lemos CA, de Souza Batista VE, Almeida DA, Santiago Júnior JF, Verri FR, Pellizzer EP. Evaluation of cement-retained versus screw-retained implant-supported restorations for marginal bone loss: A systematic review and meta-analysis. *J Prosthet Dent.* 2016;115(4):419-427.
18. Kan JYK, Rungcharassaeng K, Deflorian M, Weinstein T, Wang HL, Testori T. Immediate implant placement and provisionalization of maxillary anterior single implants. *Periodontol 2000.* 2018;77(1):197-212.

12

Management of hard tissue defects

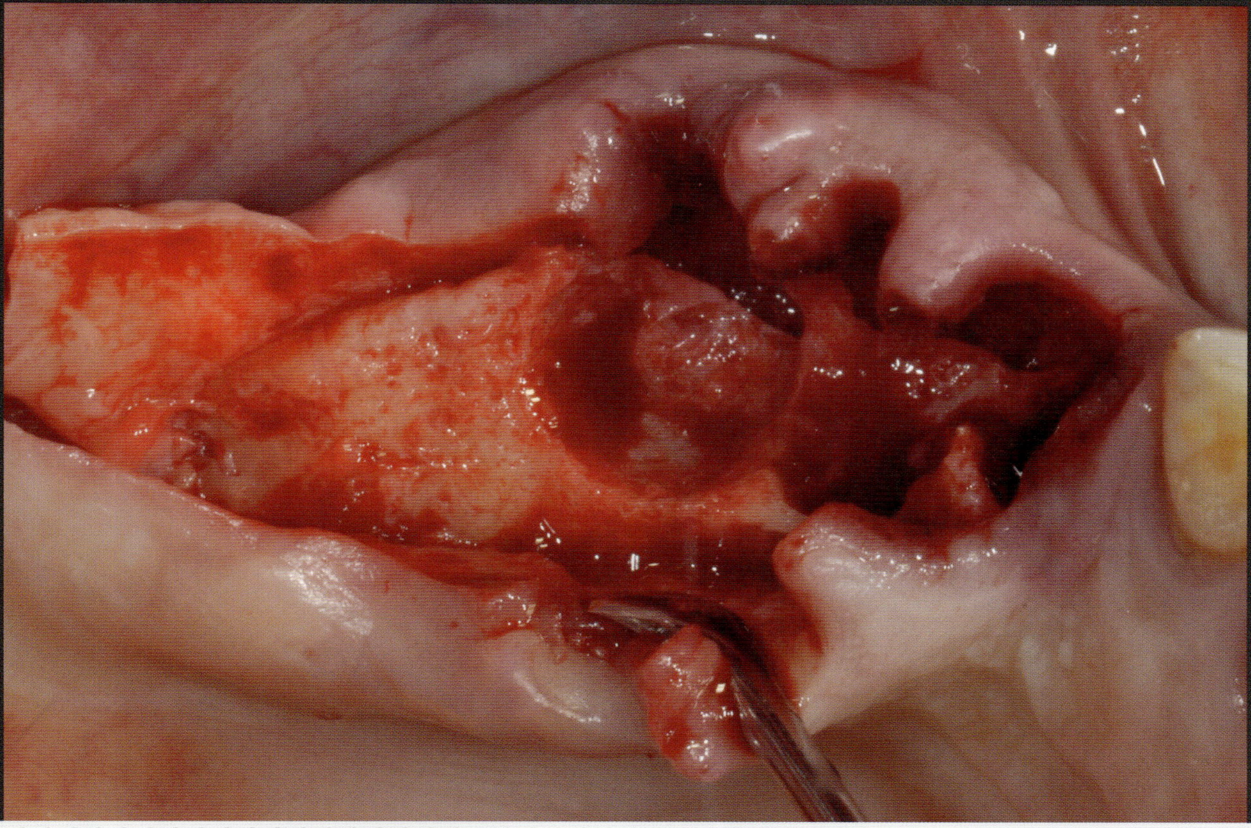

After correctly placing an implant, managing the buccal gap and the peri-implant soft tissue becomes crucial. Regarding the buccal gap, numerous scientific studies extensively discuss the management of the residual gap between the implant surface and the extraction site's internal surface during immediate implant placement. Many studies have analysed the possibility of obtaining close bone-implant surface contact in animal models. We can deduce from these studies that waiting at least 4 months allows for spontaneous bone regeneration when the maximum gap dimensions were 1-1.25 mm.

Although there is limited scientific evidence in humans, a few authors have histologically examined osteointegration levels in post-extraction implants. Paoloantonio et al.[1] observed a similar percentage of bone in direct contact with the implant surface (BIC) compared to implants placed in natural bone (70.6% for the mandible and 64.8% for the maxilla). Cases with 1-1.5 mm of inflammation-free connective tissue at the implant's coronal portion were rare. Cornelini et al.[2] reported a BIC of 61.4% and 3.2 mm of supracrestal connective tissue. Wilson et al.[3] found, in a human model, that a 1.5 mm gap presented an average BIC of 50%, with lower percentages associated with a 4 mm gap.

Contrary to previous beliefs,[4] post-extraction implants cannot prevent post-extraction bone resorption. Resorption is determined by factors related to both the extraction technique and the implant's three-dimensional placement,[5] which, if done incorrectly, can negatively affect aesthetics. To address these concerns, socket grafting has been proposed to reduce the post-extraction site's volumetric contraction. Thus, socket grafting is now considered an effective and essential procedure.[6]

In the presence of an intact buccal bone housing, determining the horizontal distance between the implant surface and the buccal bone's cortical part (referred to as IEAB, Implant-to-External sides of the Alveolar Bone) is essential to guarantee sufficient volume for peri-implant biological width formation and dimensions of the peri-implant socket space.

IEAB ≤ 3 mm

When the IEAB distance is ≤ 3 mm, it represents the most challenging clinical scenario, especially in aesthetic cases involving a thin biotype. To address this clinical situation, the recommended approach is using an Intra-Extra (allo)Graft (IEG) to achieve a minimum buccal width of 4 mm. With these initial volumes and accounting for physiological bone resorption, this should leave at least 2 mm of bone volume, which is considered sufficient for peri-implant biological width formation. Graft stabilization will require the application of a resorbable membrane covered by collagen sponges in the uncovered portion, not enveloped by the surrounding soft tissues.[7] This procedure will increase the amount of keratinized peri-implant tissue through secondary intention healing.

In cases involving multiple implants and substantial grafted material, using multiple membranes is feasible, as they can be more easily covered by the surrounding soft tissues, thereby facilitating primary intention healing. With the current advancements in flapless techniques, it is possible to exclusively perform an intra-alveolar graft together with a soft tissue width augmentation procedure, even when IEAB is ≤ 3 mm, as illustrated in the next chapter. Therefore, this procedure still allows for the placement of a healing abutment and an immediate temporary crown since the resorbable membranes are placed buccally and remain unaffected by the prosthesis.

IEAB > 3 mm

If the distance between the implant surface and external cortical bone exceeds 3 mm, managing the residual space requires consideration of the specific dental area. For implants placed in aesthetically less significant areas, finalising the graft should ensure functional aspects. This means that the graft will be placed exclusively in the residual space as an Intra (allo)Graft (IG), aiming to stabilise the blood clot, promoting the osteoconduction process and reducing buccal bone resorption. Additionally, a resorbable membrane is applied to stabilise the grafted material during the initial healing phases.

In areas of high aesthetic value, implant placement should always be accompanied by an IEG graft, creating an oversized buccal portion for an optimal aesthetic result. In this case, a resorbable membrane is placed over the graft for protection during the healing process. Although a healing abutment and immediate temporary crown may be placed, a two-step approach is preferable for aesthetically important areas. In this case, once the graft has healed, a connective tissue graft could be placed, if clinically necessary, to precisely determine the required volume of connective tissue graft.

In the absence of a partially or completely intact buccal wall, the multiple possibilities available to us must be considered, after accounting for the patient's periodontal biotype (**Figs. 12.1a,b**). For a thick biotype, surgical intervention, flapless or not, followed by a GBR with the placement of a resorbable membrane and a biomaterial graft, is necessary.

In this scenario, the same dimensional evaluations for the IEAB are still valid, with the same goal of ensuring adequate buccal bone width around the implant. Gingival recession is clinically associated with the presence of a thin periodontal biotype and the absence of cortical buccal bone. Although implant placement is still possible, a prudent approach is preferred. Therefore, the clinical protocol involves staged placement with simultaneous hard tissue (GBR) and soft tissue (CTG) corrections. The prosthodontic procedures may vary with these situations. However, immediate loaded provisional rehabilitation is recommended exclusively for cases with a thick periodontal biotype and no gingival recession.

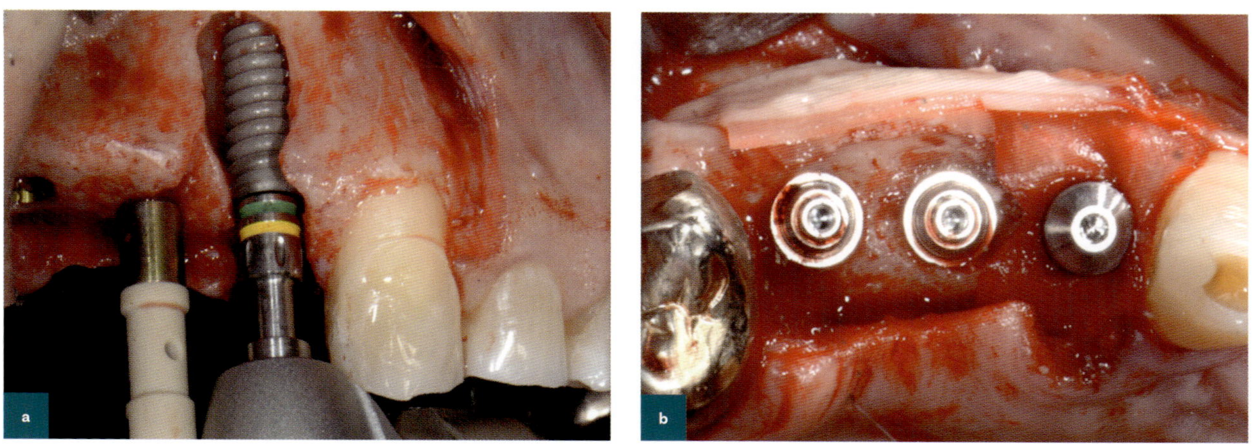

Figs. 12.1a,b ■ Immediate implant placement in the absence of buccal and palatal cortical bone. To establish the the graft's dimension, the clinician will have to respect the same dimensional evaluations relative to the IEAB and with the same goal of guaranteeing an adequate amount of buccal bone width around the implant.

INFECTED POST-EXTRACTION SITES + IMMEDIATE LOADING + PRE- AND POST-SINUS IMPLANTS

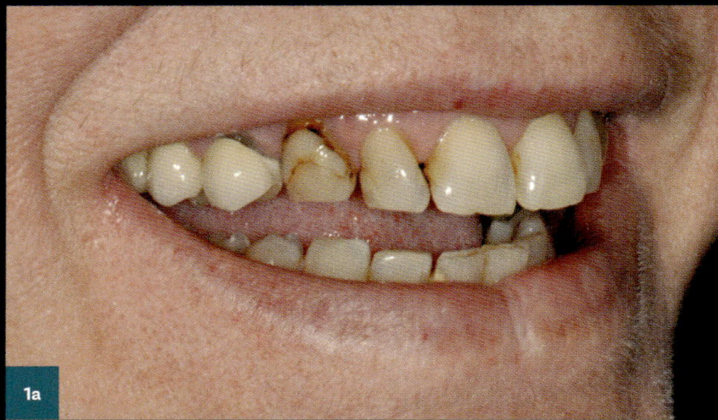

1a

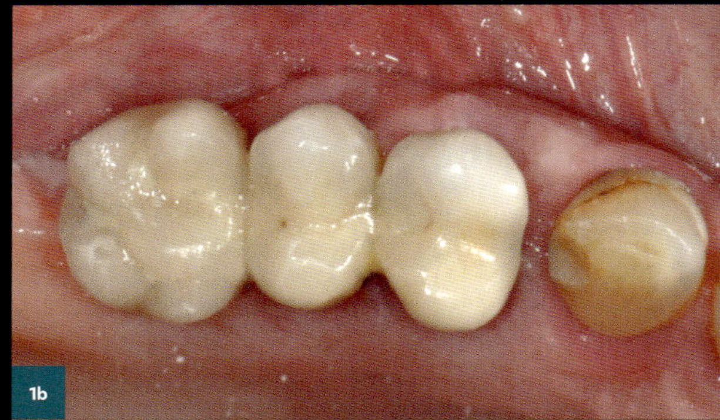

1b

Figs. 1a-c ■ Extra and intraoral images. The patient complains of mobility of the fixed rehabilitation in position 16-15-14 and tooth 13. The objective clinical examination reveals third-degree mobility in these aforementioned teeth. The periodontal probing highlights an important bone support loss despite adequate soft tissue levels related to a thick periodontal biotype. The affected teeth in question are unsavable. The patient requires a fixed rehabilitation, while avoiding a provisional removable prosthesis.

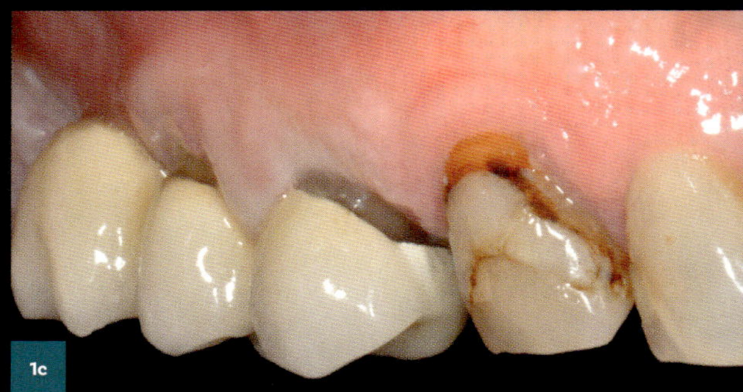

1c

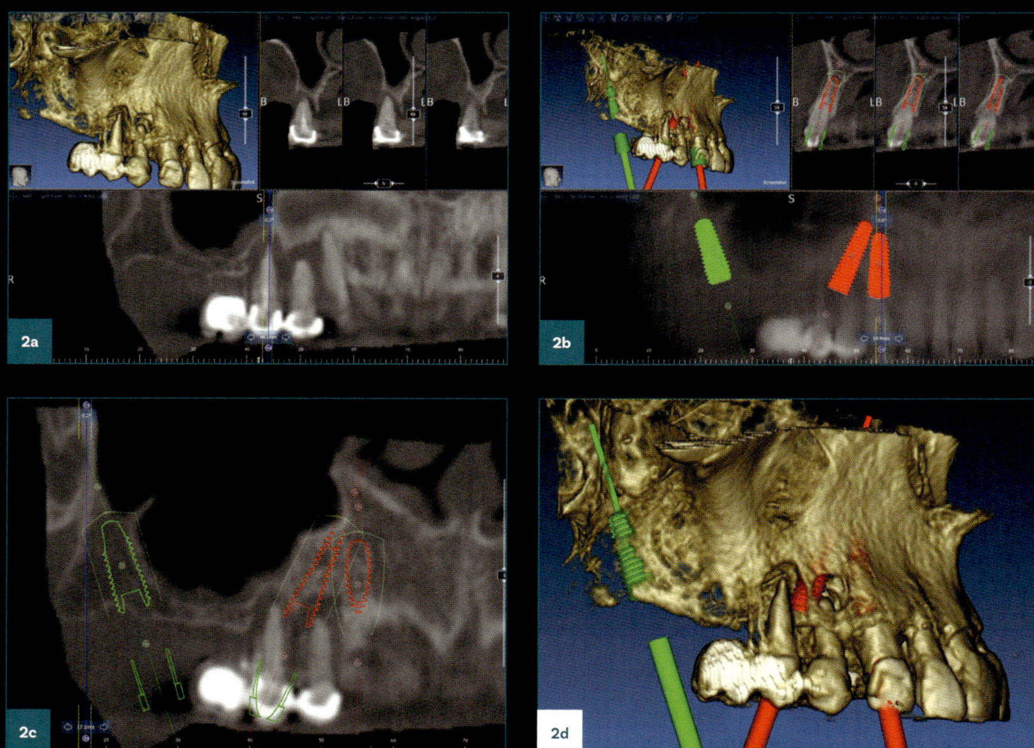

2a 2b 2c 2d

Figs. 2a-d ■ CBCT evaluation confirms extensive bone loss. The support of the literature in terms of predictability of immediate implant in infected sites and the use of dedicated software allows for accurate implant planning. Thanks to these technologies, immediate implant insertion is therefore planned in positions 13 and 15 (tilted implant) along with the positioning of an implant in the tuber maxillae, thus avoiding the need for a sinus lift.

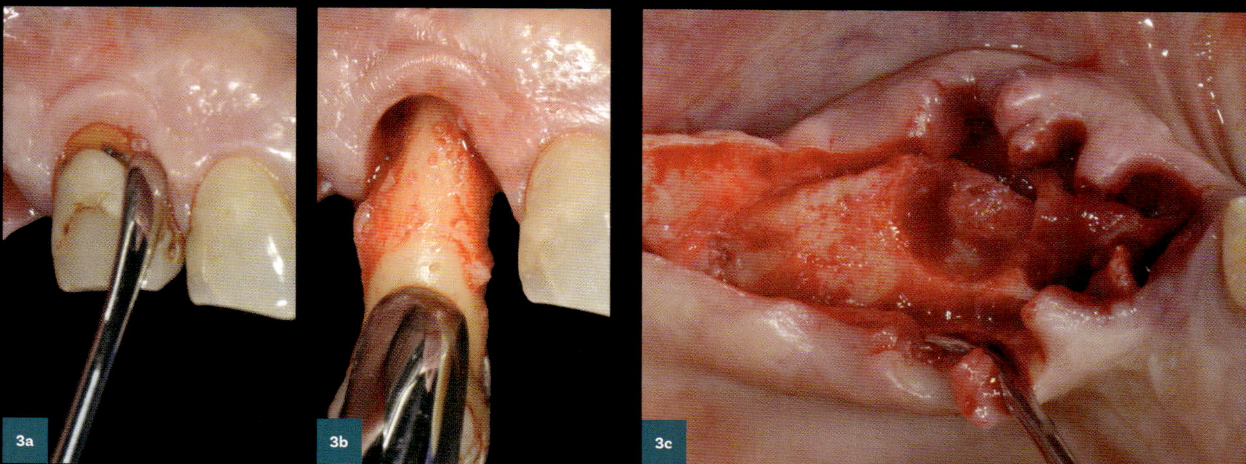

Figs. 3a-c ■ The surgical phase involves atraumatic extractions, mucoperiosteal flap elevation without vertical releasing incisions and thorough debridement of the granulation tissue. This last procedure is a fundamental condition for successful treatment in the presence of infection.

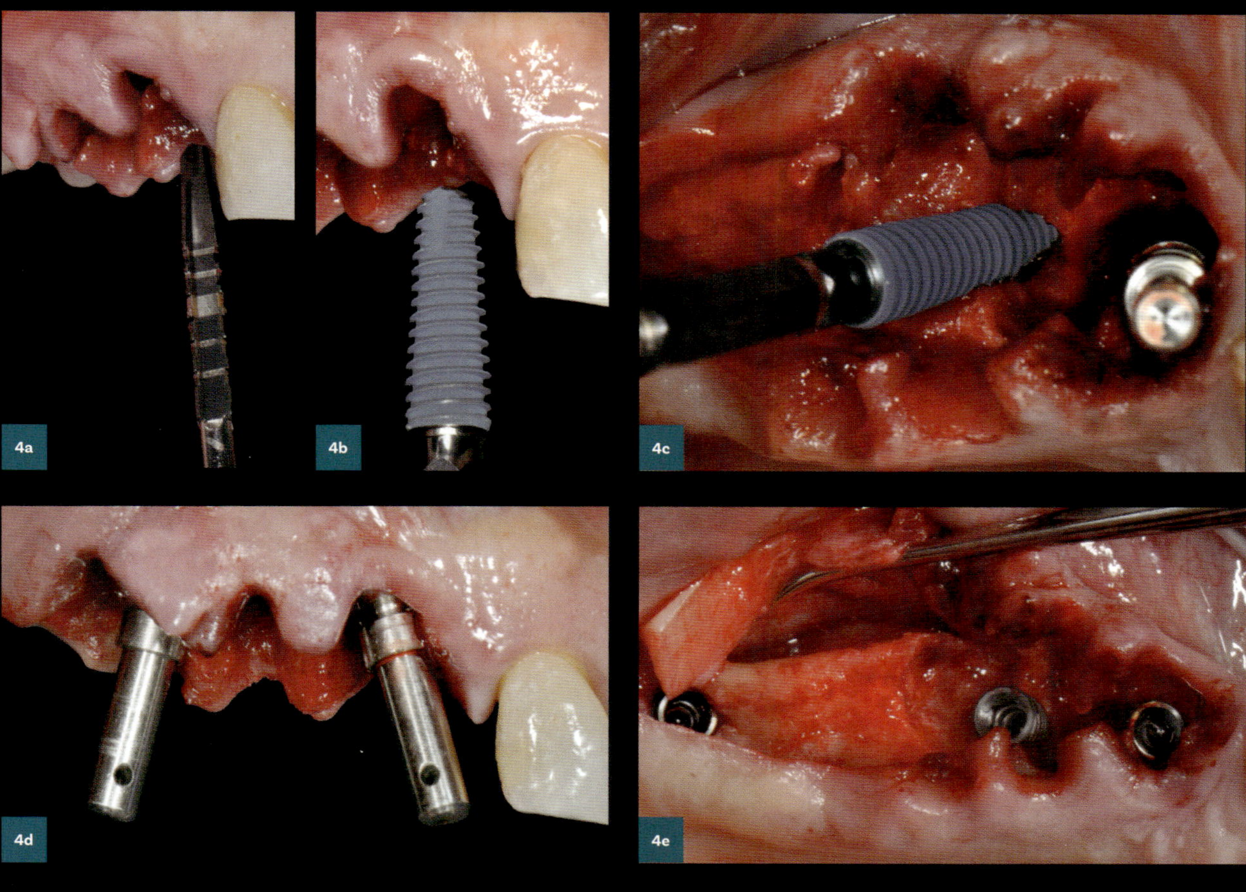

Figs. 4a-e ■ Implant placement according to the digital project.

> CONT'D

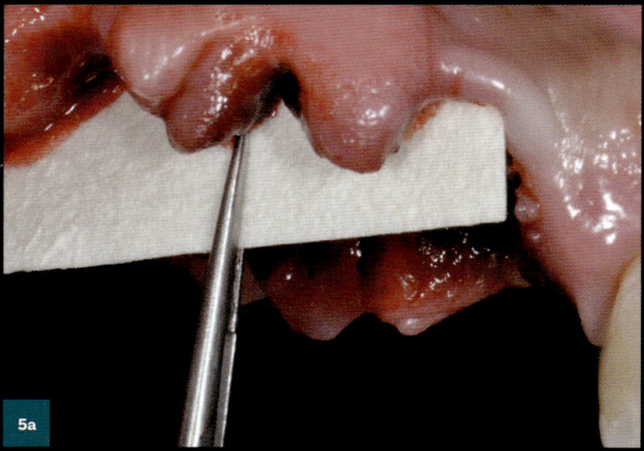

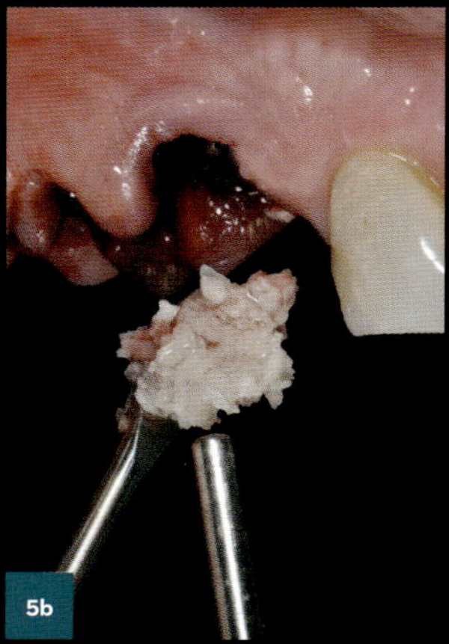

Figs. 5a,b ■ Regeneration is performed using a slow resorbing biomaterial and a resorbable collagen membrane.

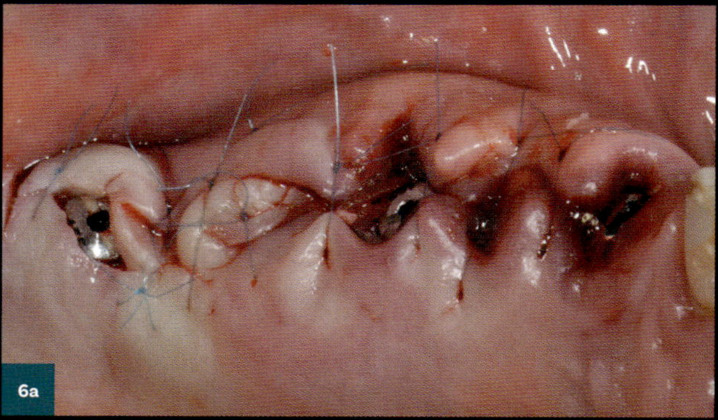

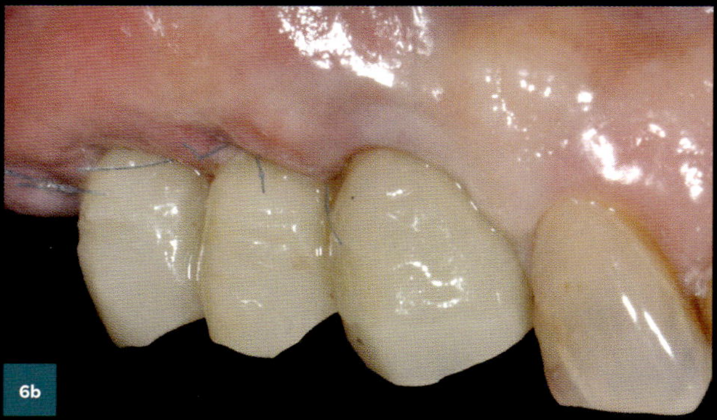

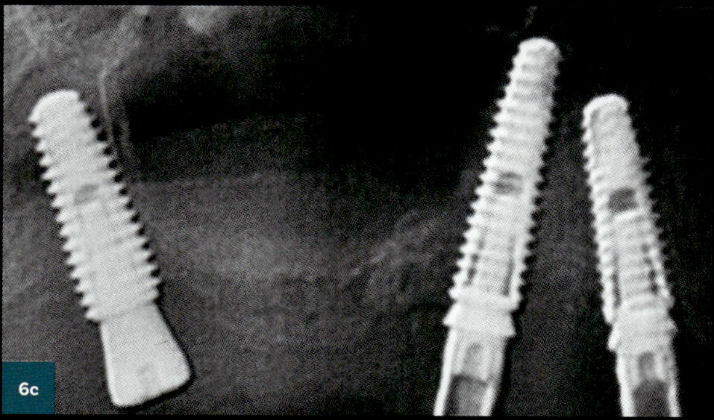

Figs. 6a-c ■ Monofilament sutures are used. The achieved insertion torque allows manufacturing of a screw retained immediate prosthesis placed on implant 13 and 15, without any contacts in centric occlusion and during excursive movements. The radiographic image shows the intact anatomical limits of the maxillary sinus.

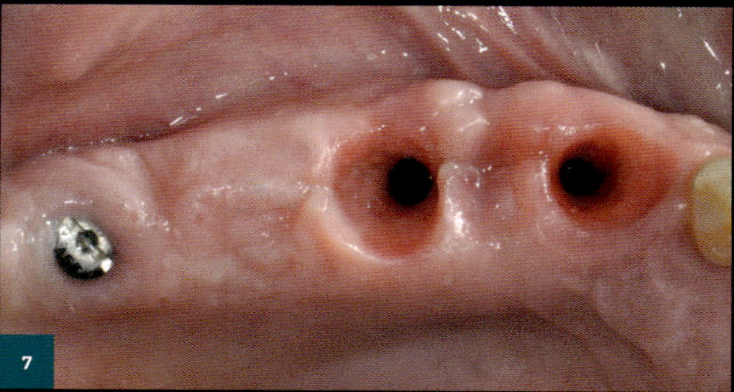

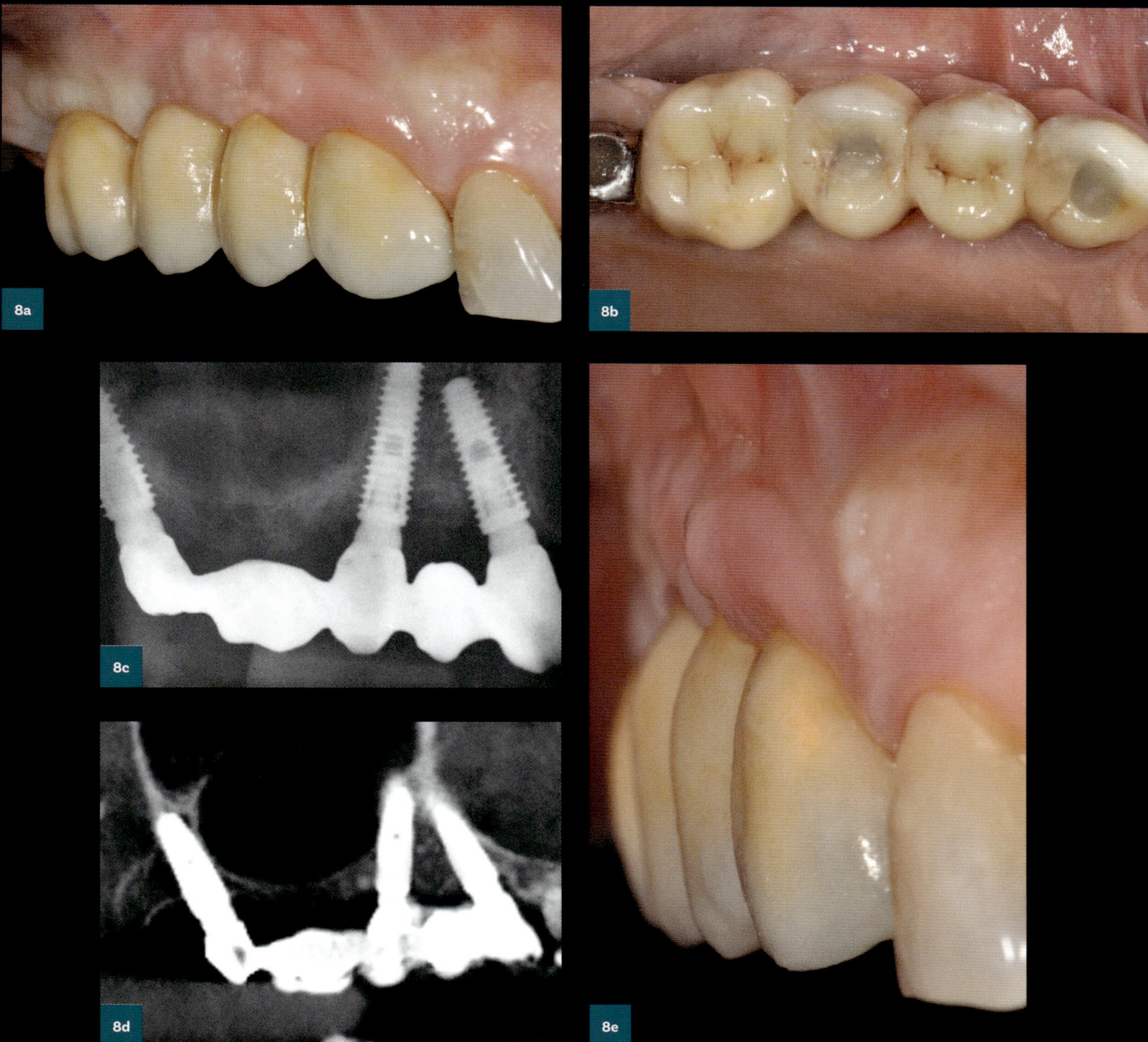

Figs. 8a-e ■ Clinical and radiographic images of the permanent screw retained metal ceramic rehabilitation, demonstrating restoration of the peri-implant tissue volumes and the maxillary sinus integrity.

Bibliography

1. Paoloantonio M, Dolci M, Scarano A, et al. Immediate implantation in fresh extraction sockets. A controlled clinical and histological study in man. *J Periodontol.* 2001;72(11): 1560-1571.
2. Cornelini R, Scarano A, Covani U, et al. Immediate one-stage postextraction implant: a human clinical and histological case report. *Int J Oral Maxillofac Implants.* 2000;15(3):432-437.
3. Wilson TG, Schenk R, Buser D, Cochran D. Implants placed in immediate extraction sites: a report of histological and histometric analysis of human biopsies. *Int J Oral Maxillofac Implants.* 1998;13(3):333-341.
4. Lazzara RJ. Immediate implant placement into extraction sites: surgical and restorative advantages. *Int J Periodontics Restorative Dent.* 1989;9(5):332-343.
5. Siegenthaler DW, Jung RE, Holderegger C, Roos M, Hämmerle CH. Replacement of teeth exhibiting periapical pathology by immediate implants. A prospective, controlled clinical trial. *Clin Oral Implants Res.* 2007;18(6):727-737.
6. Capelli M, Testori T, Galli F, et al. Implant-buccal plate distance as diagnostic parameter: a prospective cohort study on implant placement in fresh extraction sockets. *J Periodontol.* 2013;84(12):1768-1774.
7. Weng D, Bohm S. Simplify your augmentation. "What to consider at extraction to simplify the implantation. A treatment concept for extraction sockets before implantation". *Implantologie.* 2006;4:21-28.

13

Management of soft tissue defects

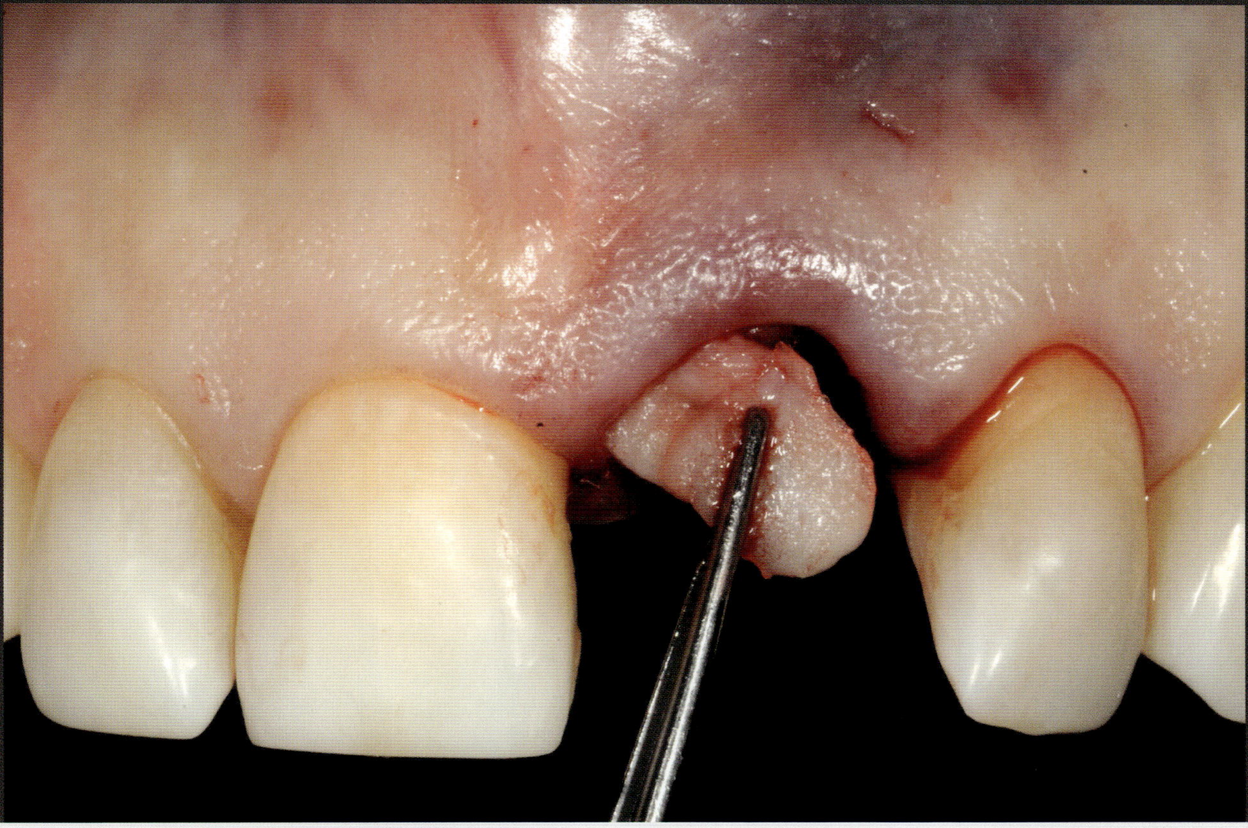

Soft tissue management is crucial in achieving effective aesthetic results in immediate post-extraction implant placement. However, this approach is often associated with soft tissue recession,[1-3] especially in cases with predisposing factors, such as the absence of buccal bone housing or thin periodontal biotype, contributing to this recession following immediate implants.[4] Achieving natural-looking implant restorations, especially in aesthetic sectors, requires the clinician to consider procedures that ensure optimal and long-lasting aesthetic outcomes. Therefore, mitigating risk factors that can lead to aesthetic problems, like gum recession, is essential. Managing peri-implant bone volume and soft tissue thickness is vital in maintaining stable soft tissue levels. The latter can be dealt using various solutions, including connective grafts using the Tunnel technique or bilaminar methods[5-7] (**Figs. 13.1a-d**). Regardless of the technique, the goal is always to create thick soft tissue. The problem has less concern in treating patients with thick biotypes as they are less prone to gingival recession.[8,9] Soft tissue augmentation is not indicated in these cases. However, patients with thin periodontal biotypes often experience resorption of the generally thin buccal bone housing[10] after tooth extraction, leading to clinically relevant soft tissue contraction.[11] Regardless of whether biomaterials are grafted into the peri-implant gap, the connective graft serves dual functions: compensating for the inevitable volumetric contraction of the post-extraction site and thickening the soft tissues. Compensating for the inevitable volumetric contraction ensures optimal aesthetics, while increasing soft tissue thickness transforms a thin periodontal biotype into a thick one, guaranteeing long-term gingival level stability. In fact, a recent literature review states that combining immediate implant loading with a connective graft could contribute to gingival margin stability and peri-implant soft tissue augmentation.[12] However, most selected studies lack a "control group" directly demonstrating the benefits of a connective graft during implant placement.

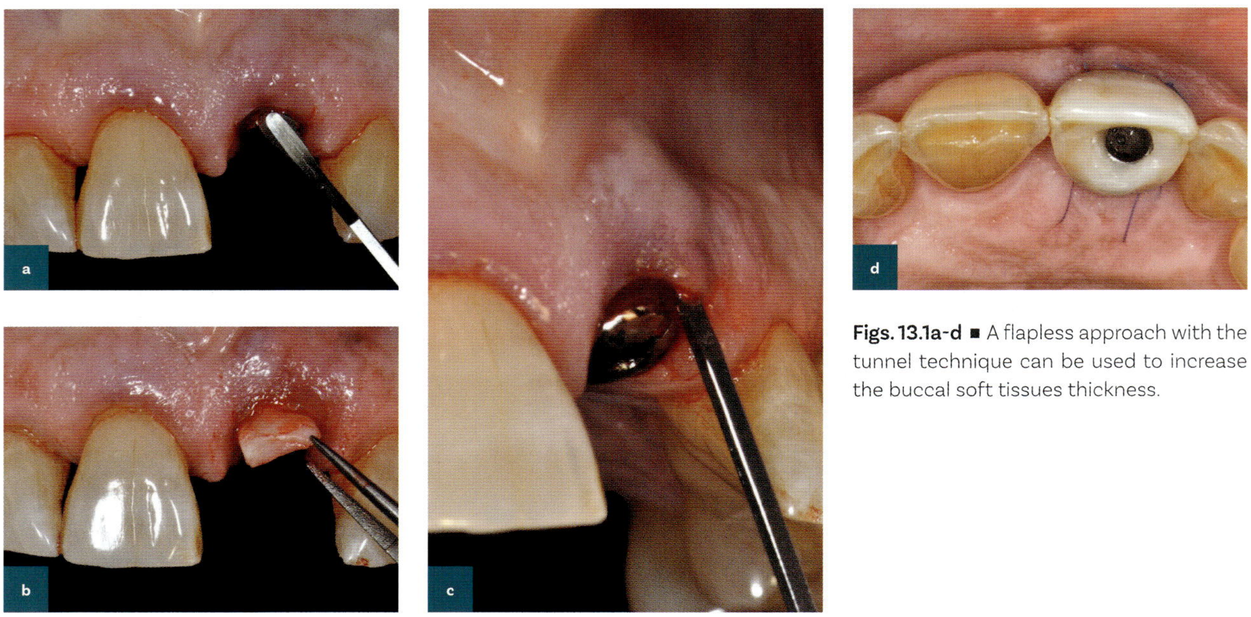

Figs. 13.1a-d ▪ A flapless approach with the tunnel technique can be used to increase the buccal soft tissues thickness.

POST EXO + IMMEDIATE LOADING + GBR + CONNETTIVE TISSUE

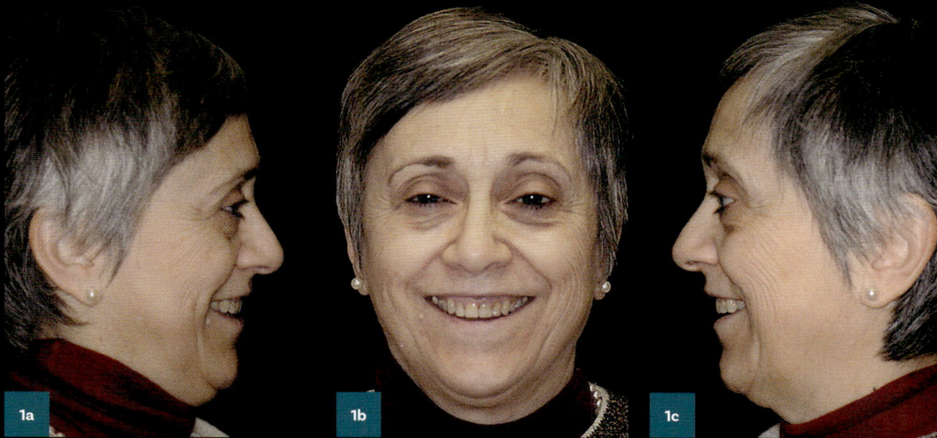

Figs. 1a-c ■ Extraoral image of the patient.

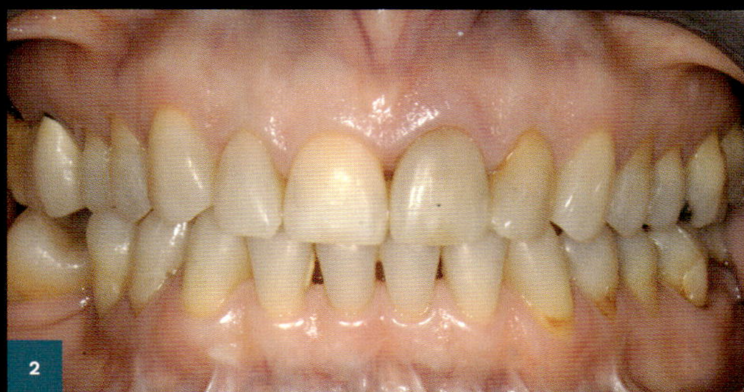

Fig. 2 ■ Frontal intraoral image of the dental arch in occlusion.

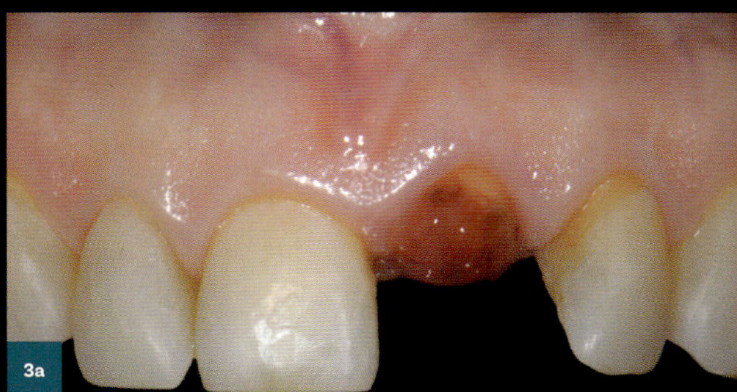

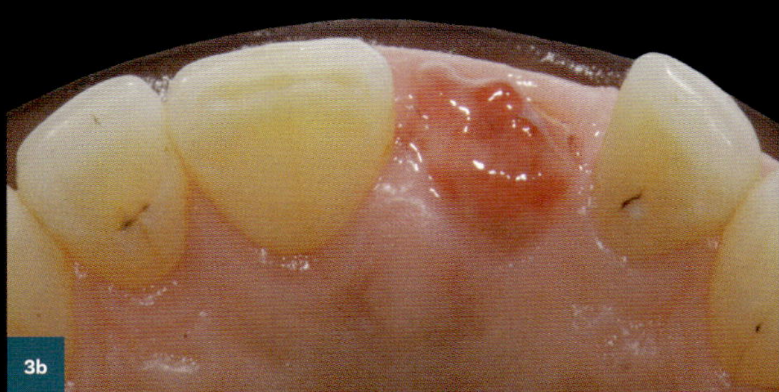

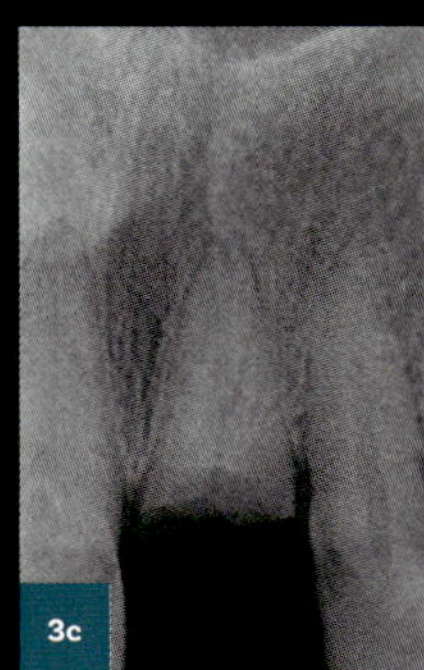

Figs. 3a-c ■ Intraoral images and intraoral radiograph of the same patient after trauma, revealing a complicated horizontal fracture of tooth 21.

> CONT'D

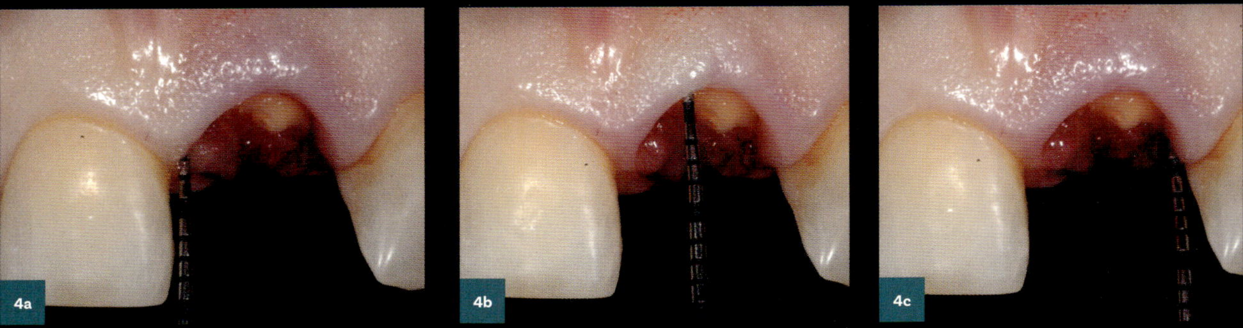

Figs. 4a-c ■ The objective clinical examination, combined with radiological findings, indicates a poor prognosis for the tooth. Consequently, tooth 21 is considered unsalvageable, and the treatment of choice is implant-prosthetic rehabilitation.

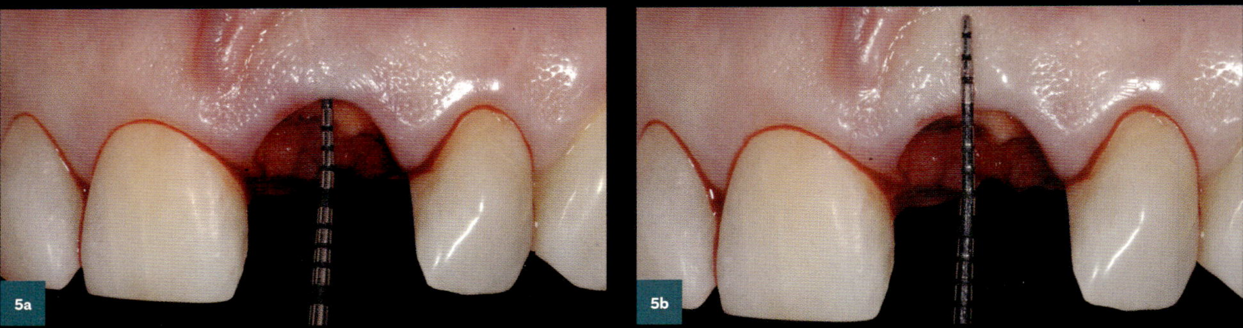

Figs. 5a,b ■ Identification and measurement of the distance between the buccal bone wall and the gingival margin.

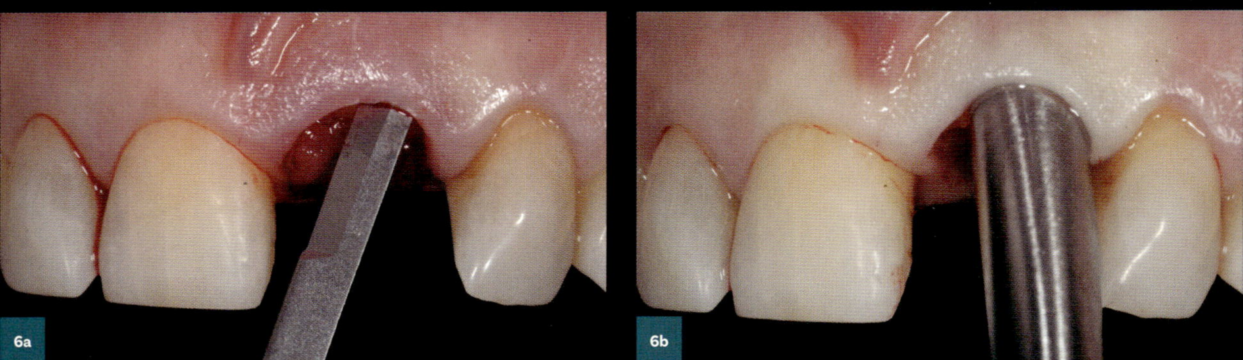

Figs. 6a,b ■ Performing fiberotomy to minimize trauma during tooth extraction.

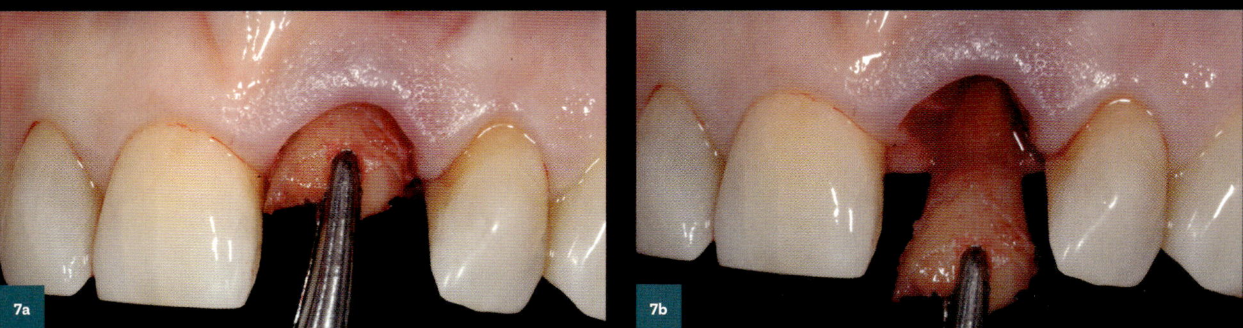

Figs. 7a,b ■ Apical placement of forceps blades to reduce the risk of root fracture during extraction manoeuvres.

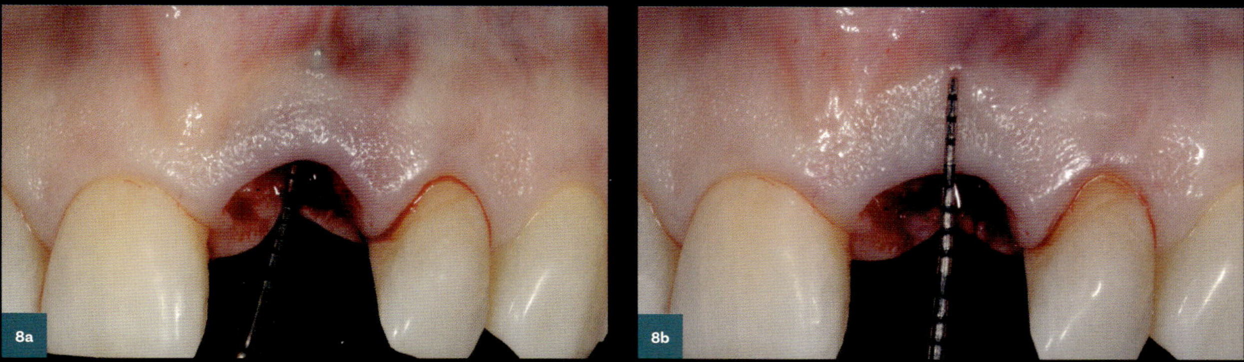

Figs. 8a,b ■ Reassessment and measurement of the distance between the buccal bone wall and the gingival margin.

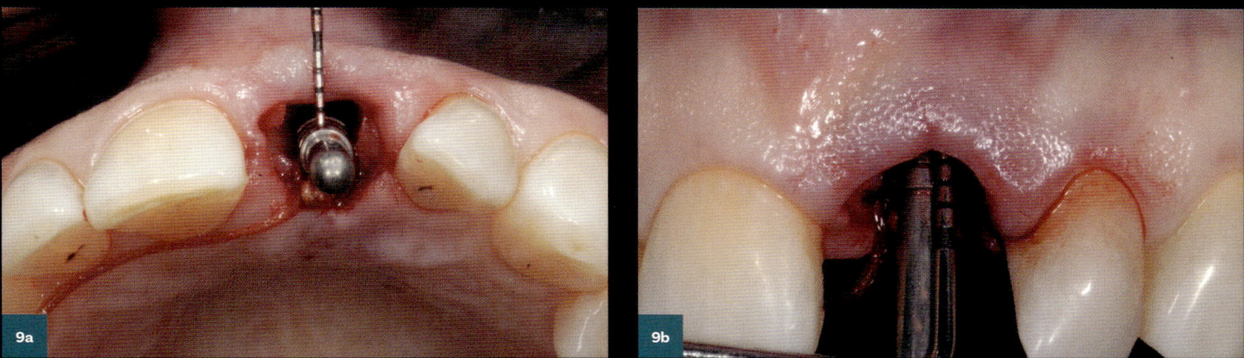

Figs. 9a,b ■ Verification of proper implant positioning inside the alveolus and its insertion axis using an implant guide pin.

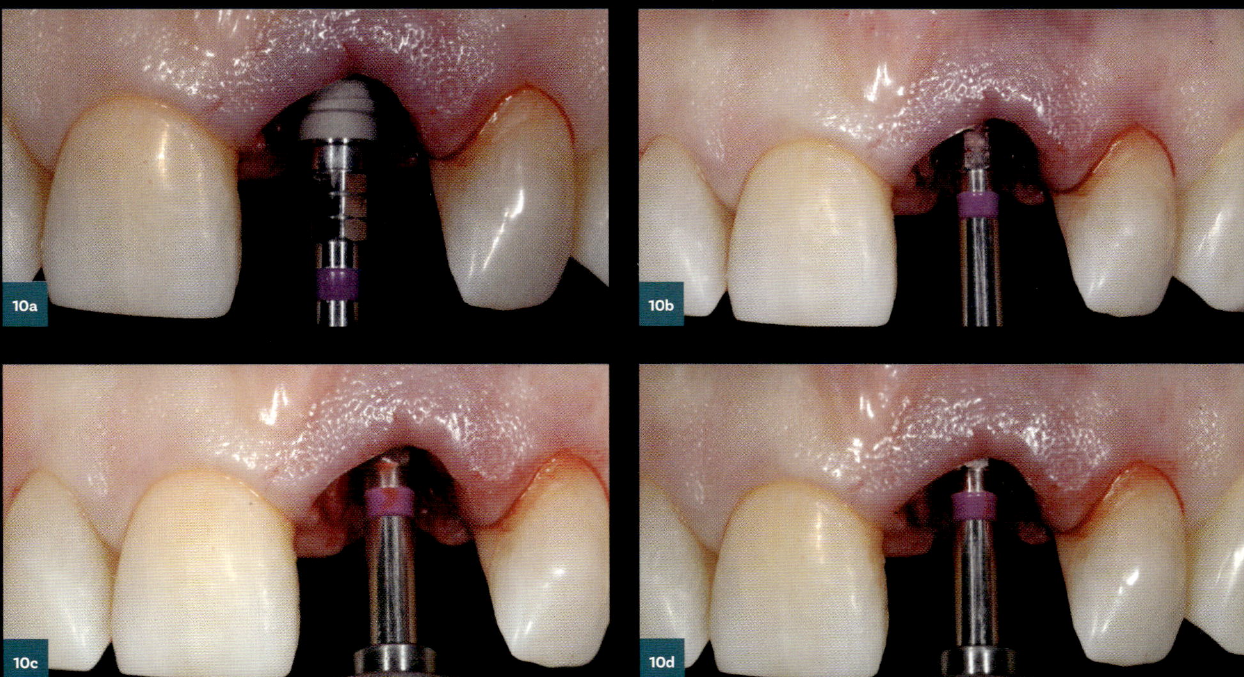

Figs. 10a-d ■ Implant placement while constantly monitoring the insertion torque.

CONT'D >

> CONT'D

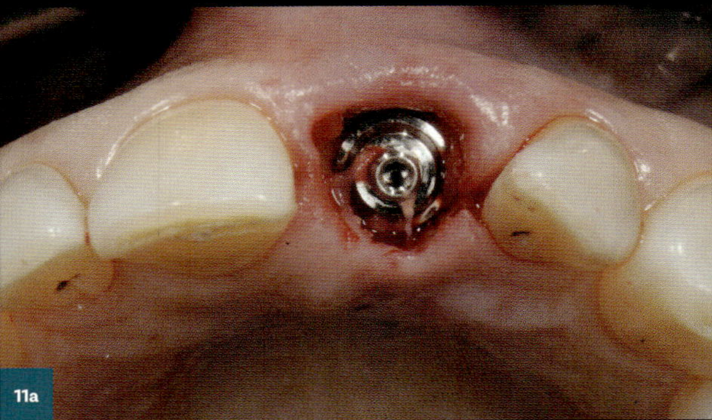

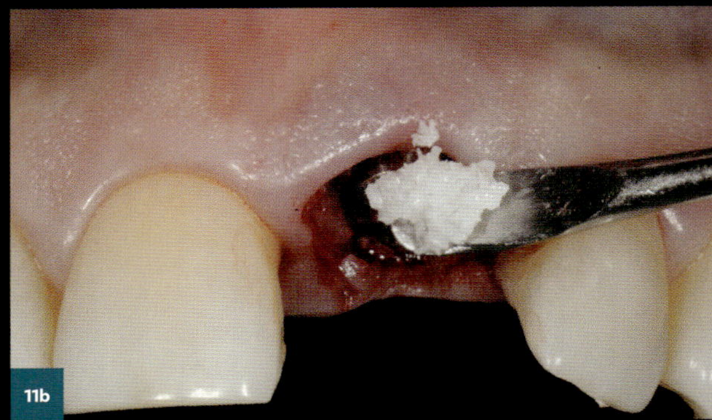

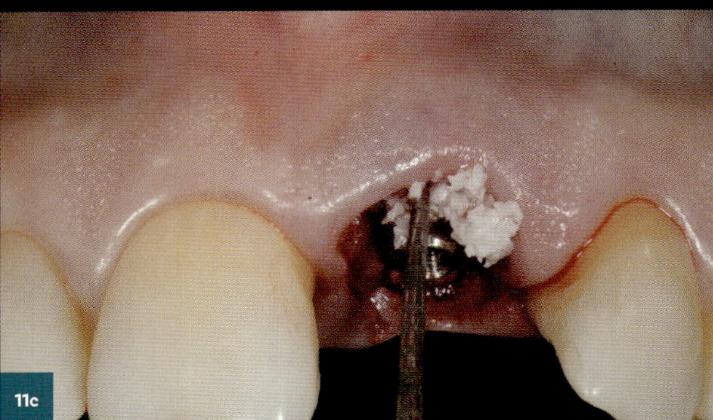

Figs. 11a-c ■ Filling the peri-implant gap with biomaterial, ensuring it does not exceed the bone crest level.

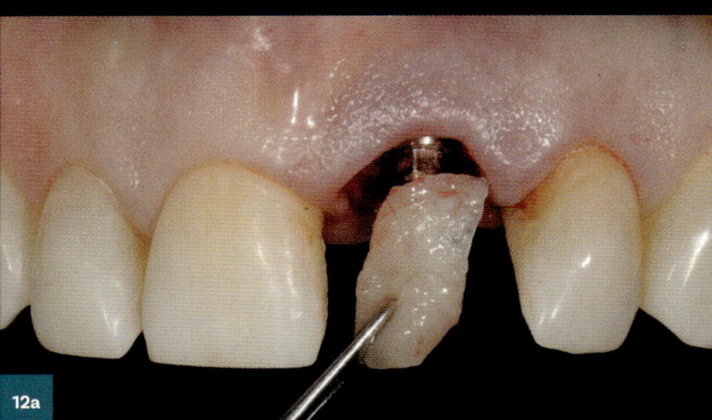

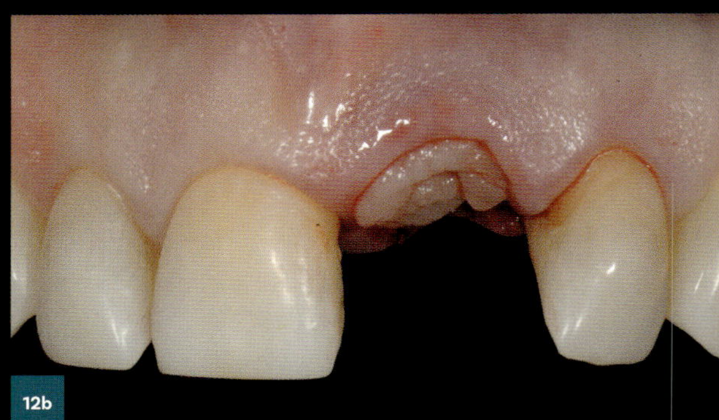

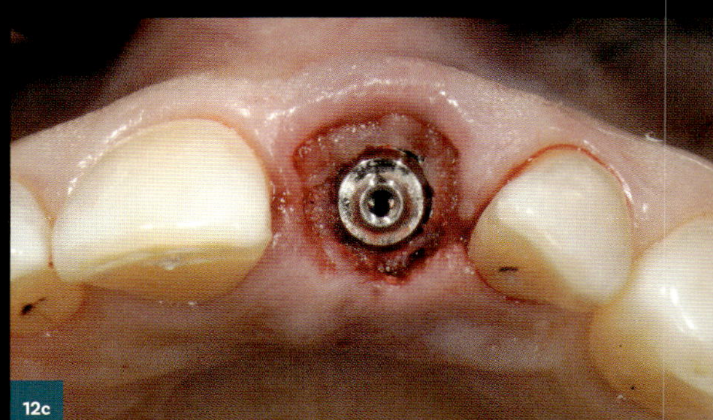

Figs. 12a-c ■ Placement of a PRF membrane to protect the graft.

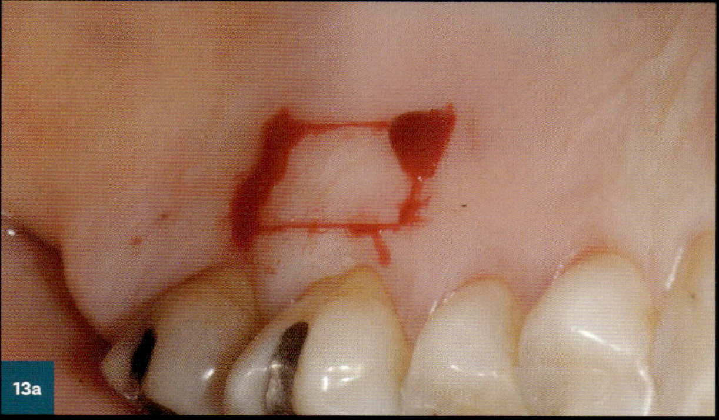

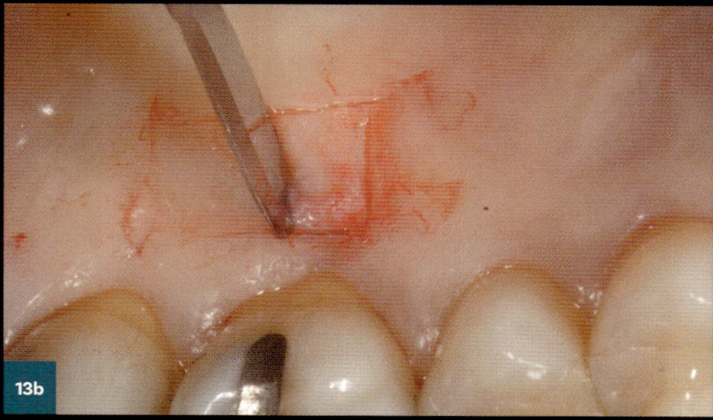

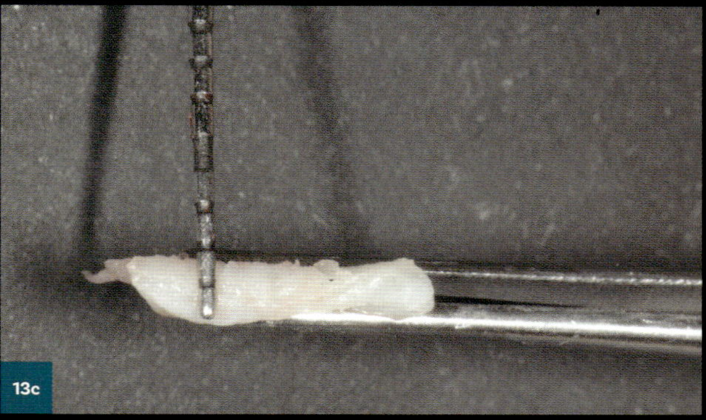

Figs. 13a-c ■ To minimize volumetric contraction of peri-implant tissues, a disepithelialized connective tissue graft from the palate is utilized.

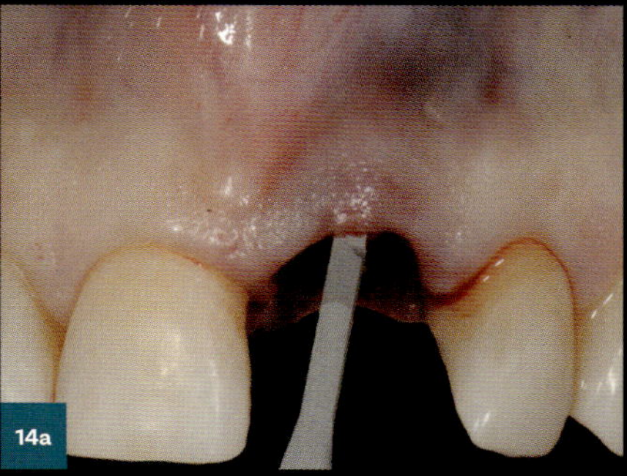

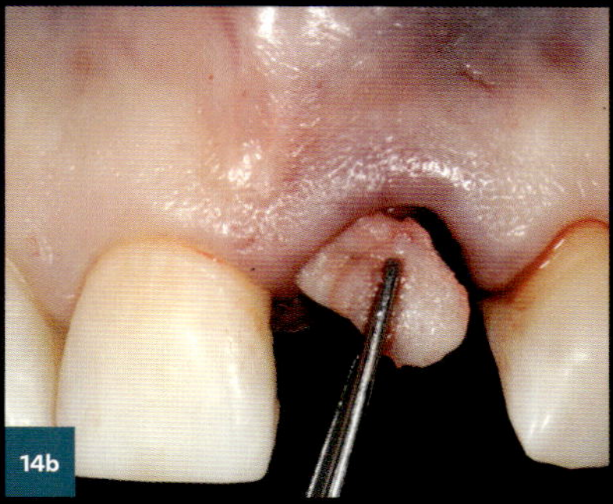

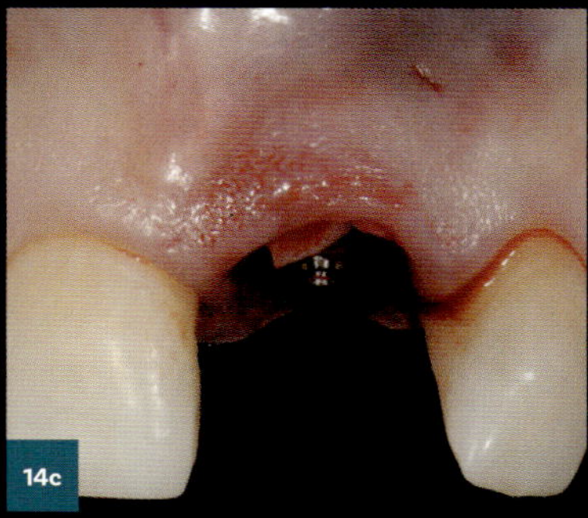

Figs. 14a-c ■ Creation of a tunnel and positioning of the connective graft after detaching the vestibular mucosa.

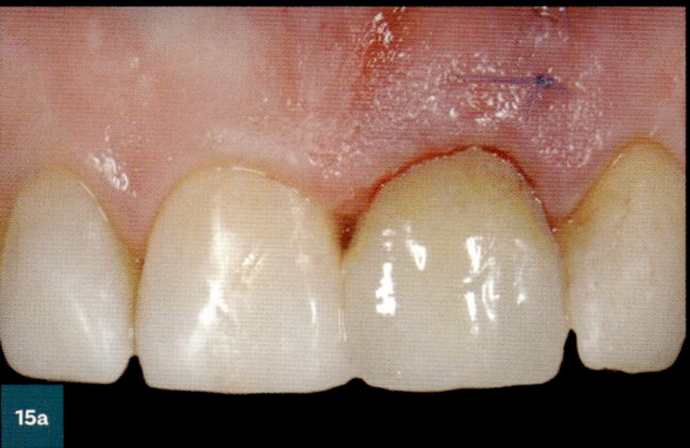

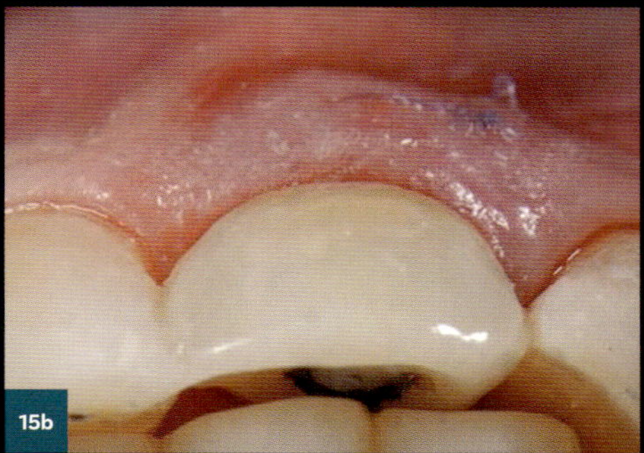

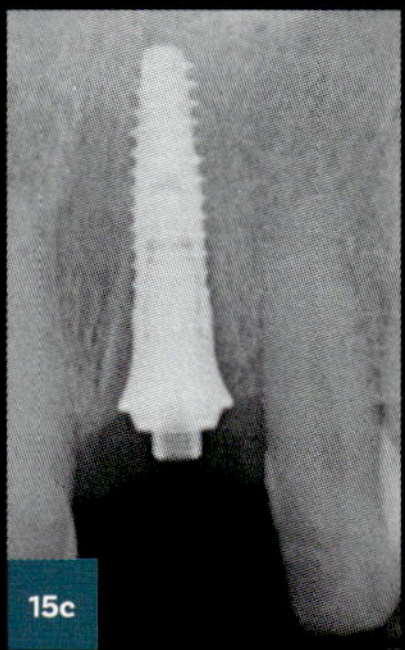

Figs. 15a-c ■ Securing the connective graft with absorbable suture and performing radiographic control. Subsequently, a temporary screw retained prosthesis without contacts in centric and excursive movements is delivered.

CONT'D >

> CONT'D

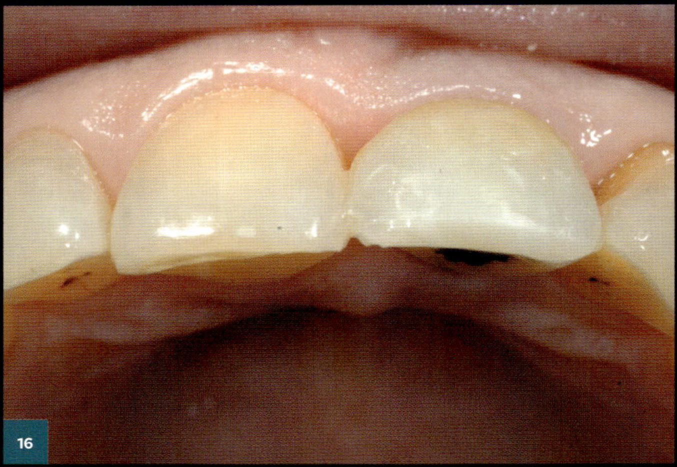

16

Fig. 16 ▪ Occlusal image of the provisional crown taken 6 months after loading.

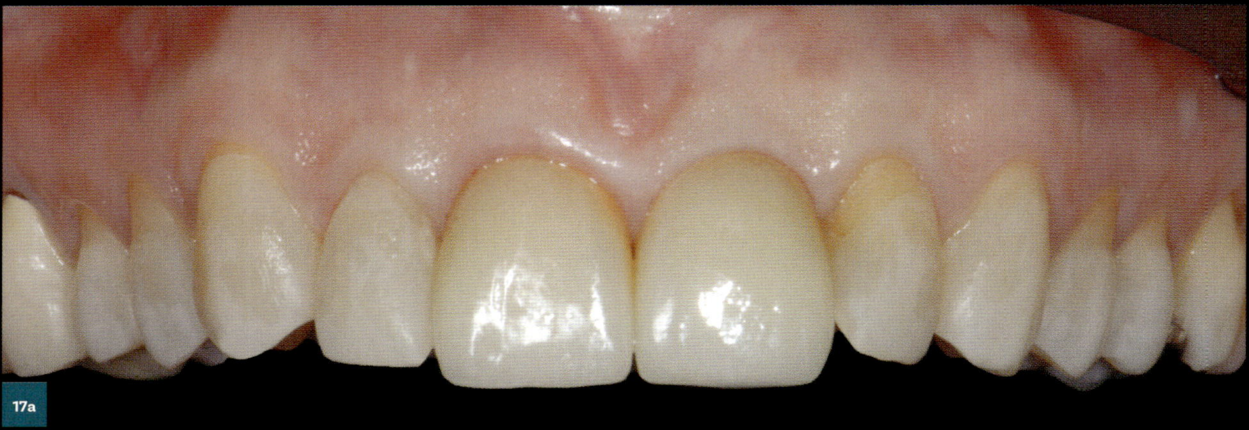

17a

Figs. 17a-c ▪ Intraoral and extraoral clinical images and intraoral radiographic control of the definitive cemented crown in zirconia ceramic.

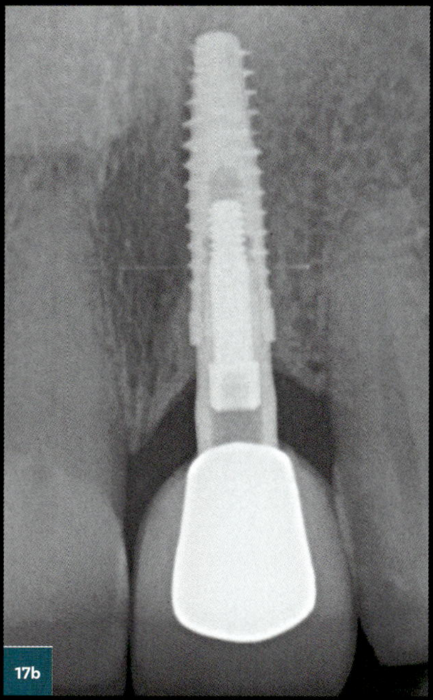

17b

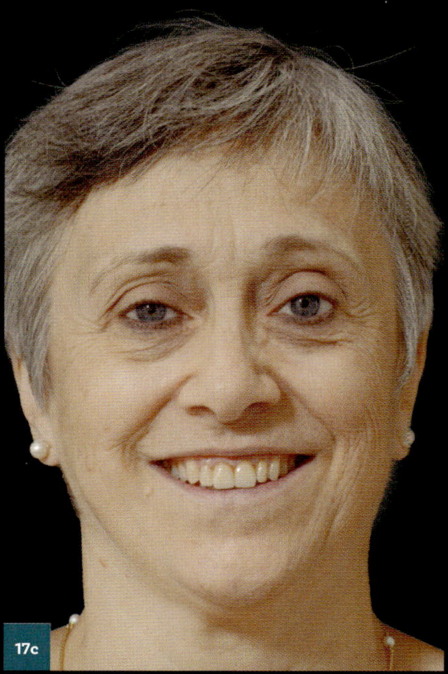

17c

Bibliography

1. Kan JY, Rungcharassaeng K, Lozada J. Immediate placement and provisionalization of maxillary anterior single implants: 1-year prospective study. *Int J Oral Maxillofac Implants.* 2003;18(1): 31-39.
2. De Rouck T, Collys K, Cosyn J. Immediate single tooth implants in the anterior maxilla: A 1-year case cohort study on hard and soft tissue response. *J Clin Periodontol.* 2008;35(7):649-657.
3. Palattella P, Toresllo F, Cordarro L. Two-year prospective clinical comparison of immediate replacement vs. immediate restoration of single tooth in the esthetic zone. *Clin Oral Implants Res.* 2008;19(11):1148-1153.
4. Kois JC, Kan JY. Predictable peri-implant gingival aesthetics: surgical and prosthodontic rationales. *Pract Proced Aesthet Dent.* 2001;13(9):691-698.
5. Zuhr O, Bäumer D, Hürzeler M. The addition of soft tissue replacement grafts in plastic periodontal and implant surgery: critical elements in design and execution. *J Clin Periodontol.* 2014;41 Suppl 15:S123-S142.
6. Cornelini R, Barone A, Covani U. Connective tissue grafts in postextraction implants with immediate restoration: a prospective controlled clinical study. *Pract Proced Aesthet Dent.* 2008;20(6):337-343.
7. Kan JY, Rungcharassaeng K, Morimoto T, Lozada J. Facial gingival tissue stability after connective tissue graft with single immediate tooth replacement in the esthetic zone: consecutive case report. *J Oral Maxillofac Surg.* 2009;67(11 Suppl): 40-48.
8. Müller HP, Eger T. Gingival phenotypes in young male adults. *J Clin Periodontol.* 1997;24(1):65-71.
9. Müller HP, Eger T, Schorb A. Gingival dimensions after root coverage with free connective tissue grafts. *J Clin Periodontol.* 1998;25(5):424-430.
10. Fu JH, Yeh CY, Chan HL, Tatarakis N, Leong DJ, Wang HL. Tissue Biotype and Its Relation to the Underlying Bone Morphology. *J Periodontol.* 2010;81:569-574.
11. Hämmerle CH, Chen ST, Wilson TG Jr. Consensus statements and recommended clinical procedures regarding the placement of implants in extraction sockets. *Int J Oral Maxillofac Implants.* 2004;19 Suppl:26-28.
12. Lee CT, Tao CY, Stoupel J. The Effect of Subepithelial Connective Tissue Graft Placement on Esthetic Outcomes After Immediate Implant Placement: Systematic Review. *J Periodontol.* 2015;87(2):156-167.

PART IV

Alternatives for replacing the compromised tooth

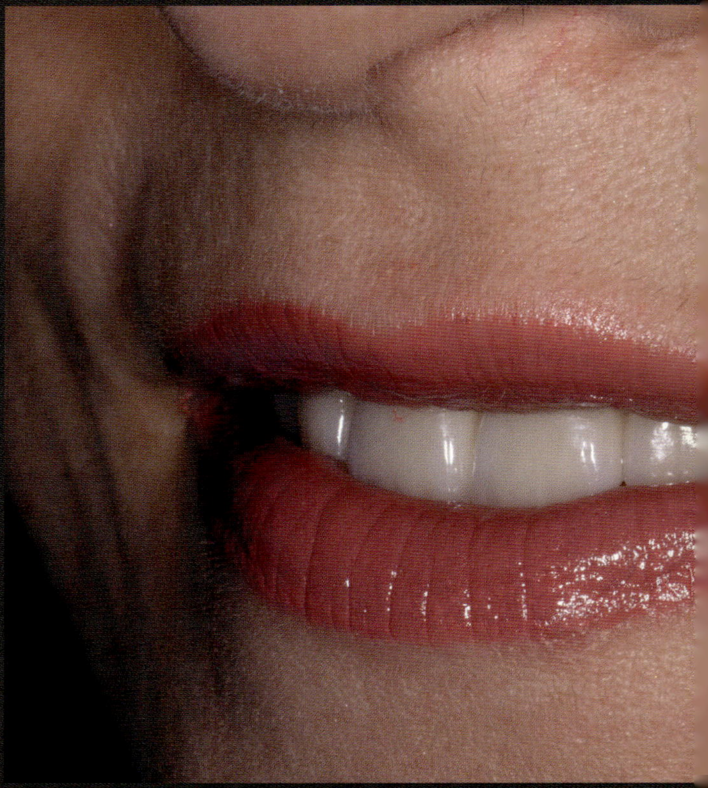

Pio **Bertani**

Paolo **Generali**

Renato **Cocconi**

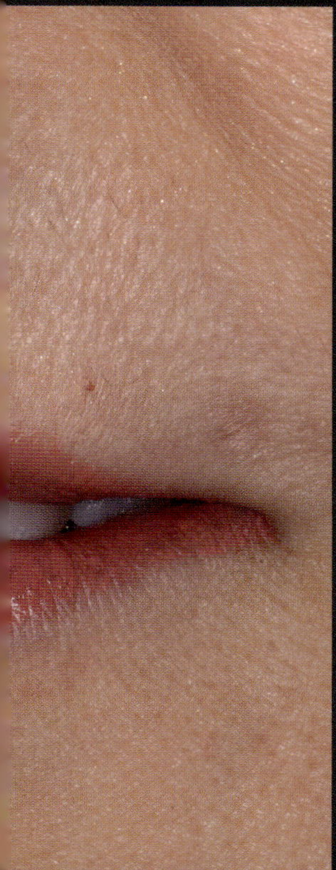

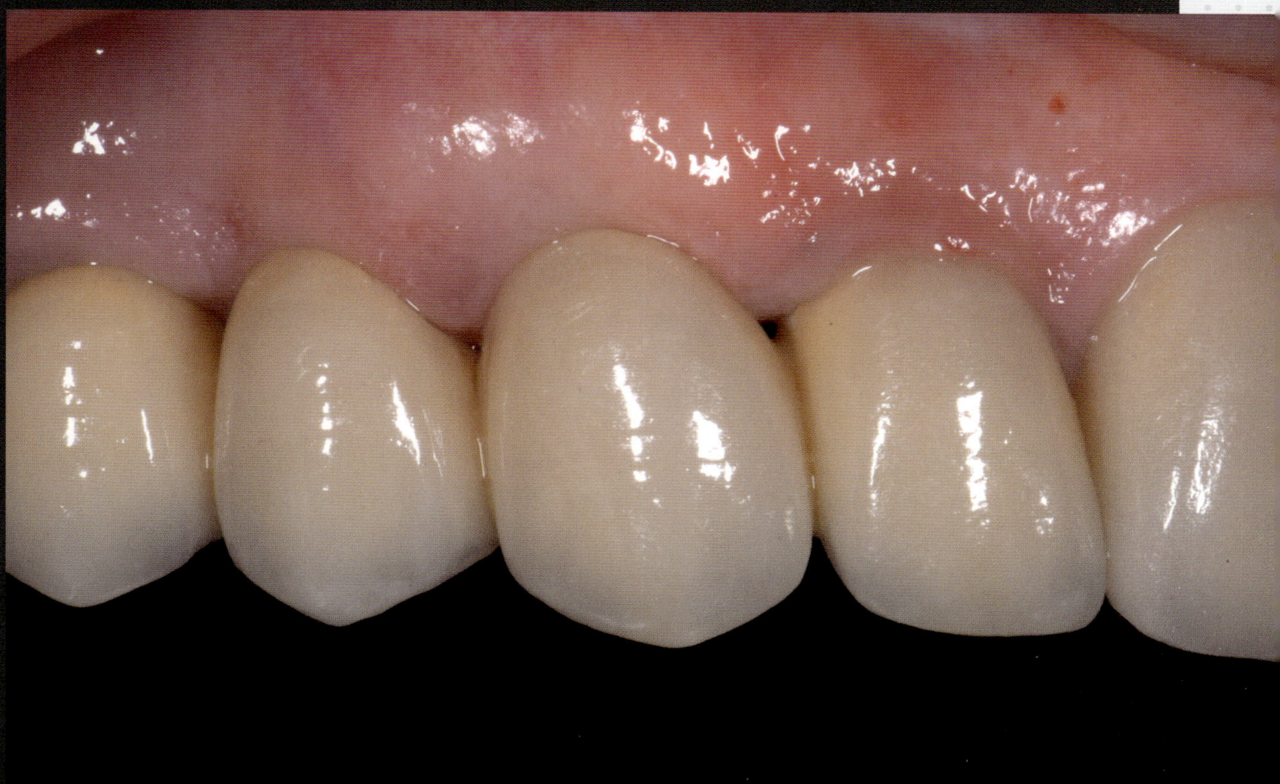

Introduction

Unfortunately, there are cases where preserving a severely compromised tooth is impossible. Sometimes, the attempt to salvage a tooth affected by a range of various pathologies may require excessive procedures, rendering it impractical.

In these cases, timely replacement of the extracted tooth intended is crucial. Immediate reduction in masticatory efficiency follows extraction, not just due to the lost tooth, but also its antagonist's reduced functionality. The patient is forced to alter his/her chewing dynamics, thus compromising dietary habits. Gingival tissue irritation at the extraction site, caused by chewing trauma, is another unpleasant consequence of the extraction.

The aesthetic impact of tooth loss is a crucial consideration. Even the absence of a single tooth, not necessarily from the frontal group, is visible when smiling and talking, thereby adversely impacting the patient's appearance.

Over time, the consequences of tooth loss worsen. Changes in chewing dynamics can dislocate the joints, potentially causing painful symptoms. Adjacent and opposing teeth's harmony is disrupted, leading to the former's inclination and rotation and the latter's overeruption. This situation can compromise their oral health, increasing vulnerability to caries and periodontal disease. Aesthetically, even a single extraction, like an upper canine, can visibly lead to supporting the atrophy of the supporting tissues, flattening the canine bump. Generally, the loss of multiple teeth accelerates premature face aging. Therefore, the replacement of compromised teeth is a priority. Currently, the implant solution is the preferred choice for single-tooth replacement, even in aesthetic regions. Implants offer better outcomes compared to a conventional fixed prosthesis, a partially fixed adhesive prosthesis and a removable prosthesis. However, complications can arise with implants, and they are not suitable for patients in the growth phase. Furthermore, implant placement does not alter the processes of remodelling and bone resorption post-extraction.

To overcome these limitations, efforts have focused on techniques like partial extraction to prevent bone resorption or streamline treatment by reducing surgery times and exploring alternatives like partial extraction techniques and implant positioning with root remnants. Another biologically oriented alternate approach, particularly suitable during all the growth phases, involves autotransplantation.

The extensive range of partial extraction techniques aims to maintain portions of roots to preserve the periodontal ligament and attached alveolar bone in extreme synthesis. This prevents resorption, thus maintaining soft tissue architecture in harmony with hard tissue. By avoiding horizontal and vertical atrophy, natural parabolas and gingival protuberances are preserved.

Implant positioning in proximity to root remnants or impacted teeth offers a less invasive alternative to procedures with potential short-term and persistent outcomes. The former involves challenging post-operative recovery, while the latter arises due to surgical access needs for deeply impacted or resorbing teeth, leading to atrophic healing orientations. This consequently requires regenerative techniques with associated morbidity and unpredictable quantitative outcomes. Under specific conditions, circumventing this lengthy and intricate therapeutic procedure can be feasible, independent of impacted elements or resorbing root removal.

Finally, autotransplantation, often misconceived, warrants further consideration across various cases as a viable therapeutic alternative. Preserving periodontal tissue and alveolar bone, enabling the orthodontic treatment, and contributing to bone segment development highlight the advantages of this technique.

14

Partial extraction technique for saving tissue

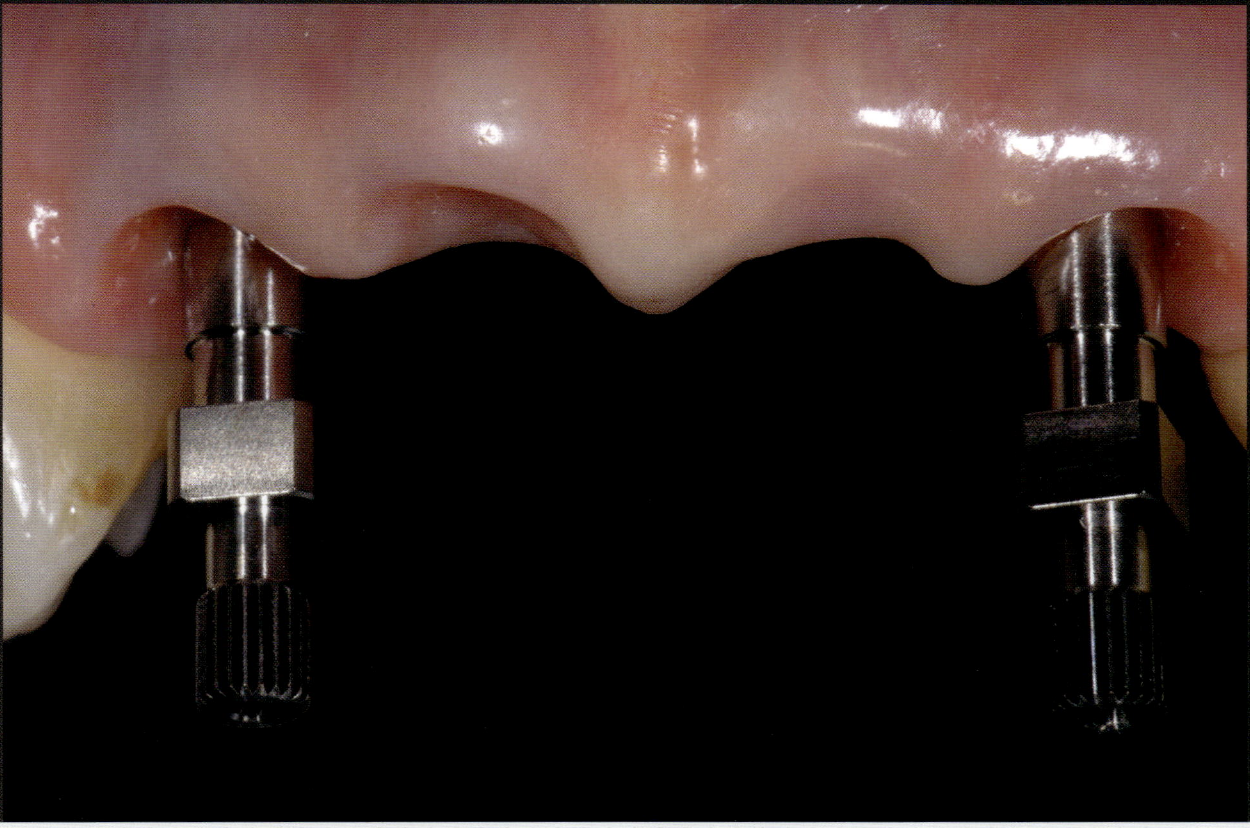

Outcome of extractions

Following each tooth extraction, the alveolar bone undergoes varying degrees of remodelling,[1] with greater resorption occurring on the buccal side.[2]

This phenomenon leads to diverse negative consequences, including changes in soft tissue profile, reduction of bone tissue necessary for potential implant positioning, and loss of perioral tissue support, resulting in facial profile alteration.[3] To mitigate these negative consequences, various socket-preserving techniques have been proposed based on the guided bone regeneration principles, using autologous bone or bone substitutes. These materials are often protected and enclosed by a membrane, which may be resorbable or removed in a subsequent surgical step. The membrane can be reinforced to maintain a pre-determined shape.

In some guided bone regeneration procedures, bone block grafts or metal grids fixed with osteosynthesis devices may be utilized. While these techniques can increase hard tissue volume, they have limitations, including heightened morbidity and technical complications that demand highly experienced operators.

These factors lead to extended dental treatment times and elevated costs due to the need for sophisticated, expensive, and sometimes scarce materials. Furthermore, they carry the risk of crestal bone reduction in both vertical and horizontal components, as well as potential loss of interdental papillae.[4] Even when placing an intermediate pontic for a bridge without an implant, extraction-induced resorption unavoidably alters the crestal profile, posing challenges for achieving ideal aesthetics.

Partial extraction techniques

These assessments introduce a set of techniques described and classified by Gluckman et al. in 2016[5] as "Partial Extraction Therapies" (PET). PET comprises procedures to prevent alveolar tissue collapse by preserving parts of the tooth, including the root and its periodontal attachment. This preservation of the alveolar bone-ligament complex, with its vascular support, is achieved by retaining portions of the root. The techniques within PET include Submergence, Socket Shield and Pontic Shield, and several related variations.

Conserving submerged roots beneath removable prostheses to prevent alveolar ridge atrophy is a widespread practice. A 1980 review[6] confirmed the clinical and histological evidence for coronal bone tissue development around non-infected roots submerged below the crest. Even without coronal bone development, the submerged root can help maintain alveolar ridge width, avoiding the need for bone grafting.[7] The technique, initially developed by Bjorn[8] in animals and subsequently in humans in 1965, mandates a specific site and the prerequisites of the root to be submerged for successful implementation. These prerequisites encompass the absence of occlusal loads and the presence of a non-infected and endodontically treated root with decoronation executed 1-2 mm below the bone crest.

Full root coverage with soft tissue is achieved using connective grafts if necessary. After 3 months of healing, the gradual application of an aesthetically optimizing compressive intermediate pontic becomes feasible.[9,10]

However, this technique has limitations, including the potential for apical complications and the need for endodontic treatment. Additionally, if applied with overdentures, there is a risk of soft tissue fenestration, leading to root exposure and root caries. Detailed iconographic illustration of this technique, along with the clinical case images, is shown on page 168.

Socket Shield

The Socket Shield, introduced by Hurzeler and Zuhr in 2010[11] through animal experiments, involves partial extraction of a tooth followed by immediate implant placement. This method leaves the buccal coronal third of the root intact during extraction, acting as a protective shield against buccal bone resorption. This preserves the soft tissue profile and enhances aesthetics.

Creating this "shield" involves a delicate and complex procedure. The entire treatment requires highly experienced operators well-versed in immediate and atraumatic surgery, extraction, implantation and crafting immediate provisionals with good soft tissue management.[12] The apical third of the root must be completely removed, leaving the middle and coronal portions on the buccal side, with thickness adjusted to not interfere with implant placement. The shield must remain immobile post-preparation, typically with a sufficient 1.5 mm thickness. Its shape should align with buccal bone curvature while reducing the occlusal surface to the bone crest level.

Numerous variations have been proposed over the years compared to the original technique. These include the "Proximal Socket Shield", where the intentionally left fragment is interproximal to maintain the papilla level.[13] The Glocker technique deferred implant positioning.[14] The "Root Membrane Technique" has direct root fragment contact with the implant.[15] The "C-Shaped Socket Shield" extends the shield to interproximal areas, aiming to preserve the interdental papillae height, but with increased risk of implant-shield contact for multiple adjacent implants.[16] The "Pontic Shield Technique" involves the same sectioning and partial root extraction as the Socket Shield. The root fragment is then left under the bridge pontic, and a bone graft/substitute can be placed in the socket. This avoids the possibility of endodontic complications occuring with root submergence. It preserves the soft tissue contour and bone crest, thereby preventing resorption. Clinical case images on page 173 depict the technique.

Indications and contraindications

Partial extraction techniques (**Fig. 14.1**) are applicable when stable teeth cannot be prosthetically reconstructed with healthy periodontium. An endodontic lesion does not necessarily contraindicate this technique; it involves removing the apical third. If complete periapical lesion curettage is possible, immediate implant placement becomes feasible.[17] In other cases, implant placement might need to be postponed following the Glocker technique. Adequate palatal and apical bone is crucial for immediate implant stability; a minimum of 3-5 mm of healthy bone beyond the root apex to be replaced[18] is necessary. Finally, the immediate provisional placement ability is also essential. The contraindications arise from lacking the prerequisites mentioned earlier, particularly the presence of periodontal lesions and mobility discourage partial extraction. Furthermore, insufficient horizontal bone volume hinders good primary implant stability, especially palatally, and endangers shield stability if anchored to a small bone plate, thus risking dislocation during site preparation or implant placement. Therefore, this technique is not recommended for malpositioned or discoloured roots.

The possible complications arising from implant therapy extend beyond the procedural errors, or the undesirable effects of post-implant therapy mainly include mobility, migration, exposure or infection of the retained root fragment.

Mobility and infection of the shield necessitate its removal, followed by addressing any resulting soft tissue defects. Exposure can be managed by re-preparing the exposed margin, allowing for spontaneous soft tissue coverage for minor exposure. However, significant exposure necessitates a connective tissue graft after re-preparation.

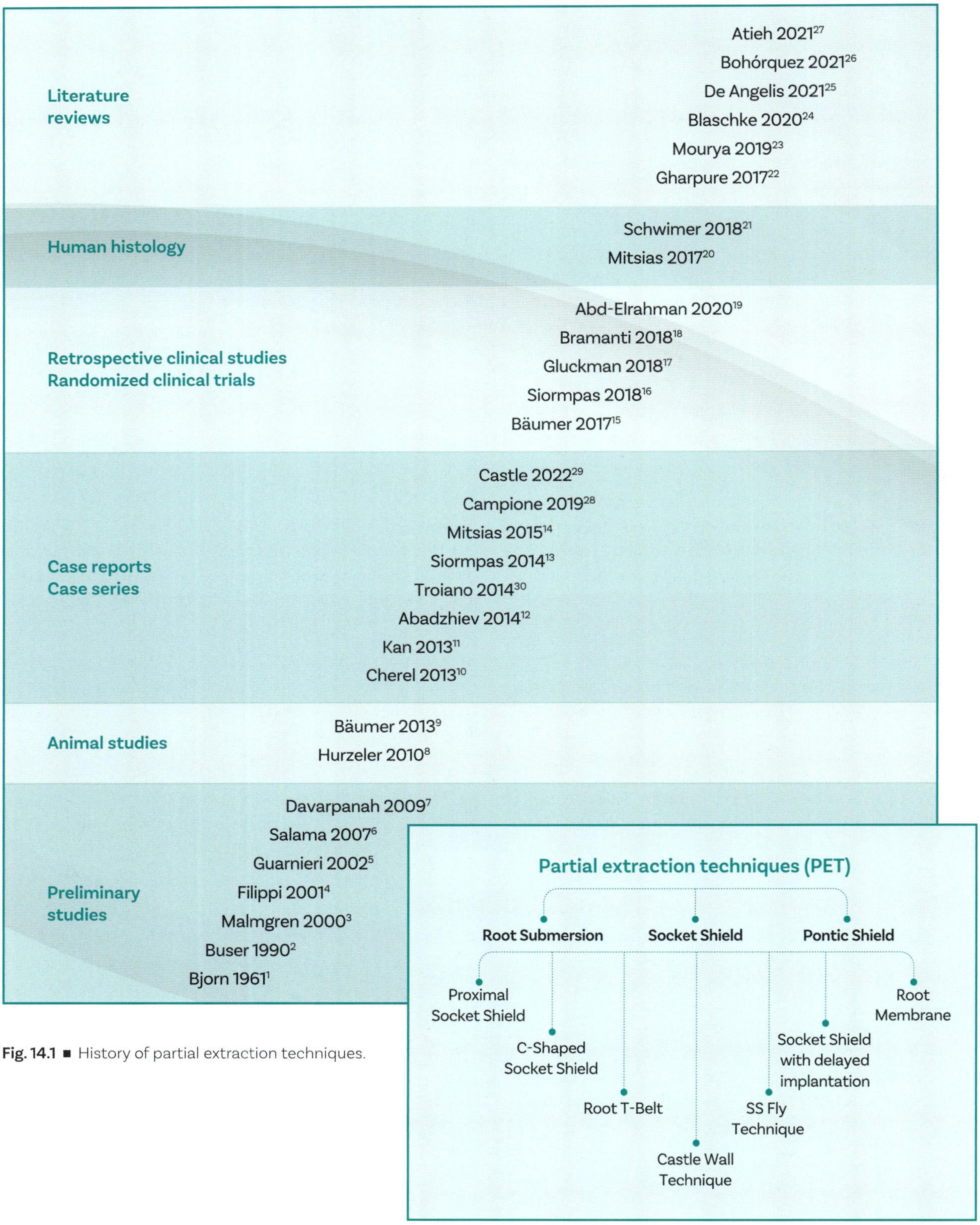

Fig. 14.1 ■ History of partial extraction techniques.

Bibliography Fig. 14.1

1. Bjorn H. Experimental studies on reattachment. *Dent Pract.* 1961;11:351-354.
2. Buser D, Warrer K, Karring T. Formation of a periodontal ligament around titanium implants. *J Periodontol.* 1990;61(9):597-601.
3. Malmgren B. Decoronation: how, why, and when? *J Calif Dent Assoc.* 2000;28(11):846-854.
4. Filippi A, Pohl Y, von Arx T. Decoronation of an ankylosed tooth for preservation of alveolar bone prior to implant placement. *Dent Traumatol.* 2001;17(2):93-95.
5. Guarnieri R, Giardino L, Crespi R, Romagnoli R. Cementum formation around a titanium implant: a case report. *Int J Oral Maxillofac Implants.* 2002;17(5):729-732.
6. Salama M, Ishikawa T, Salama H, Funato A, Garber D. Advantages of the root submergence technique for pontic site development in esthetic implant therapy. *Int J Periodontics Restorative Dent.* 2007;27(6):521-527.
7. Davarpanah M, Szmukler-Moncler S. Unconventional implant treatment: I. Implant placement in contact with ankylosed root fragments. A series of five case reports. *Clin Oral Implants Res.* 2009;20(8):851-856.
8. Hürzeler MB, Zuhr O, Schupbach P, Rebele SF, Emmanouilidis N, Fickl S. The socket shield technique: A proof-of-principle report. *J Clin Periodontol.* 2010;37(9):855-862.
9. Bäumer D, Zuhr O, Rebele S, Schneider D, Schupbach P, Hürzeler M. The socket-shield technique: first histological, clinical, and volumetrical observations after separation of the buccal tooth segment - a pilot study. *Clin Implant Dent Relat Res.* 2015;17(1):71-82.
10. Cherel F, Etienne D. Papilla preservation between two implants: a modified socket-shield technique to maintain the scalloped anatomy? A case report. *Quintessence Int.* 2014;45(1):23-30.
11. Kan JY, Rungcharassaeng K. Proximal socket shield for interimplant papilla preservation in the esthetic zone. *Int J Periodontics Restorative Dent.* 2013;33(1):e24-31.
12. Abadzhiev M, Nenko P, Velcheva P. Conventional immediate implant placement and immediate placement with socket-shield technique - Which is better. *Int J Clin Med Res.* 2014;1(5):176-180.
13. Siormpas KD, Mitsias ME, Kontsiotou-Siormpa E, Garber D, Kotsakis GA. Immediate implant placement in the esthetic zone utilizing the "root-membrane" technique: clinical results up to 5 years postloading. *Int J Oral Maxillofac Implants.* 2014;29(6):1397-1405.
14. Mitsias ME, Siormpas KD, Kontsiotou-Siormpa E, Prasad H, Garber D, Kotsakis GA. A Step-by-Step Description of PDL-Mediated Ridge Preservation for Immediate Implant Rehabilitation in the Esthetic Region. *Int J Periodontics Restorative Dent.* 2015;35(6):835-841.
15. Bäumer D, Zuhr O, Rebele S, Hürzeler M. Socket Shield Technique for immediate implant placement - clinical, radiographic and volumetric data after 5 years. *Clin Oral Implants Res.* 2017;28(11):1450-1458.
16. Siormpas KD, Mitsias ME, Kotsakis GA, Tawil I, Pikos MA, Mangano FG. The Root Membrane Technique: A Retrospective Clinical Study With Up to 10 Years of Follow-Up. *Implant Dent.* 2018;27(5):564-574.
17. Gluckman H, Salama M, Du Toit J. A retrospective evaluation of 128 socket-shield cases in the esthetic zone and posterior sites: Partial extraction therapy with up to 4 years follow-up. *Clin Implant Dent Relat Res.* 2018;20(2):122-129.
18. Bramanti E, Norcia A, Cicciù M, et al. Postextraction Dental Implant in the Aesthetic Zone, Socket Shield Technique Versus Conventional Protocol. *J Craniofac Surg.* 2018;29(4):1037-1041.
19. Abd-Elrahman A, Shaheen M, Askar N, Atef M. Socket shield technique vs conventional immediate implant placement with immediate temporization. Randomized clinical trial. *Clin Implant Dent Relat Res.* 2020;22(5):602-611.
20. Mitsias ME, Siormpas KD, Kotsakis GA, Ganz SD, Mangano C, Iezzi G. The Root Membrane Technique: Human Histologic Evidence after Five Years of Function. *Biomed Res Int.* 2017;2017:7269467.
21. Schwimer C, Pette GA, Gluckman H, Salama M, Du Toit J, et al. Human Histologic Evidence of New Bone Formation and Osseointegration Between Root Dentin (Unplanned Socket-Shield) and Dental Implant: Case Report. *Int J Oral Maxillofac Implants.* 2018;33(1):e19-e23.
22. Gharpure AS, Bhatavadekar NB. Current Evidence on the Socket-Shield Technique: A Systematic Review. *J Oral Implantol.* 2017;43(5):395-403.
23. Mourya A, Mishra SK, Gaddale R, Chowdhary R. Socket-shield technique for implant placement to stabilize the facial gingival and osseous architecture: A systematic review. *J Investig Clin Dent.* 2019;10(4):e12449.
24. Blaschke C, Schwass DR. The socket-shield technique: a critical literature review. *Int J Implant Dent.* 2020;6(1):52.
25. De Angelis N, Signore A, Alsayed A, et al. Immediate Implants in the Aesthetic Zone: Is Socket Shield Technique a Predictable Treatment Option? A Narrative Review. *J Clin Med.* 2021;10(21):4963.
26. Velasco Bohórquez P, Rucco R, Zubizarreta-Macho Á, et al. Failure Rate, Marginal Bone Loss, and Pink Esthetic with Socket-Shield Technique for Immediate Dental Implant Placement in the Esthetic Zone. A Systematic Review and Meta-Analysis. *Biology (Basel).* 2021;10(6):549.
27. Atieh MA, Shah M, Abdulkareem M, AlQahtani HA, Alsabeeha NHM. The socket shield technique for immediate implant placement: A systematic review and meta-analysis. *J Esthet Restor Dent.* 2021;33(8):1186-1200.
28. Campione F, SS Fly. A therapy for root reimplantation. *Dent Health Curr Res.* 2019;5.
29. Castle C. A Novel Approach to Immediate Implants: The CastleWall Surgical Technique. *Dent J. (Basel).* 2022;10(4):62.
30. Troiano M, Benincasa M, Sanchez, P, Calvo-Guirado JL. Bundle bone preservation with Root-T-Belt: Case Study. *Ann Oral Max Surg.* 2014;2(1):7.

Complex prosthetic rehabilitation, with morphological rebalancing thanks to the Root Submergence Technique

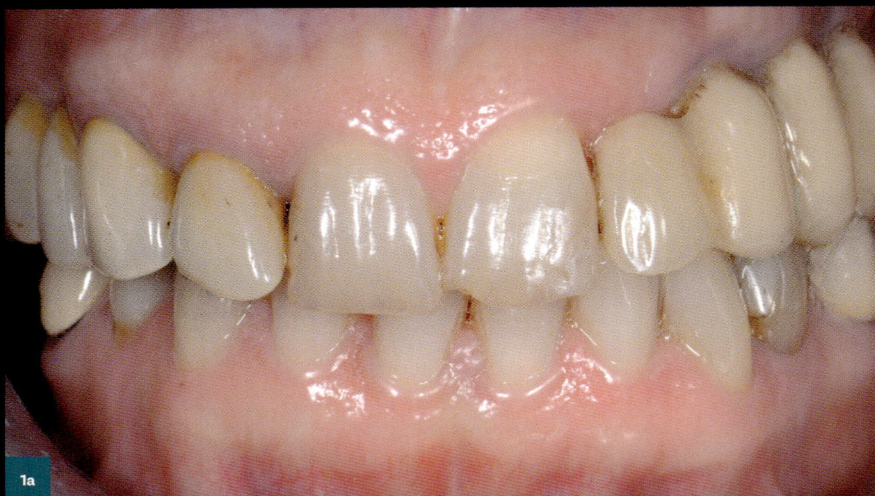

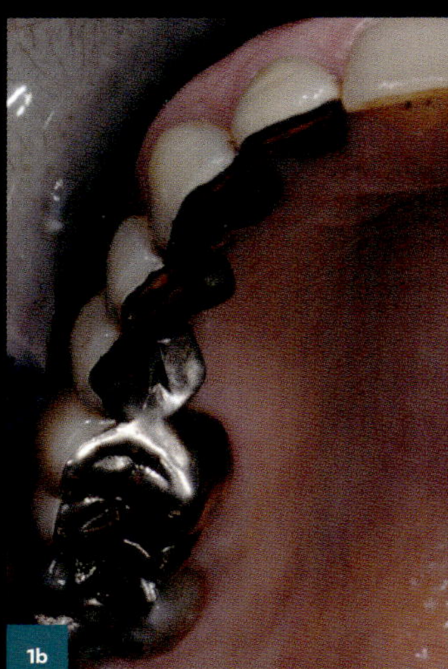

Figs. 1a,b ■ The 47-year-old patient C.A. complains of severe dysfunctional symptoms, which worsened following an implant-borne prosthetic treatment performed elsewhere. He also complained of an asymmetry of the area overlying the left corner of the mouth, presumably due to the flattening of the left canine bump. **a**: frontal view; **b**: occlusal view of the upper arch.

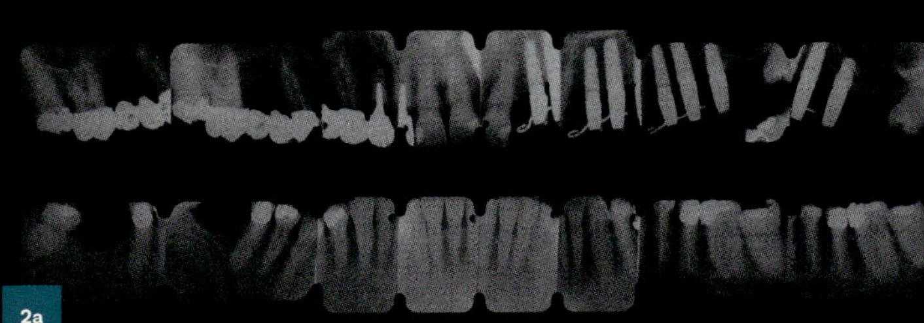

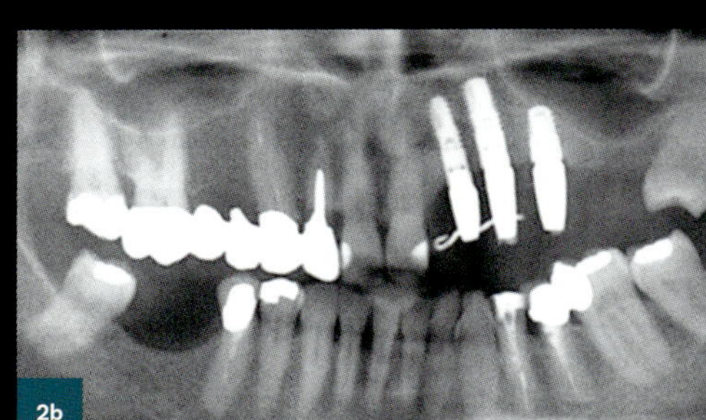

Figs. 2a,b ■ Radiographic status and orthopantomography.

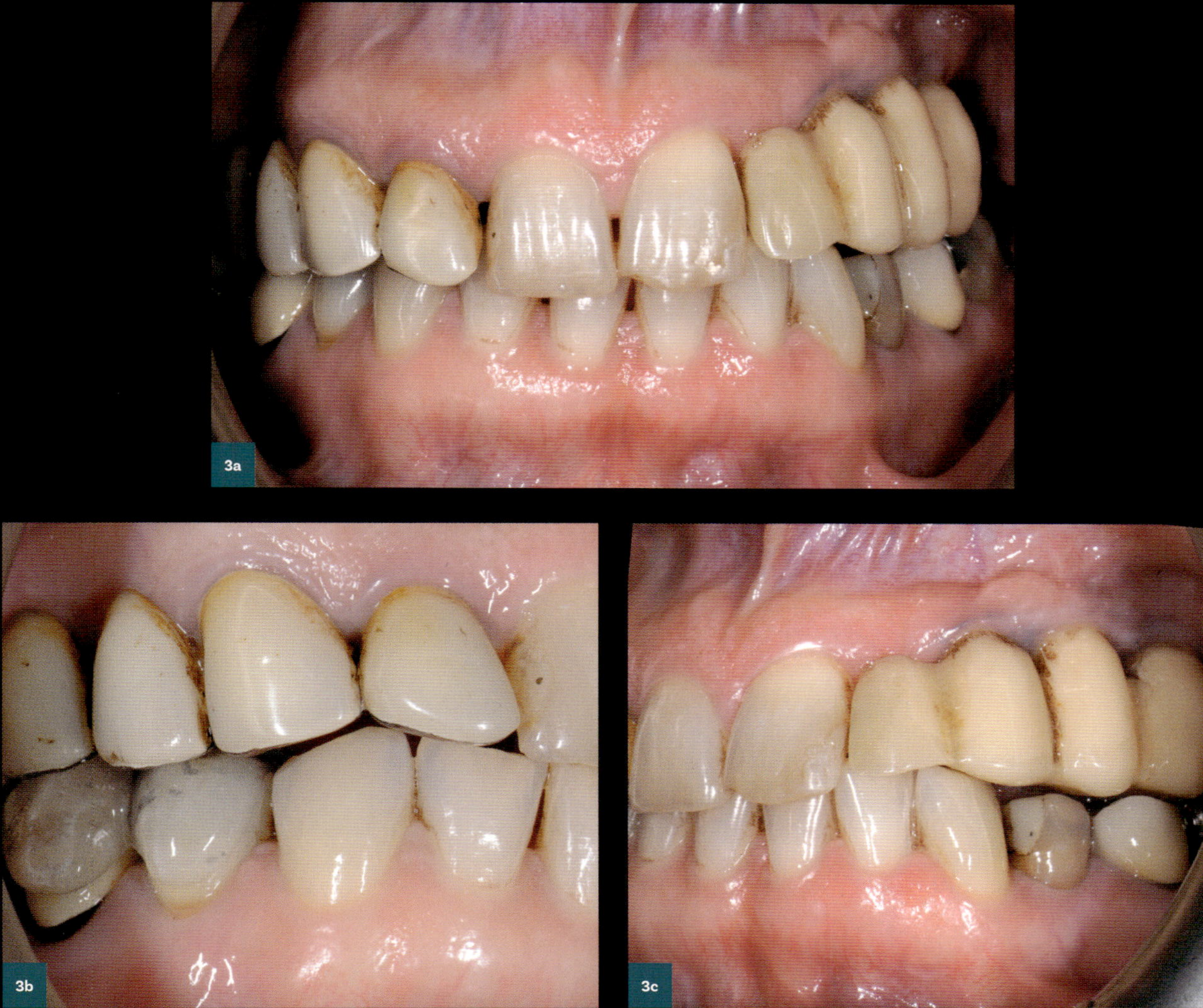

Figs. 3a-c ■ Intermaxillary relationship. Frontal and lateral vision.

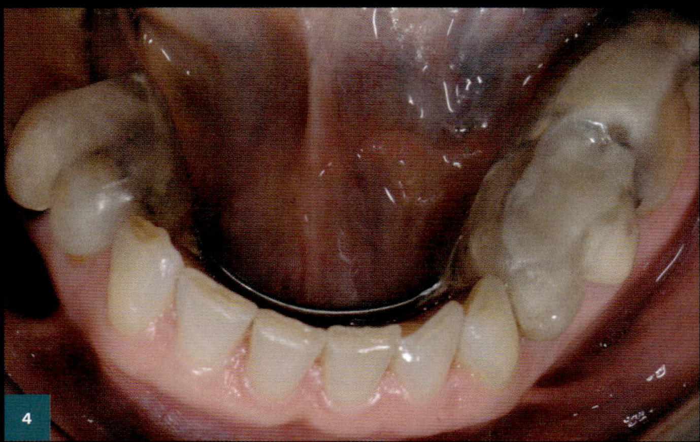

> *CONT'D*

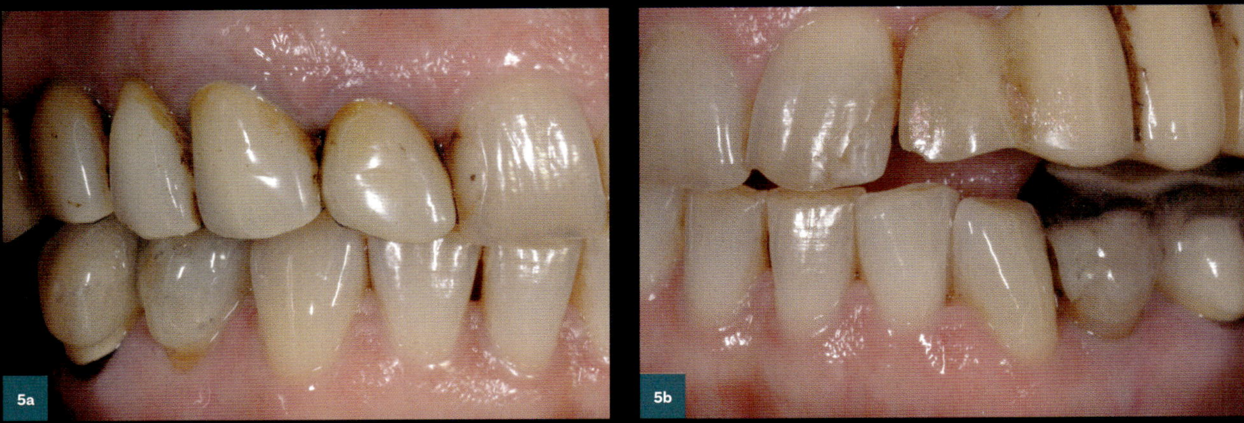

Figs. 5a,b ■ The lateral view shows a significant increase in the vertical dimension. The dysfunctional symptoms were resolved.

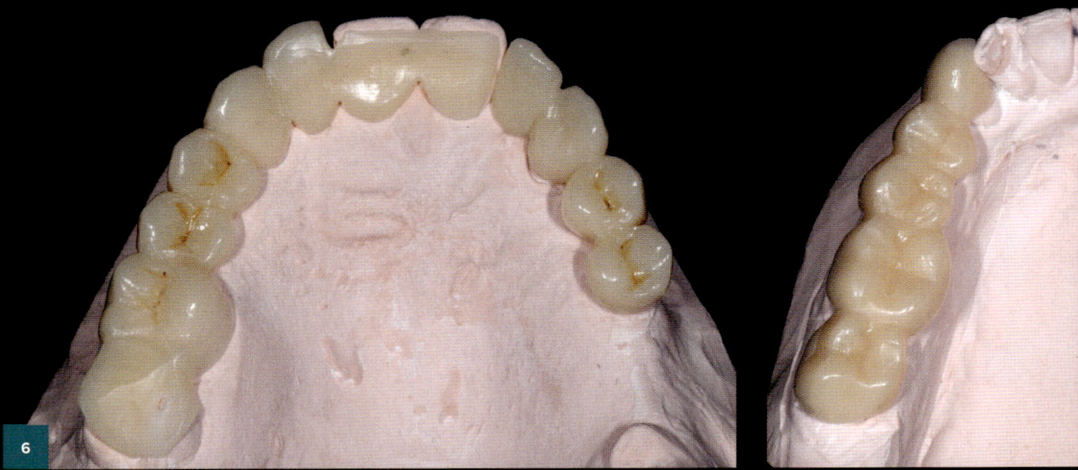

Fig. 6 ■ Provisionals to stabilize the patient in the correct and functional intermaxillary relationship.

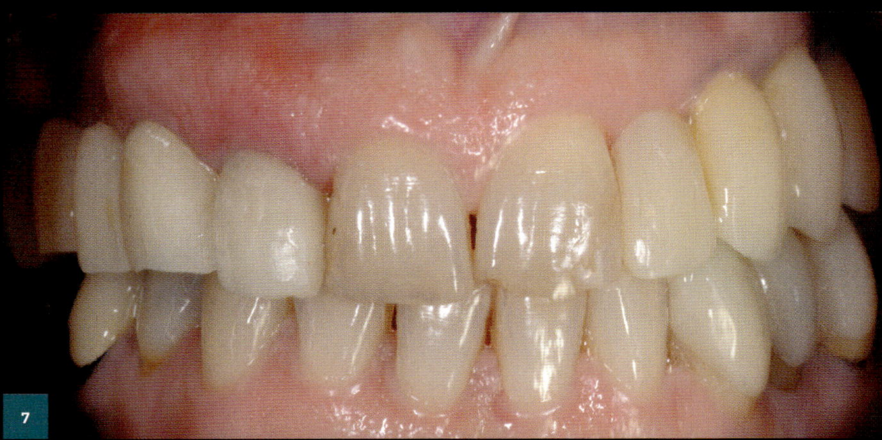

Fig. 7 ■ Provisionals in place.

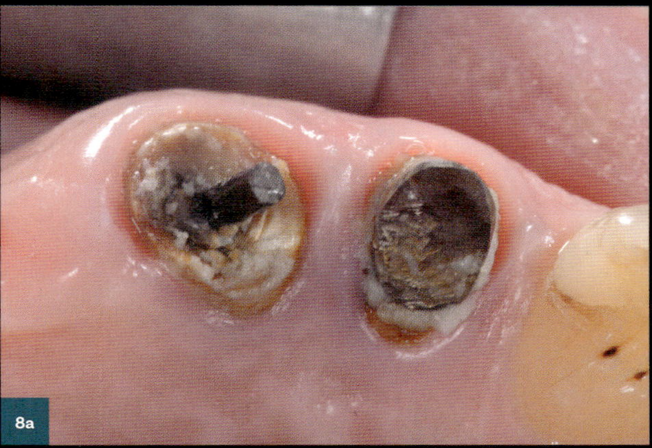

Fig. 8a ■ The right upper canine and lateral roots have root caries, making it impossible to use them as prosthetic abutments.

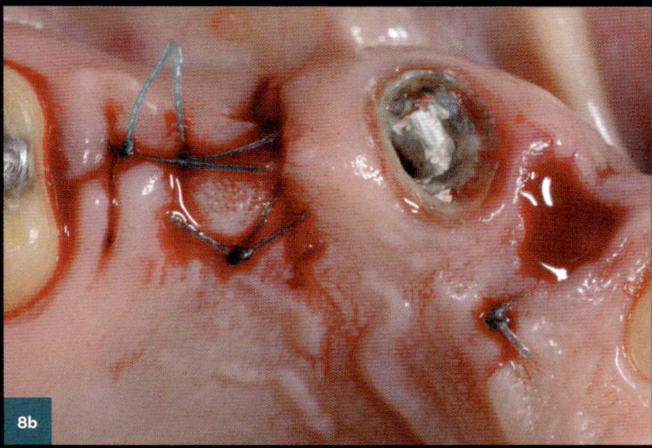

Fig. 8b ■ The 12 is extracted, and implants are placed in the sites 12 and 15. The root of the 13 is kept to support the provisional and will then be submerged to maintain the volume of the canine bulge.

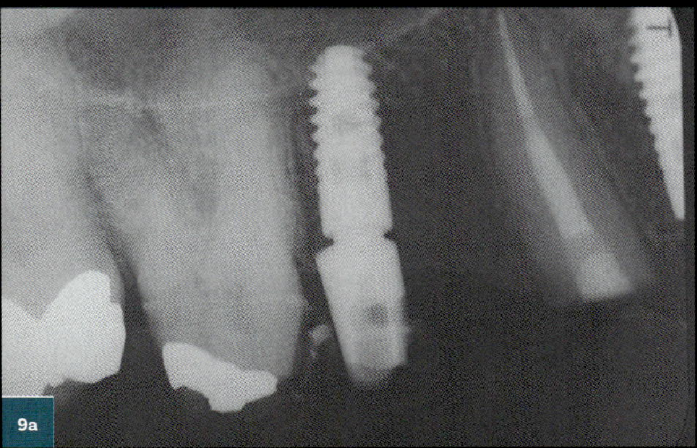

Fig. 9a ■ Rx after placement of a new provisional on the implant.

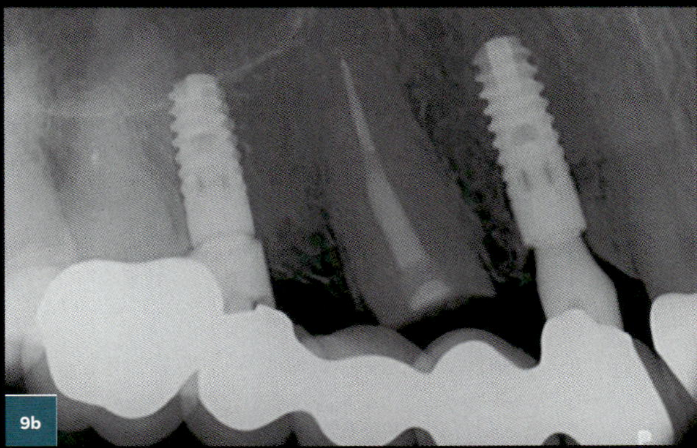

Fig. 9b ■ Rx of the definitive bridge and submerged root of tooth 13.

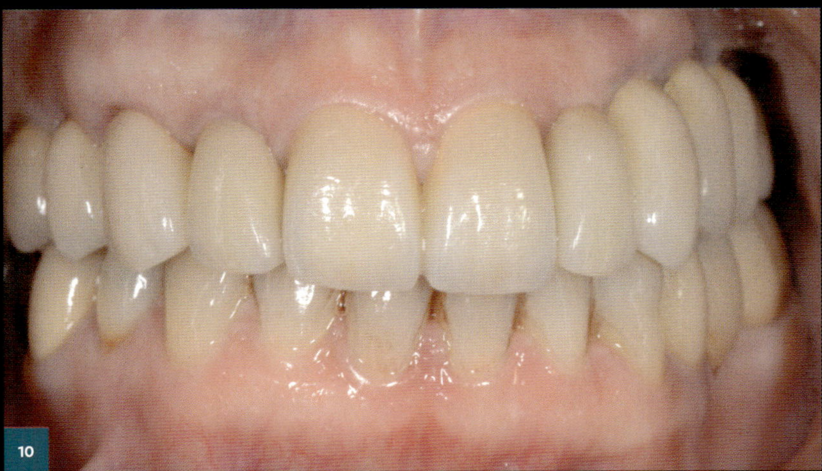

Fig. 10 ■ Definitive prostheses positioned in both arches.

CONT'D

CONT'D

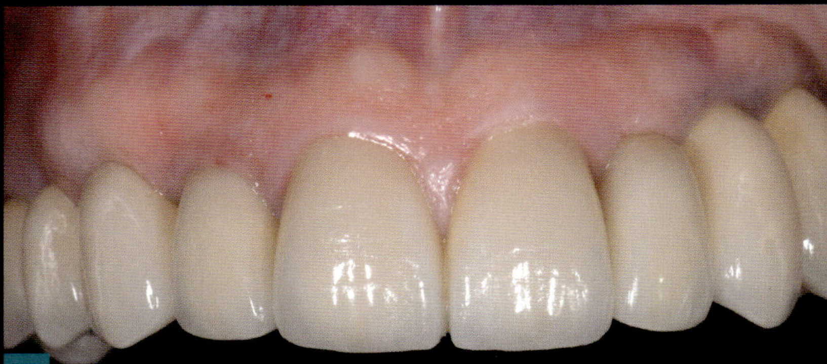

11a

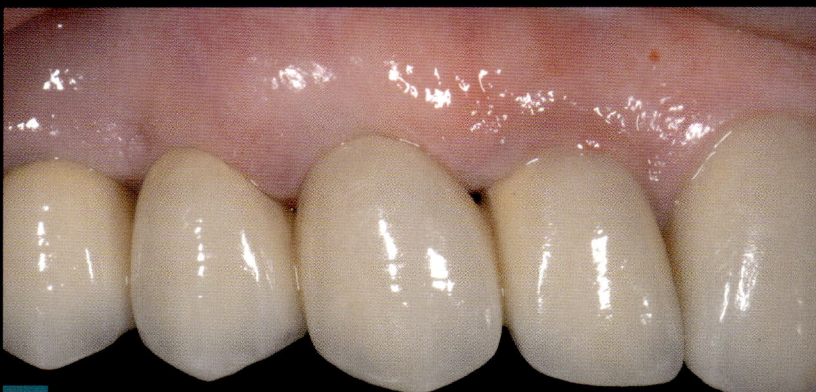

11b

Figs. 11a,b ▪ Check-up after one year in which the preservation of the volume and morphology of the canine bump is also appreciated.

Aesthetic rehabilitation with conservation of the parabola through use of the Socket Shield and Pontic Shield Techniques

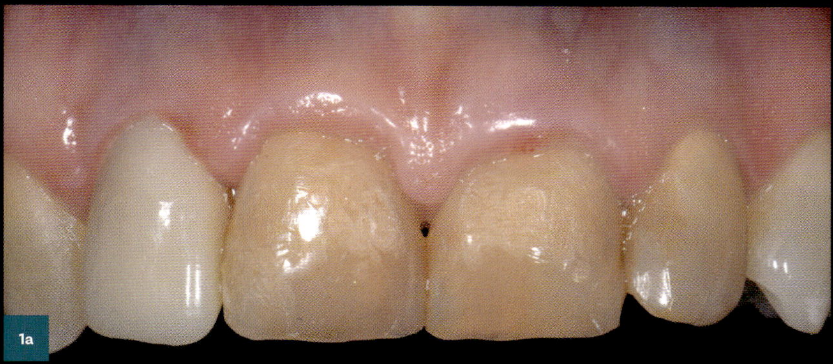

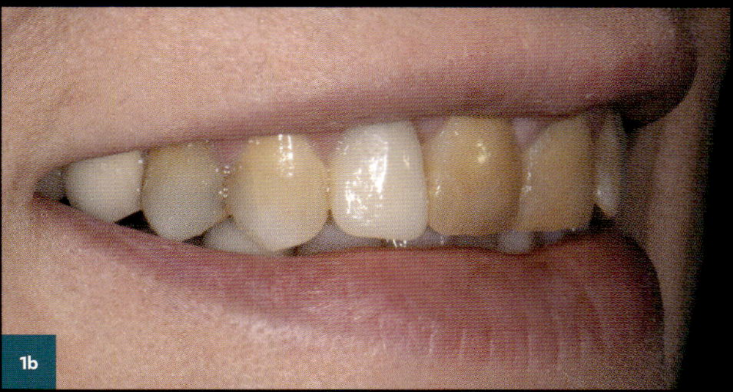

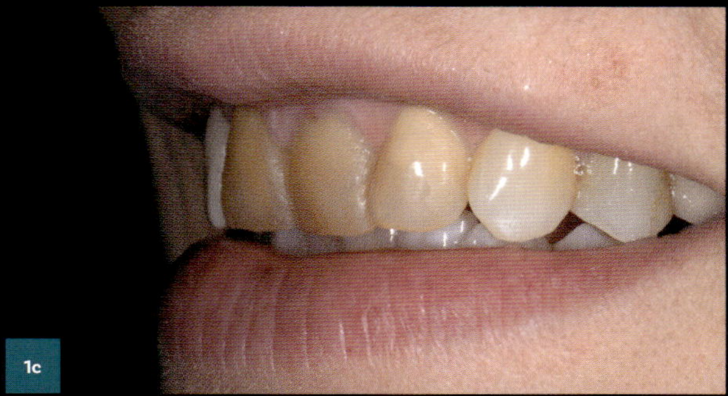

Figs. 1a-c ■ The 52-year-old patient, C.A., attends a consultation complaining of recurrent abscesses affecting the upper incisors. She also declares herself seriously dissatisfied with the aesthetic aspect. Upon clinical examination, the incisors appear repeatedly and variously restored, with notable differences in colour and shape.

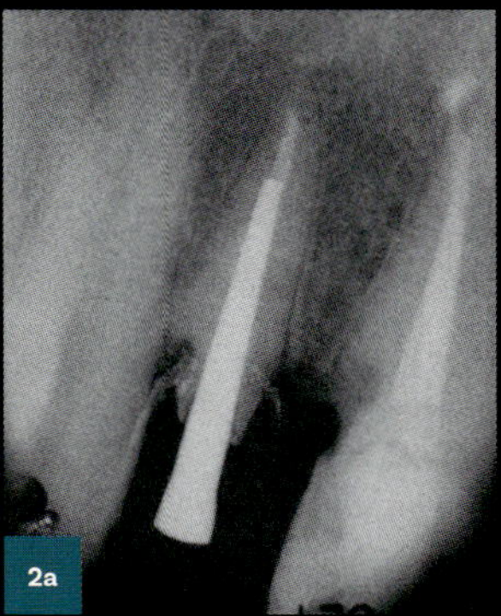

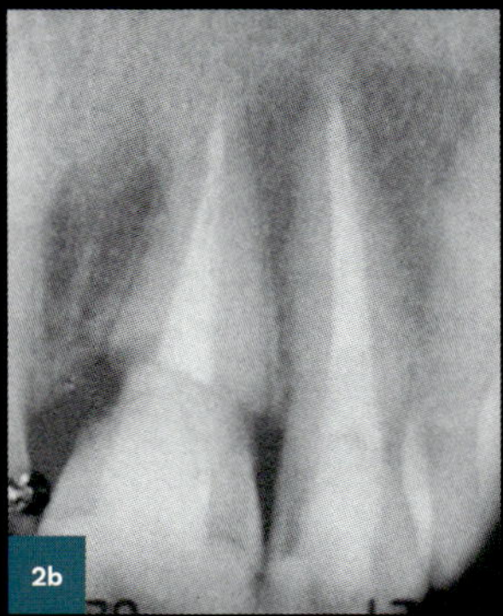

Figs. 2a,b ■ The intraoral X-rays show cervical resorption of 11, root caries below the bone crest of 12, horizontal coronal-root fracture of 21, and periradicular lesion of 22. Since the four elements were unsuitable for conservative treatment, it was decided to use a fixed prosthesis on implants. Given the visibility of the papillae and parabolas during the natural smile, it was planned to partially extract the compromised elements, maintaining buccal portions of the roots to support and stabilize the architecture of the hard and soft tissues.

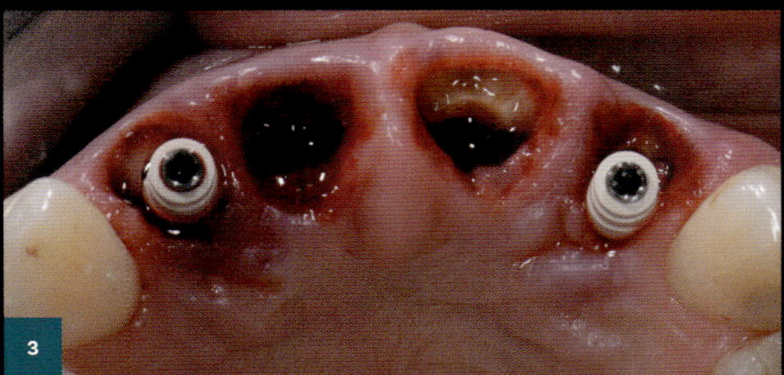

Fig. 3 ■ Partial extractions are performed according to the "Socket Shield" technique for the laterals and "Pontic Shield" for the centrals. Two implants are placed in positions 12 and 22.

> *CONT'D*

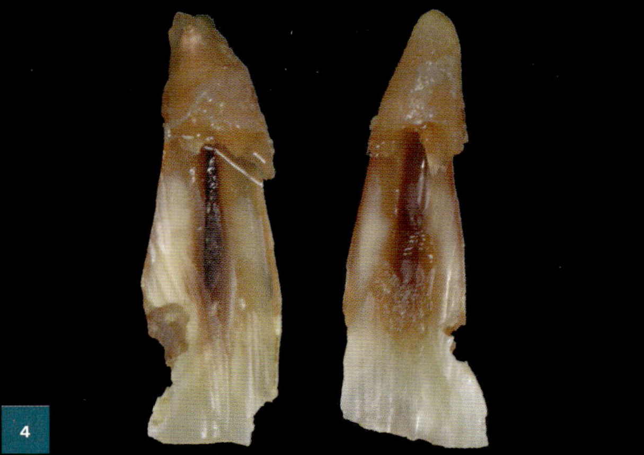

4

Fig. 4 ■ The removed fragments must include the apical third and the root canal to avoid endodontic problems.

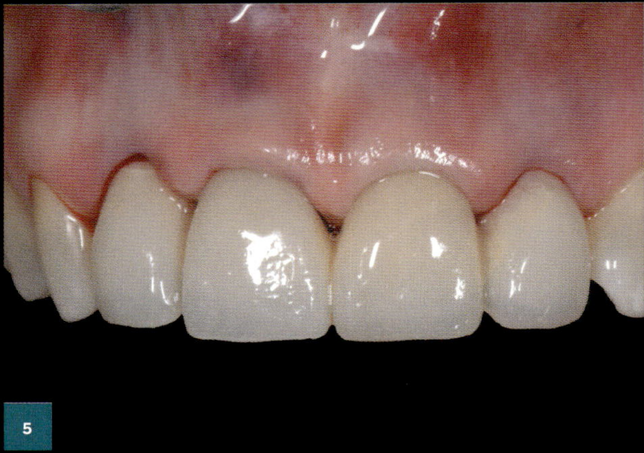

5

Fig. 5 ■ Immediate provisional.

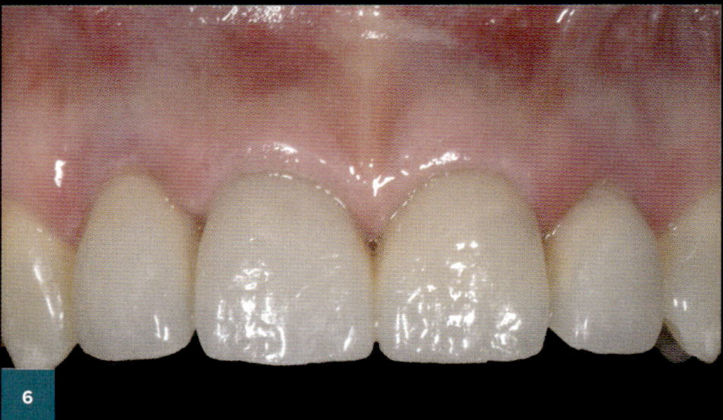

6

Fig. 6 ■ Check-up after 48 hours.

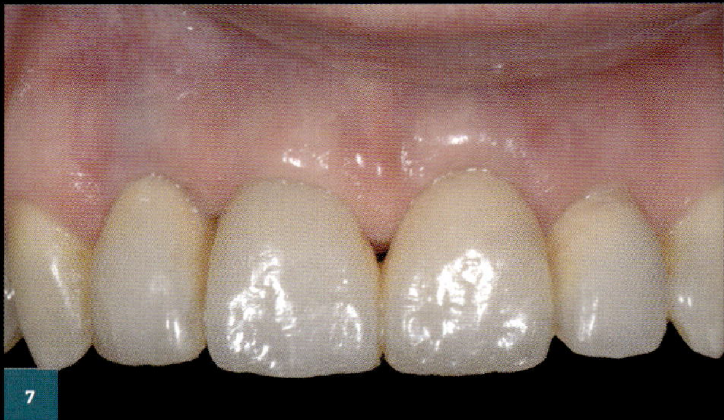

7

Fig. 7 ■ Check-up at three months.

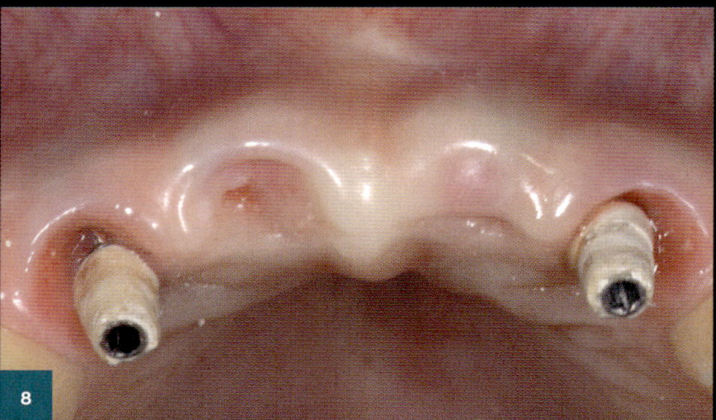

8

Fig. 8 ■ Note the good tissue conditioning and the lack of exposure of the root fragments.

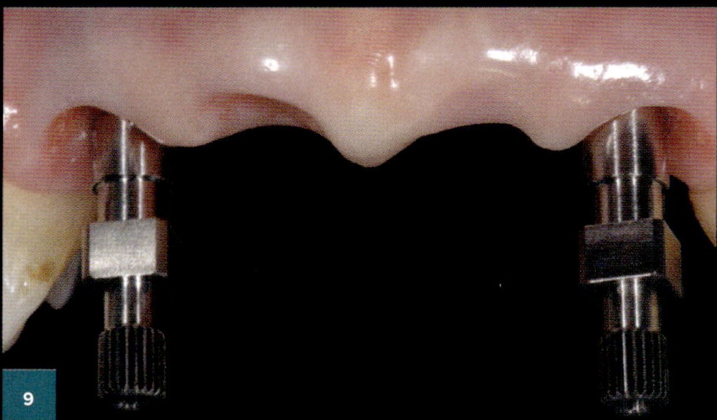

9

Fig. 9 ■ Impression transfers for constructing customized abutments and the definitive product.

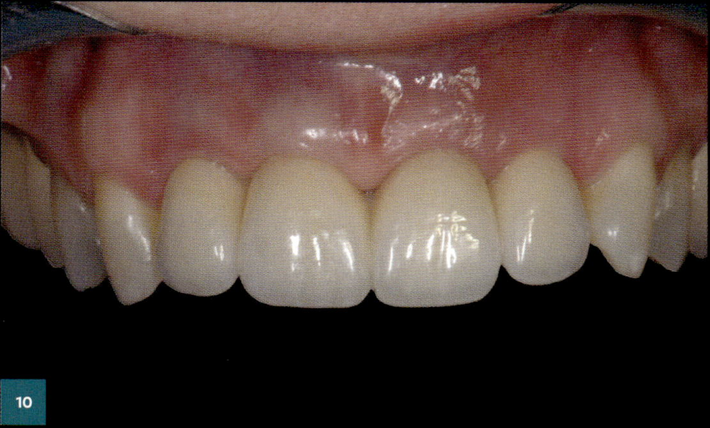

Fig. 10 ■ Try in of the four-unit bridge.

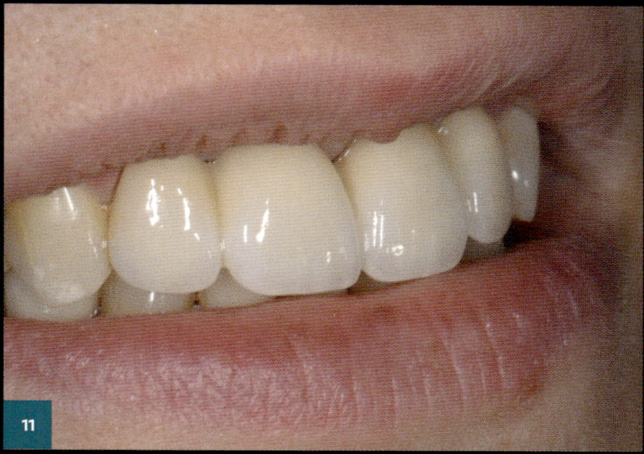

Fig. 11 ■ The aesthetic and functional adaptation of the prosthesis is verified.

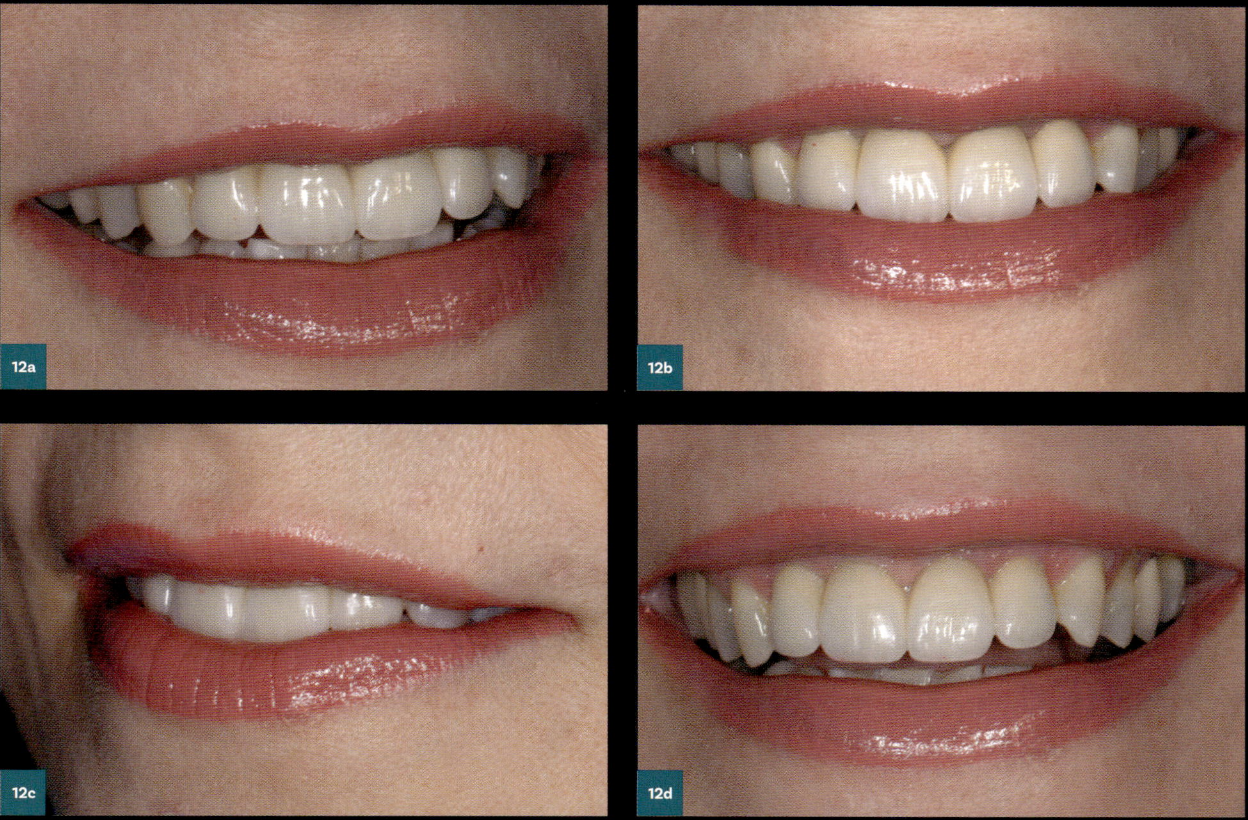

Figs. 12a-d ■ Maintaining the gingival architecture allows for perfect integration of the restoration.

Bibliography

1. Amler M, Johnson P, Salsman I. Histologic and histochemical investigation of human alveolar socket healing in undisturbed extraction wounds. *J Am Dent Assoc*. 1960;61:32-44.
2. Pietrokovski J, Massler M. Alveolar ridge resorption following tooth extraction. *J Prosthet Dent*. 1967;17(1):21-27.
3. Comut A, Mehra M, Saito H. Pontic Site Development with a Root Submergence Technique for a Screw Retained Prosthesis in the Anterior Maxilla. *J Prosthet Dent*. 2013;110(5):337-343.
4. Salama M, Ishikawa T, Salama H, Funato A, Garber D. Advantages of the root submergence technique for pontic site development in esthetic implant therapy. *Int J Periodontics Restorative Dent*. 2007;27(6):521-527.
5. Gluckman H, Salama M, Du Toit J. Partial Extraction Therapies (PET) Part 1: Maintaining Alveolar Ridge Contour at pontic and immediate implant sites. *Int J Periodontics Restorative Dent*. 2016;36(5):681-687.
6. Casey DM, Lauciello FR. A Review Of Submerged-Root Concept. *J Prosthet Dent*. 1980;43(2):128-132.
7. Wong KM, Chneh CM, Ang CW. Modified root submergence technique for multiple implant-supported maxillary anterior restorations in a patient with thin gingival biotype: A clinical report. *J Prosthet Dent*. 2012;107(6):349-352.
8. Bjorn H. Experimental studies on reattachment. *Dent Pract*. 1961;11:351-354.
9. O'Neal R, Gound T, Levin MP, del Rio BCE. Submergence of roots for alveolar bone preservation.I. Endodontically treated roots. *Oral Surg Oral Med Oral Pathol*. 1978;45(5):803-810.
10. Plata RL, Kelln EE. Intentional retention of vital submerged roots in dogs. *Oral Surg Oral Med Oral Pathol*. 1976;42(1):100-108.
11. Hürzeler MB, Zuhr O, Schupbach P, Rebele SF, Emmanouilidis N, Fickl S. The socket shield technique: A proof-of-principle report. *J Clin Periodontol*. 2010;37(9):855-862.
12. Kher, U, Tunkiwala, A. Partial Extraction Therapy in Implant Dentistry. Cham, Springer International Publishing 2020.
13. Kan JY, Rungcharassaeng K. Proximal socket shield for interimplant papilla preservation in the esthetic zone. *Int J Periodontics Restorative Dent*. 2013;33(1):e24-31.
14. Glocker M, Attin T, Schmidlin PR. Ridge Preservation with Modified "Socket-Shield" Technique: A Methodological Case Series. *Dent. J*. 2014;2(1):11-21.
15. Siormpas KD, Mitsias ME, Kontsiotou-Siormpa E, Garber D, Kotsakis GA. Immediate implant placement in the esthetic zone utilizing the "root-membrane" technique: clinical results up to 5 years postloading. *Int J Oral Maxillofac Implants*. 2014;29(6):1397-405.
16. Kumar PR, Kher U. Shield the socket: procedure, case report and classification. *J Indian Soc Periodontol*. 2018;22(3):266-272.
17. Lee CT, Chuang SK, Stoupel J. Survival analysis and other clinical outcomes of immediate implant placement in sites with periapical lesions: systematic review. *Int J Oral Maxillofac Implants*. 2015;30(2):268-278.
18. Kan JY, Rungcharassaeng K. Immediate placement and provisionalization of maxillary anterior single implants: a surgical and prosthodontic rationale. *Pract Periodontics Aesthet Dent*. 2000;12(9):817-824.

15

Replacement of severely resorbed teeth and implants in contact with root remnants

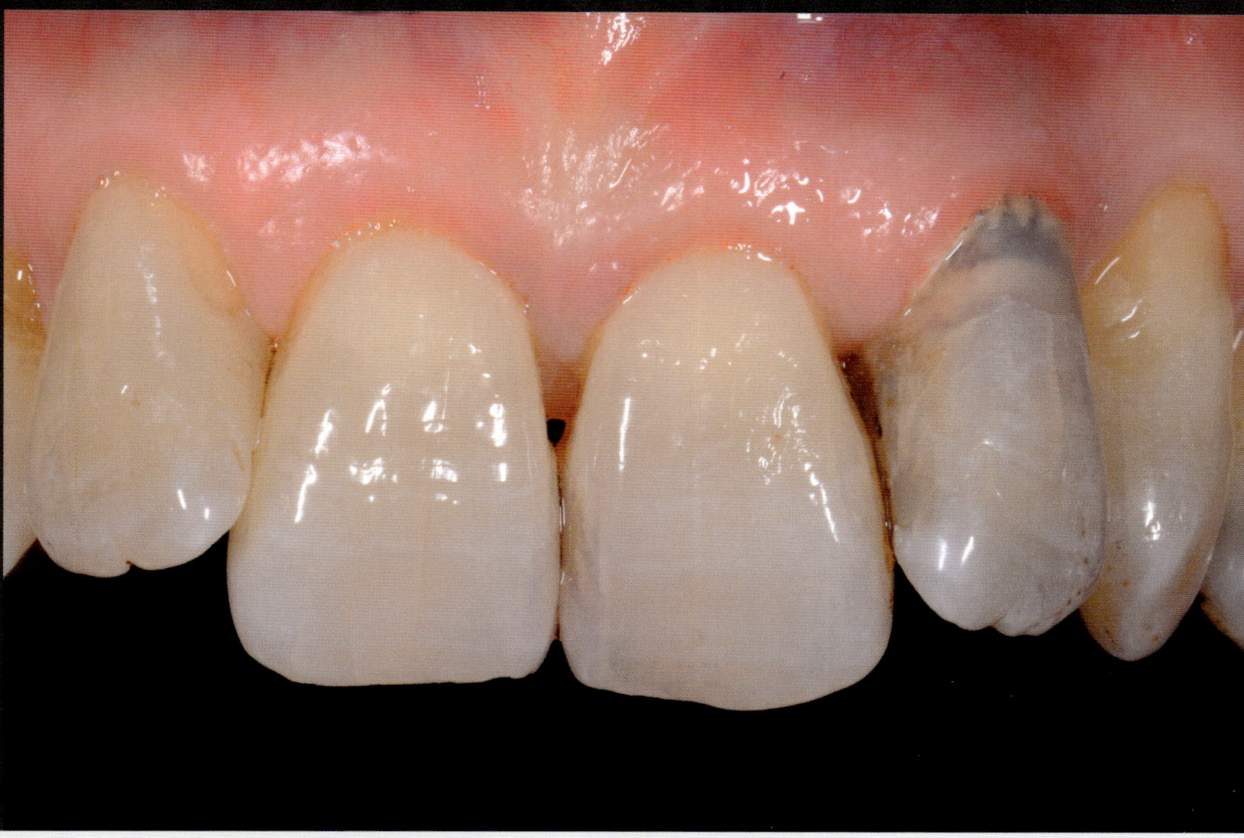

Root resorptions are more frequently diagnosed now due to improved and widely available radiological examinations, increased clinician awareness, and a gradual reduction of teeth loss from caries or periodontal disease.[1]

Treatment of root resorption

When promptly diagnosed, root resorption in any form can be successfully treated using endodontic, restorative and periodontal procedures or by pausing orthodontic treatment.[2] Therefore, it is important to remember that external apical resorption induced by orthodontic movements might not lead to clinically relevant problems, even in cases with severe resorption. Considering that the cervical third of a root bears over half the occlusal loading, while the apical third only bears only 10%, limited orthodontically induced resorption in the apical area of a root does not pose problems in maintaining these teeth. Endodontic therapy is not indicated in these cases, as the resorption does not originate from the pulp.[3]
Mobility in teeth with a short residual root may have other causes, including the recent orthodontic appliance removal or excessive occlusal loading.[4]
The presence of short roots might not always relate to resorption-independent factors. Short Root Anomaly, first described by Lind in 1972,[5] presents root underdevelopment that may simulate external root resorption. However, this anomaly develops without trauma or orthodontic movement. It principally impacts upper central incisors, with potential effects on other teeth. This could raise doubts about performing the necessary orthodontic procedures.[6]
However, orthodontics is not completely contraindicated in these cases, but should be performed with caution. This is possible, by minimizing or avoiding movements of the affected teeth and conducting radiographic check-ups every 4-6 months to intercept potential resorption. Additionally, vitamin D deficiencies might lead to teeth and root developmental abnormalities, including rare genetic cases of hypophosphatemic rickets.

Properly performed endodontic treatment can halt internal inflammatory resorption. Here, careful irrigation and ultrasonic activation of the irrigant, along with intermediate phase of medication with calcium hydroxide[7] are important. Early-stage invasive cervical resorption can be treated through surgical flap exposure of the lesion. This is achieved by cauterizing with trichloroacetic acid, granulation tissue removal, and a conservative composite resin reconstruction, as described by Heitersay in 2007.[8]
This technique was also described in a video by Style Italiano Endodontics[9] on Facebook. Accessing the lesion through endodontic spaces might be preferable in certain cases, as shown in another video by the same group.[10]

Replacement of resorbed teeth

Due to the asymptomatic nature of the pathology, diagnosis often occurs when the tooth is irreparably compromised. This determines a series of complex problems tied to the patient's age, especially if young individuals, compromised tooth location, especially in the anterior aesthetic zone, or the potential difficulty of performing extractions.

Patient's age

Resorption, whether idiopathic, traumatic or carious origin tends to affect younger patients. Severe resorption leading to tooth loss complicates its replacement due to tooth eruption and arch development, which hinder artificial tooth attachment to the adjacent teeth. Root loss disrupts the normal and symmetrical development of alveolar bone.

Location

Frontal teeth most commonly impacted by resorption, causing aesthetic and functional problems that patients struggle with. Therefore, swift replacement of compromised tooth becomes essential.

Difficulty of extraction

The extraction of resorbed teeth can be a complex procedure that causes significant alveolar bone loss. This necessitates various regenerative procedures for proper implant placement or even the intermediate bridge element, ensuring both function and aesthetics are maintained.[11]

Implants in contact with root remnants

Implant selection for resorbed tooth replacement is often the preferred solution, albeit one with distinct peculiarities. Challenges linked to replacing roots with advanced resorption are intertwined with those stemming from persistent root remnants in sites designated for osseointegrated implants. This common scenario complicates treatment planning and execution, especially with root remnant extraction.

Considering the current implantology paradigm of osteointegration—direct bone-implant contact[12]—it is evident that any intervening structure between the bone and implant contradicts this discipline's foundations. Therefore, in cases of root remnants, the clinician faces two options. First, tilting the implant for insertion path adjustment, avoiding the root remnant. This is achievable under specific anatomical conditions with thin roots and ample available bone. The second option involves root remnant removal, followed by bone defect filling, healing, and subsequent implant placement. However, this approach can be highly invasive, at times necessitating complex guided bone regeneration procedures that increase costs and treatment duration while diminishing outcome predictability.[13]

The patient might benefit from a more direct solution involving implant placement, irrespective of any remaining root remnants. Although this approach challenges implantology principles, numerous international publications support its feasibility.

In 1990, Buser et al. published histological data on the possible formation of a periodontal ligament around implants adjacent to root remnants.[14] In 2004, Gray and Vernino[15] analysed histological data from implants unintentionally placed near root remnants in experimental animals, showing no adverse effects. From 2009 onwards, Davarpanah and Szmuckler-Moncler documented a series of clinical cases intentionally involving implant placement in contact with or through retained dental structures, including ankylosed root fragments[16] or impacted teeth.[17] The reported success rates were comparable to conventional techniques.[18]

This approach can effectively shorten treatment times[19] and is particularly relevant for patients with age-related concerns or systemic diseases. This strategy minimizes invasiveness and becomes essential when extraction surgery could cause more harm than benefit. The growing number of publications in this field is evident, with systematic literature reviews shedding light on its significance. Labidi et al. introduced the concept of "mineral integration" for implants in 2019[20], while Perez-Gonzales et al.'s recent comprehensive review in 2021[21] considered studies with a minimum 12-month follow-up. Their analysis involved 44 patients who received 62 implants, boasting an average survival rate of over 90%. Notably, some studies reported a remarkable 100% success rate over 7-9 years. For specific cases, survival rates stood at 76% for implants placed in residual roots and 97.5% for implants placed through impacted teeth. Among the examined cases, only 6 implants failed. Five of these were unintentionally placed in contact with root remnants, while one failed due to intentional placement through an upper impacted canine. Late failures reported by Nevins et al.[22] and Langer et al.[23] were probably due to bacterial colonies and calculus on implant surfaces when placed near retained roots. This may account for the relatively lower success rates compared to implant placement through impacted teeth, where there is no risk of infection. Davarpanah et al.[24] and Amato et al.[25] proposed comprehensive guidelines for case selection and management. They recommended the complete inclusion of impacted teeth with a minimum of 5 mm of coronal bone and implant positioning outside the pulp space. For cases involving retained roots, they advised the thorough removal of any existing endodontic filling material. However, it is evident that from a clinical point of view, this last situation has no practical value. To summarize, for effective utilization of this technique, we should place the implant in the most clinically favourable position, even if it necessitates the inclusion of coronal portions of the impacted tooth, while ensuring no pulp involvement.

The systematic literature review by Perez-Gonzales concludes with a positive evaluation of implant placement through impacted teeth and a more uncertain evaluation for placements in contact with retained roots.[21]

Implants and root resorption

In cases involving root resorption, implant placement is an exceptional case, bearing resemblance to severe dental trauma cases in growing children. This trauma often causes ankylosis of the affected tooth and subsequent infraocclusion. The suitable approach for such instances is tooth decoronation.[26] This technique involves raising a mucoperiosteal flap, eliminating the crowns of the affected teeth, and sectioning ankylosed roots 2 mm below the bone level. The root canals are then irrigated with saline solution and allowed to fill up with blood before suturing the flap. This allows normal alveolar bone growth, creating an optimal environment for subsequent implant placement.[27] Following complete bone development, implant placement becomes feasible without concern for any root undergoing resorption.[28] The decoronation technique followed by implant placement is a well-documented procedure that treats ankylosed and resorbing roots as bone tissue, allowing implant placement to align with prosthetic choice[29] (**Fig. 15.1**). While tooth extraction due to resorption may be traumatic and destructive, it can necessitate various regenerative surgical procedures,[30] an alternative, less invasive and faster alternative exists. With proper caution, considering this unconsolidated procedure built upon a series of case reports, one can bypass extraction and proceed with implant placement adjacent to the root remnants.[31-33] (**Fig. 15.1**).

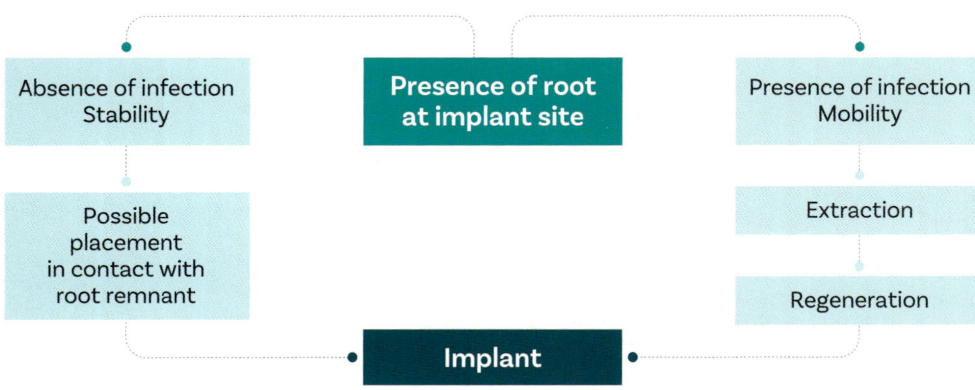

Fig. 15.1 ■ Algorithmic evaluation for the possibility of maintaining a root or parts of it.

Implant placement through the root of an impacted canine, which the patient refuses to extract

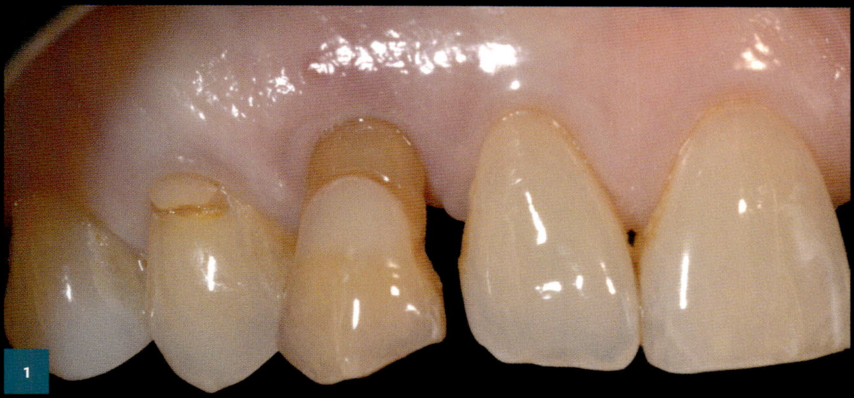

Fig. 1 ■ The patient, S.B., aged 63, complains of high mobility of the upper right deciduous canine.

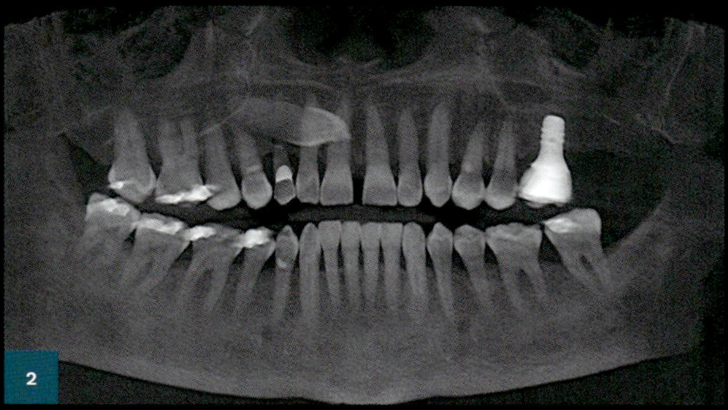

Fig. 2 ■ The OPG shows the presence of the retained permanent canine. The patient refuses the extraction of the impacted tooth and still requests a fixed prosthesis.

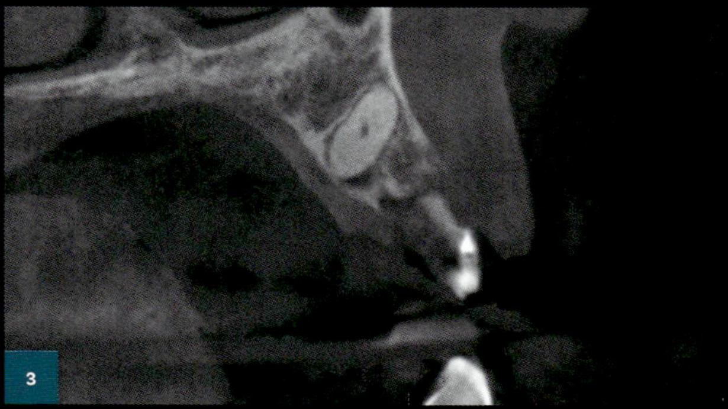

Fig. 3 ■ The CBCT confirms the impossibility of placing a short implant, given the presence of only a few millimetres of bone coronal to the impacted root. It is, therefore, proposed to place the implant despite the presence of the canine. The buccal-lingual section demonstrates the possibility of planning the inevitable invasion of the impacted tooth's radicular dentine, carefully avoiding the involvement of the pulp tissue.

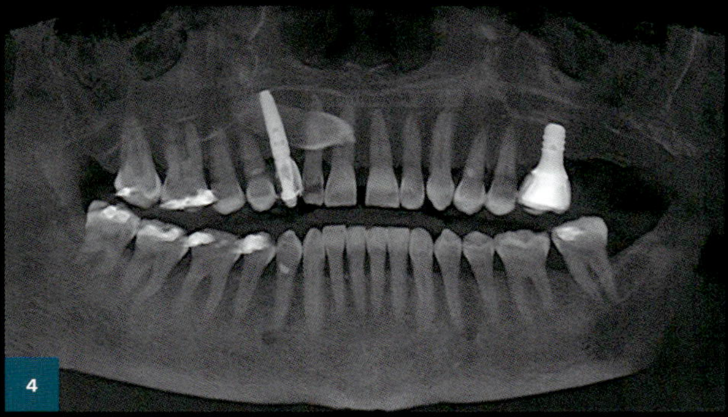

Fig. 4 ■ CBCT after implant placement.

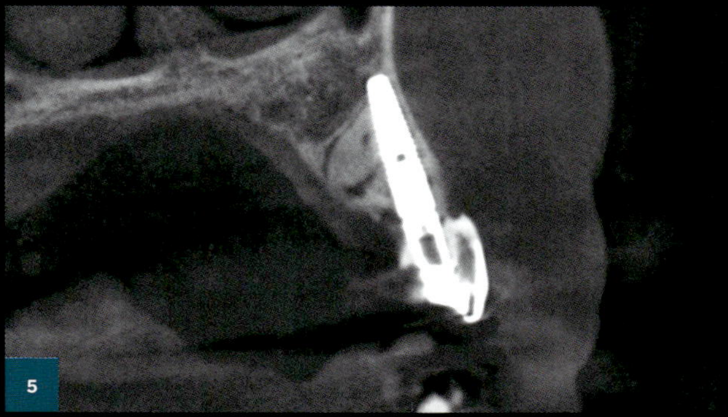

Fig. 5 ■ Buccal-palatal section to confirm the absence of invasion of the pulp.

CONT'D >

> *CONT'D*

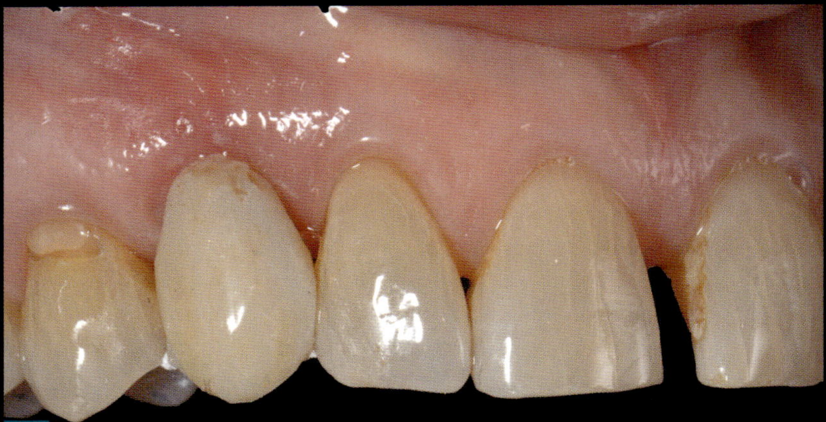

6

Fig. 6 ■ Immediate provisional crown.

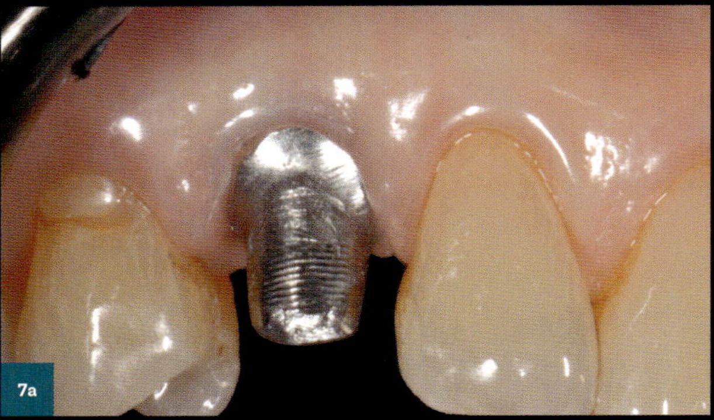

7a

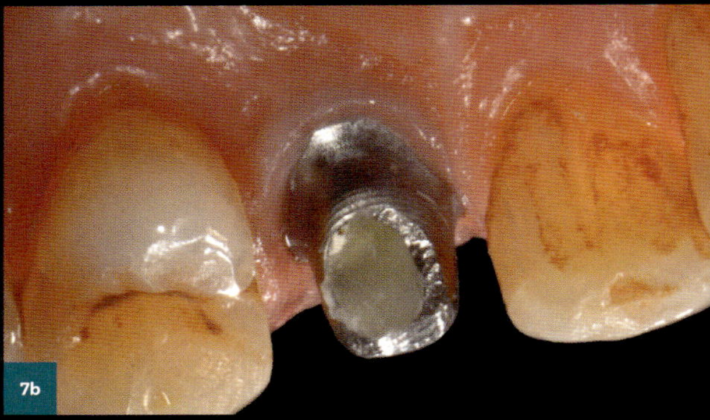

7b

Figs. 7a,b ■ Three months after placement, a scan is performed to produce a customized abutment.

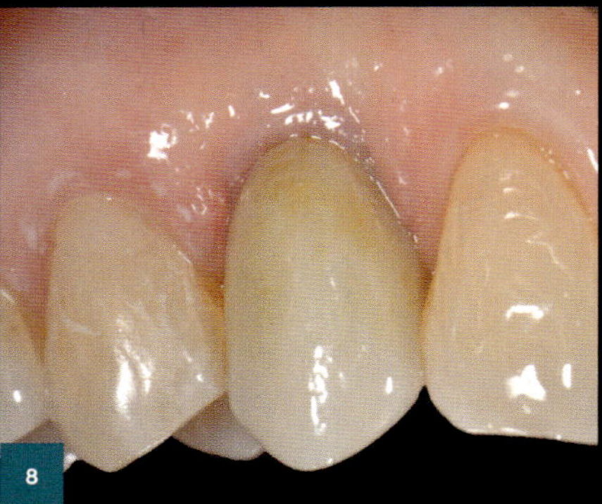

8

Fig. 8 ■ All ceramic crown positioned.

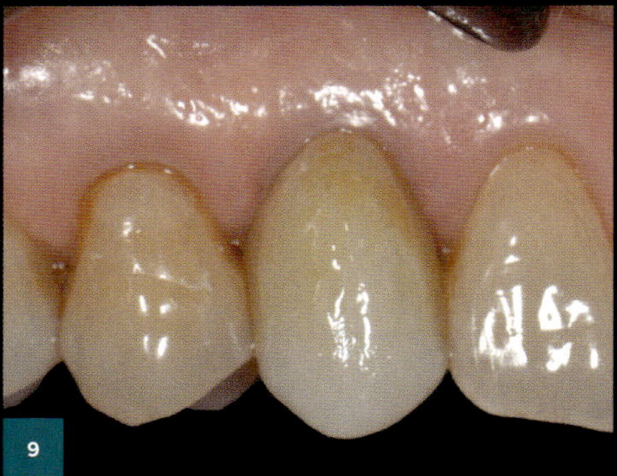

9

Fig. 9 ■ Clinical follow-up at 2 years.

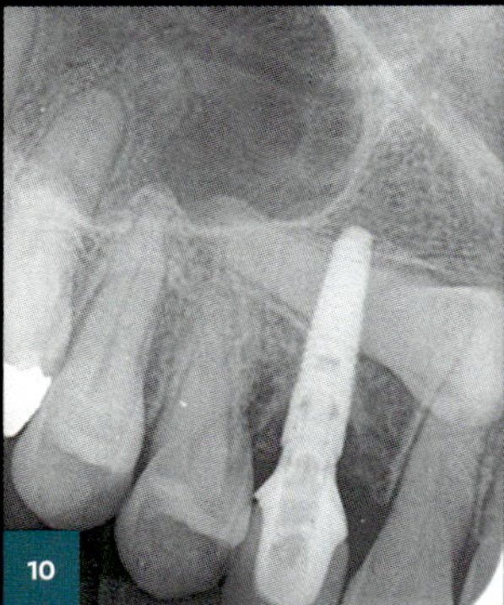

10

Fig. 10 ■ Radiographic follow-up at 2 years.

CLINICAL CASES

Implant placement through severely resorbed root, with considerable simplification of the procedure

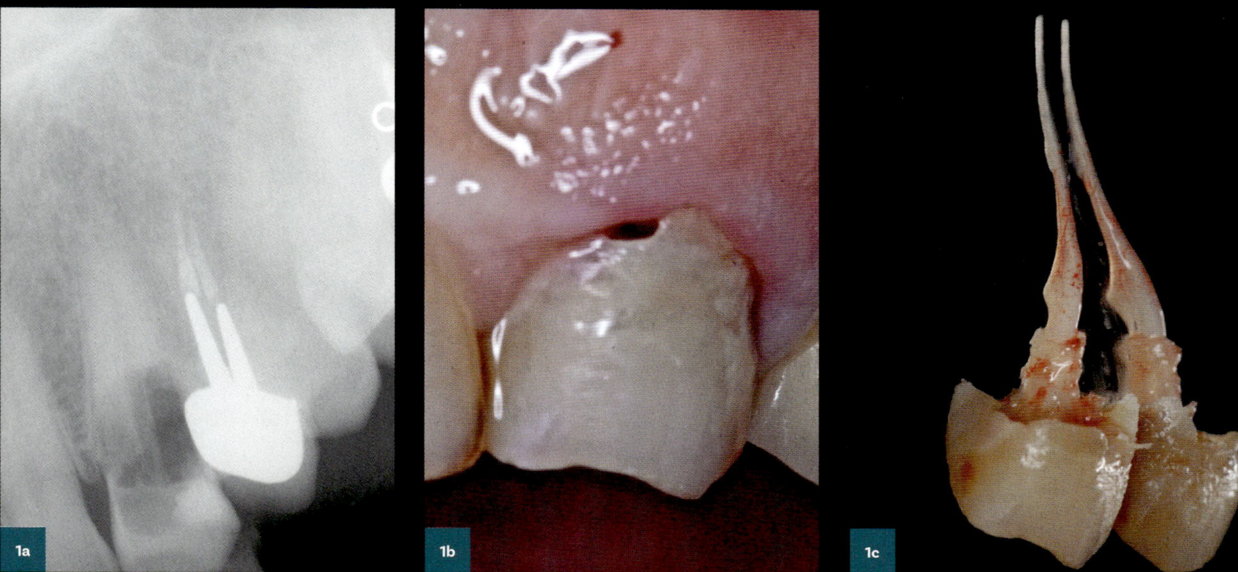

Figs. 1a-c ■ The patient P.V., aged 62, complains of mobility of the upper left canine and pain perceived not as acute but constant, such as to make chewing difficult and hygiene procedures impossible. **a**: periapical radiograph showing Heitersay grade 4 invasive cervical resorption. **b**: clinical image; **c**: removal of the coronal fragment drags all the pulp tissue with it.

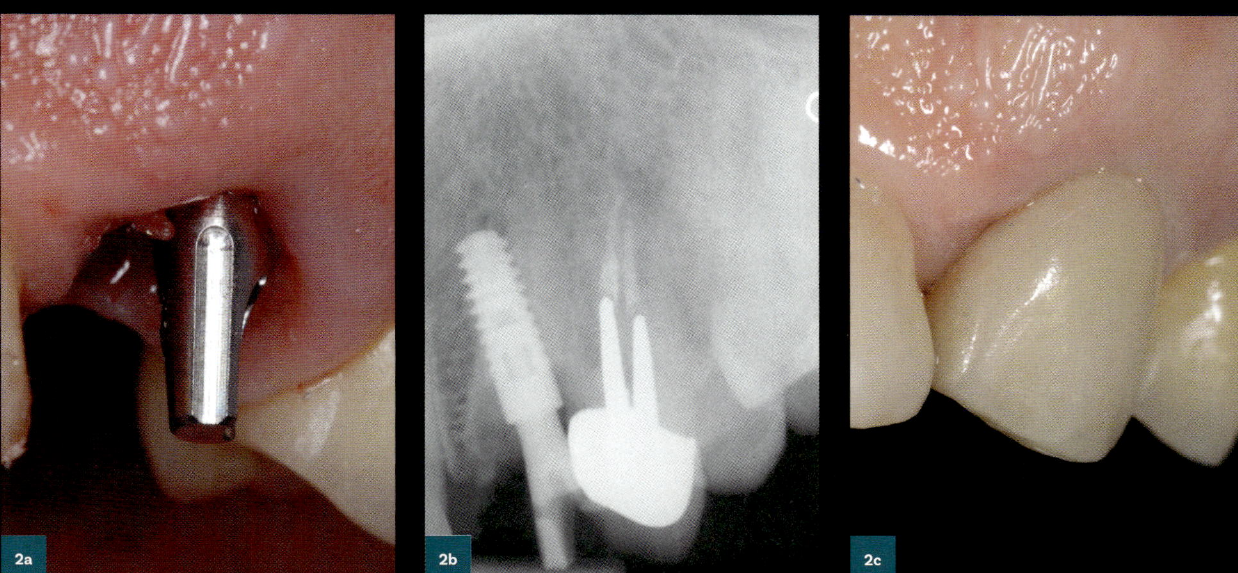

Figs. 2a-c ■ An immediate implant is performed while intentionally keeping a mesio-buccal portion of the root dentin to maintain tissue stability. **a**: implant positioned with abutment; **b**: radiograph that highlights the portion of the root capable of supporting the correct morphology of the tissues; **c**: immediate provisional crown.

CONT'D

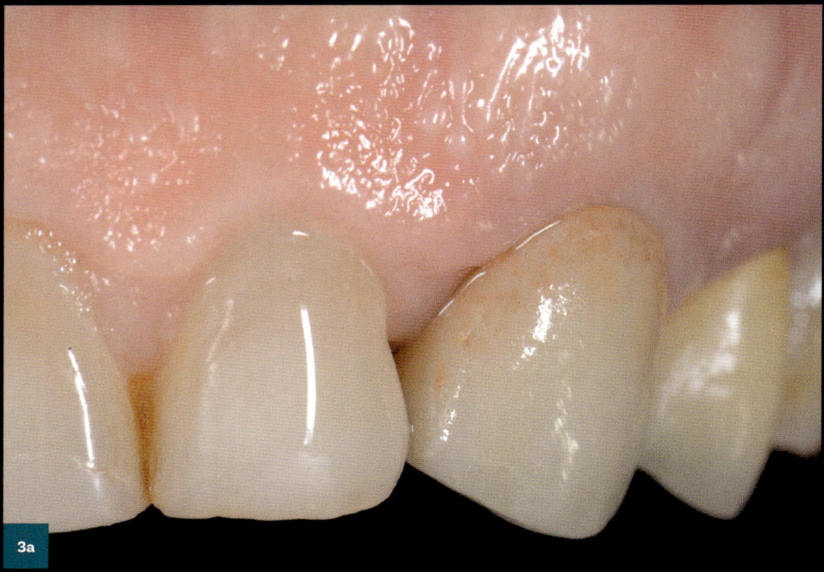

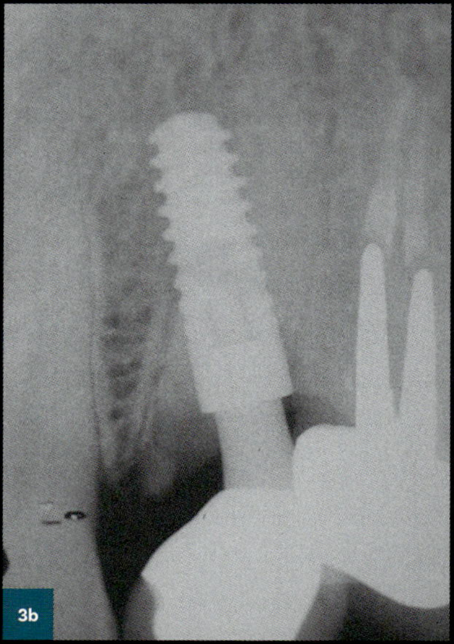

Figs. 3a,b ▪ All ceramic crowns. **a**: 10-year clinical follow-up; **b**: 10-year radiographic follow-up. One can appreciate the excellent volumetric stability of the mesial papilla of tooth 13, which was achieved by intentionally preserving a portion of the mesial root to support the surrounding soft tissues.

Placement of an implant in correspondence with a root in resorption

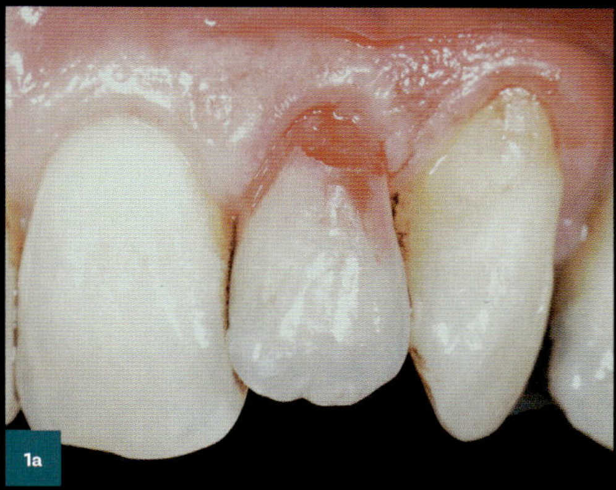

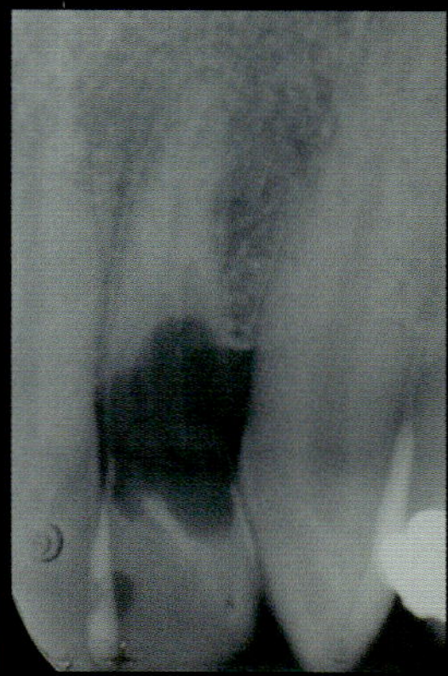

Figs. 1a,b ■ The patient, Z.P.A., aged 40, presents an invasive cervical resorption of the left upper lateral incisor, along with an angle 2, division 2 malocclusion, with retroclined upper central incisors and proclined and rotated mesio-buccally lateral incisors, bilaterally.

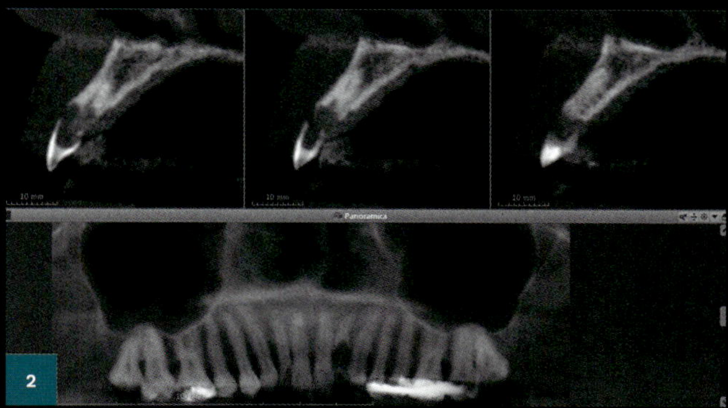

Fig. 2 ■ CBCT, performed before tooth loss, shows severe invasive cervical resorption. The extraction of the apical root fragment would most likely result in the loss of the buccal bone and require extensive regeneration to achieve an aesthetically and functionally acceptable outcome. The patient requires a less invasive alternative to avoid using removable provisional devices.

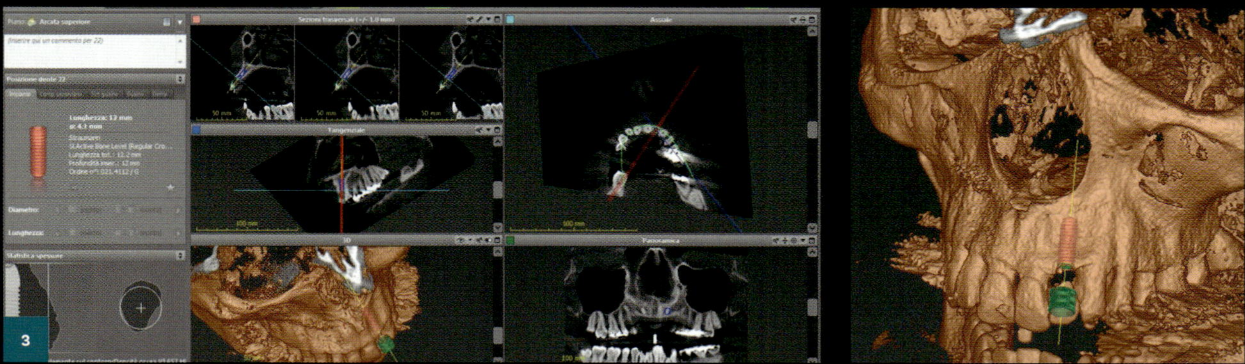

Fig. 3 ■ Using planning software, the implant positioning is programmed in such a way as to occupy most of the space that is currently taken up by parts of the root that are affected by resorption, minimizing the amount of residual root tissue, and trying to obtain maximum contact between the bone tissue and implant. This results in an uncommon positioning of the implant, more buccal and apical than usual, to obtain the best symmetry.

CONT'D >

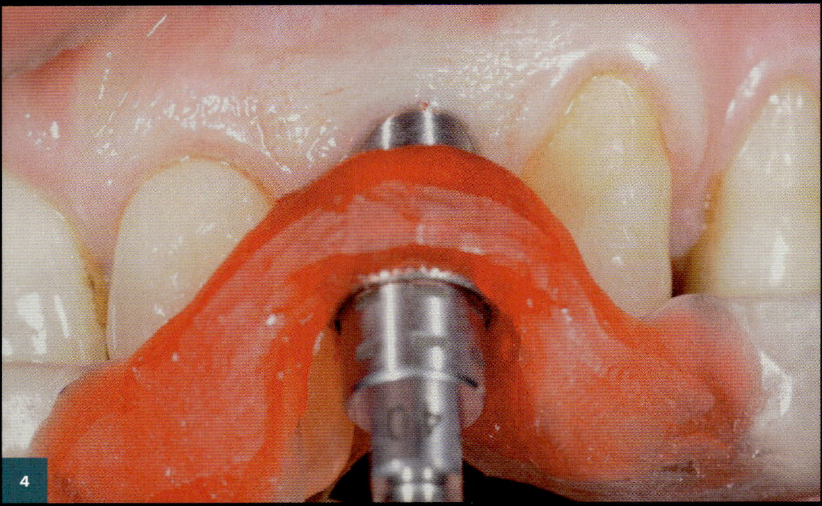

Fig. 4 ■ The implant was placed with a surgical guide, allowing for precise site preparation despite tissues with different consistencies.

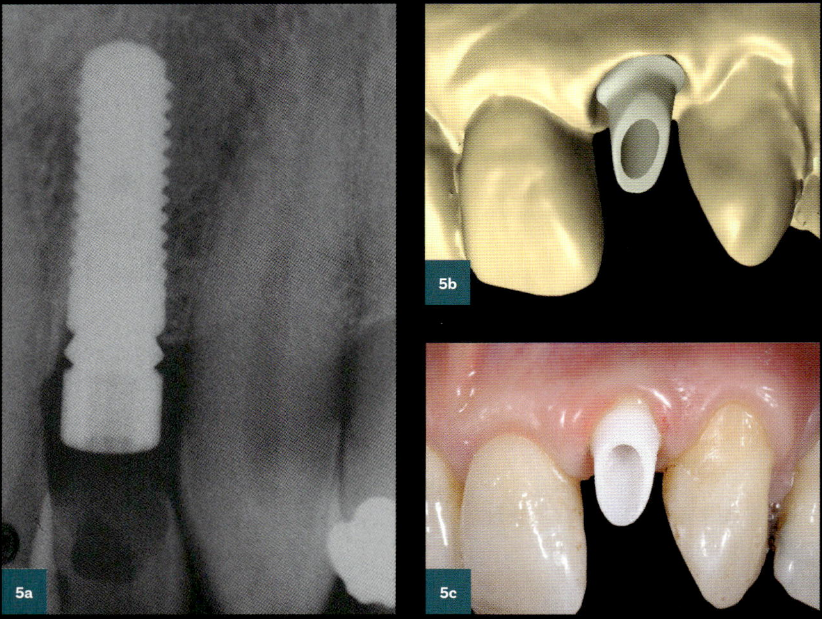

Figs. 5a-c ■ **a:** Post-operative periapical radiograph. The lost tooth was used as an immediate provisional. **b**: scan and design of the aesthetic abutment; **c**: ceramic abutment screwed onto the implant.

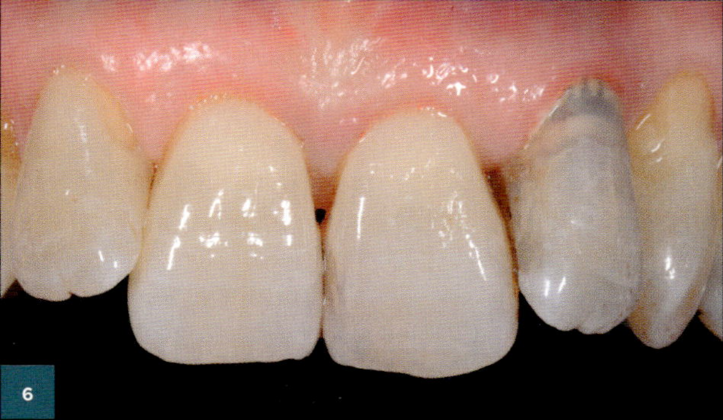

Fig. 6 ■ Initial situation. The malposition of lateral incisors is evident, but the patient prefers to respect his original aspect.

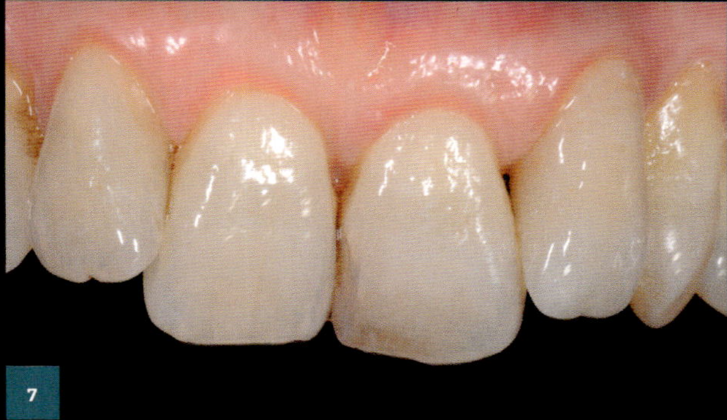

Fig. 7 ■ 1-year clinical follow-up. The implant and the crown were designed to respect the symmetry of contralateral tooth and the position of the natural tooth that has been lost, and to allow the maximum bone-implant contact, without extracting the resorbed root.

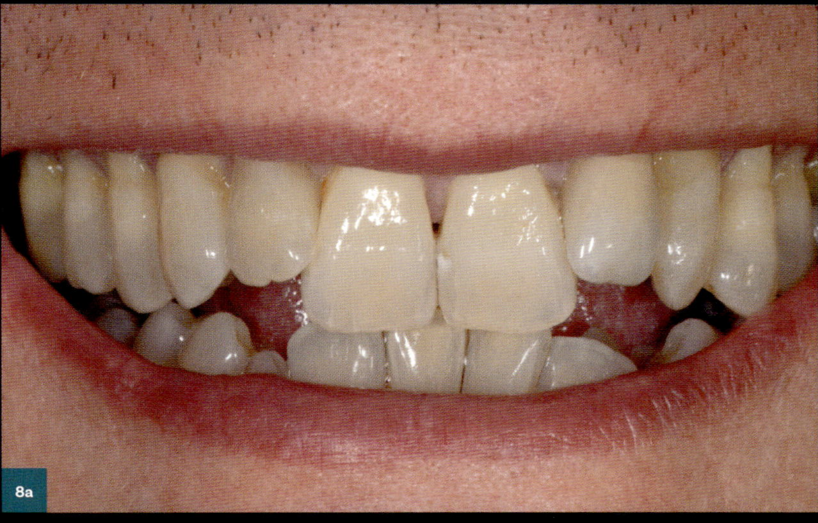

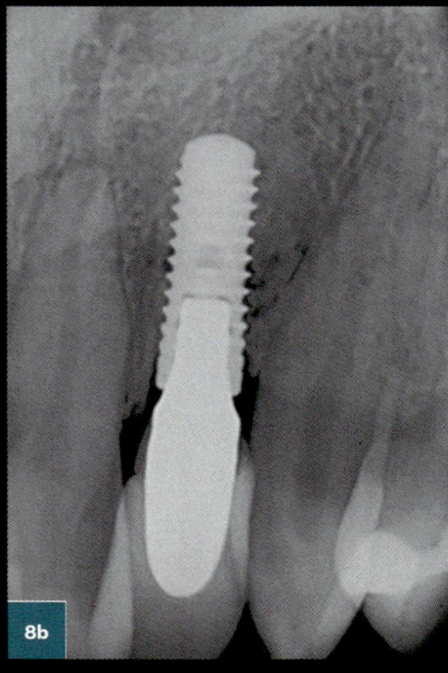

Figs. 8a,b ■ **a:** 12-year clinical follow-up; **b**: 12-year radiographic follow-up. Mesial to the implant, note the portion of root intentionally left in place to improve support of the soft tissues.

Bibliography

1. Consolaro A. External cervical resorption: diagnostic and treatment tips. *Dental Press J Orthod.* 2016;21(5):19-25.
2. Pop Dentistry, 2019, 16 maggio. Management of internal and external resorptions - Clinical case. Video YouTube: www.youtube.com/watch?v=RY5mal5npNk.
3. Malmgren O, Goldson L, Hill C, Orwin A, Petrini L, Lundberg M. Root resorption after orthodontic treatment of traumatized teeth. *Am J Orthod.* 1982;82(6):487-491.
4. Consolaro A, Furquim LZ. Extreme root resorption associated with induced tooth movement: a protocol for clinical management. *Dental Press J Orthod.* 2014;19(5):19-26.
5. Lind V. Short root anomaly. *Scand J Dent Res.* 1972;80(2):85-93.
6. Valladares Neto J, Rino Neto J, de Paiva JB. Orthodontic movement of teeth with short root anomaly: Should it be avoided, faced or ignored? *Dental Press J Orthod.* 2013;18(6):72-85.
7. Nilsson E, Bonte E, Bayet F, Lasfargues JJ. Management of internal root resorption on permanent teeth. *Int J Dent.* 2013;2013:929486.
8. Heithersay GS. Management of tooth resorption. *Aust Dent J.* 2007;52(1 Suppl.):S105-S121.
9. Style Italiano Endodontics, 2018, 30 maggio. Invasive tooth resorption. The video. Video Facebook: www.facebook.com/styleitalianoendodontics/videos/1974568739522544.
10. Style Italiano Endodontics, 2018, 5 dicembre. Female 27 yrs old - Invasive external cervical resorption. Video Facebook: https://www.facebook.com/styleitalianoendodontics/videos/669138393481026.
11. Javaheri DS, Garibaldi JA. Forceps extraction of teeth with severe internal root resorption. *J Am Dent Assoc.* 1997;128(6);751-754.
12. Brånemark PI, Hansson BO, Adell R, et al. Osseointegrated implants in the treatment of the edentulous jaw. Experience from a 10-year period. *Scand J Plast Reconstr Surg Suppl.* 1977;16:1-132.
13. Szmukler-Moncler S, Davarpanah M, Davarpanah K, et al. Unconventional Implant Placement Part III: Implant Placement Encroaching upon Residual Roots - A Report of Six Cases. *Clin Implant Dent Relat Res.* 2015;17 Suppl 2:e396-405.
14. Buser D, Warrer K, Karring T. Formation of a periodontal ligament around titanium implants. *J Periodontol.* 1990;61(9):597-601.
15. Gray JL, Vernino AR. The interface between retained roots and dental implants: a histologic study in baboons. *J Periodontol.* 2004;75(8):1102-1106.
16. Davarpanah M, Szmukler-Moncler S. Unconventional implant treatment: I. Implant placement in contact with ankylosed root fragments. A series of five case reports. *Clin Oral Implants Res.* 2009;20(8):851-856.
17. Davarpanah M, Szmukler-Moncler S. Unconventional implant placement. 2: Placement of implants through impacted teeth. Three case reports. *Int J Periodontics Restorative Dent.* 2009;29(4):405-413.
18. Szmukler-Moncler S, Davarpanah M, Davarpanah KK, Rajzbaum P, Capelle-Ouadah N, Demurashvili G. Implants in contact with tissues other than bone. Is there room for a potential paradigm shift? *Swiss Dent J.* 2014;124(2):149-164.
19. Mazor Z, Segal P, Levin L. Computer-guided implant placement for rehabilitation of the edentulous maxilla with two impacted canines: an approach without extraction of the impacted teeth. *Int J Periodontics Restorative Dent.* 2015;35(1):93-97.
20. Labidi A, Bekri S, Mansour L, Ghoul-Mazgar S. Implants Placement in Contact with Dental Tissue: A Potential Paradigm Shift? Systematic Literature Review. *Eur J Dent.* 2019;13(4):642-648.
21. Pérez-González F, Sánchez-Labrador L, Molinero-Mourelle P, et al. Dental implant placement through impacted teeth or residual roots as an alternative to invasive extraction surgeries: a systematic literature review. *Br J Oral Maxillofac Surg.* 2021;59(10):1120-1129.
22. Nevins ML, Langer L, Schupbach P. Late dental implant failures associated with retained root fragments: case reports with histologic and SEM analysis. *Int J Periodontics Restorative Dent.* 2018;38(1):9-15.
23. Langer L, Langer B, Salem D. Unintentional root fragment retention in proximity to dental implants: a series of six human case reports. *Int J Periodontics Restorative Dent.* 2015;35(3):305-313.
24. Davarpanah M, Szmukler-Moncler S, Rajzbaum P, Davarpanah K, Capelle-Ouadah N, Demurashvili G. Unconventional implant placement. V: Implant placement through impacted teeth; results from 10 cases with an 8- to 1-year follow-up. *Int Orthod.* 2015;13(2):164-180.
25. Amato F, Macca U, Amato G, Mirabella D. Immediate loading of implants inserted through impacted teeth in the esthetic area: a series of 10 cases with up to 7 years of follow-up. *Int J Periodontics Restorative Dent.* 2019;39(3):325-332.
26. Malmgren B. Decoronation: how, why, and when? *J Calif Dent Assoc.* 2000;28(11):846-854.
27. Cohenca N, Stabholz A. Decoronation - a conservative method to treat ankylosed teeth for preservation of alveolar ridge prior to permanent prosthetic reconstruction: literature review and case presentation. *Dent Traumatol.* 2007;23(2):87-94.
28. Malmgren B. Ridge preservation/decoronation. *J Endod.* 2013;39(3 Suppl):S67-S72.
29. Consolaro A, Ribeiro Júnior PD, Cardoso MA, Miranda DAO, Salfatis M. Decoronation followed by dental implants placement: fundamentals, applications and explanations. *Dental Press J Orthod.* 2018;23(1):24-36.
30. Tischler M. Grafting the anterior maxilla after tooth loss from external resorption. A case report. *Dent Today.* 2002;21(4):90-93.
31. Scheuber S, Bosshardt D, Brägger U, von Arx T. Implantattherapie nach Frontzahntrauma. Eine neue Methode zum Erhalt des Alveolarkammes nach posttraumatischer Ankylose und externer Wurzelresorption. *Schweiz Monatsschr Zahnmed.* 2013;123(5):417-439.
32. Sapir S, Kalter A, Sapir MR. Decoronation of an ankylosed permanent incisor: alveolar ridge preservation and rehabilitation by an implant supported porcelain crown. *Dent Traumatol.* 2009;25(3):346-349.
33. Checchi V, Bertani P, Generali P, Generali L. Computer-guided implant placement in contact with root remnants in the esthetic area. *Quintessence Int.* 2021;52(2):132-137.

16

Autotransplantation

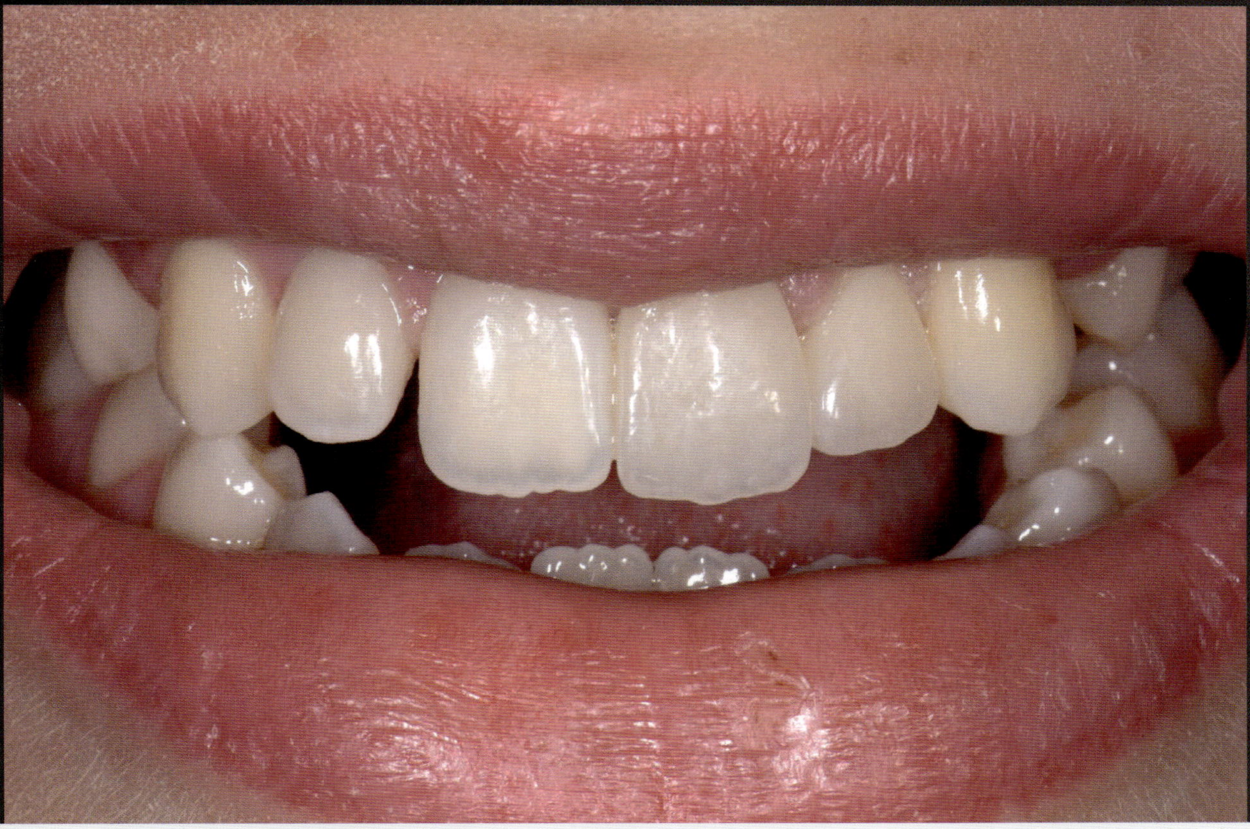

Introduction

The prognosis of a natural tooth, even when compromised by periodontal or endodontic diseases, remains more reliable and lasting than a potentially replacing implant. However, certain cases necessitate immediate extraction of a severely compromised tooth. In these situations, dental autotransplantation is among the available options.

Dental autotransplantation, or autogenous transplantation, refers to repositioning a tooth within the same patient's mouth. This may involve moving impacted or erupted teeth to post-extraction sites or surgically prepared sites.[1,2]

This technique offers numerous advantages. It maintains the periodontal ligament, ensuring proprioception and supporting dento-facial development and jaw growth. Furthermore, the transplanted tooth remains adaptable for orthodontic adjustments. When the donor tooth has incomplete root development, it allows for pulp vitality preservation and ongoing root development. Finally, an autotransplanted tooth sustains bone volume, facilitating potential future implant restoration in adults.[3]

History

The origins of this practice can be traced to ancient Egypt, where slaves offered their healthy teeth as gifts to pharaohs who had lost their teeth.[4] In the 18th and 19th centuries, multi-person dental transplants were prevalent in specialized dental facilities in London. Surprisingly, these allografts had an average lifespan of six years. However, compatibility issues led to the abandonment of this technique, which was subsequently replaced by autotransplantation. The technique's precise description was first provided by Hale in 1956, and the principles outlined remain applicable.[5]

Indications, contraindications and prognosis

In young patients, compromised first molars predominantly warrant third molar autotransplantation. Additionally, restoratively or endodontically compromised second molars are suitable candidates. Since the end of the 1950s, Scandinavian countries have employed premolar autotransplantation of premolars in the frontal regions, particularly post-trauma. Ectopic canines can also necessitate autotransplantation.[6] Currently, due to consistently reliable long-term results, autotransplantation stands as a viable therapeutic option,[7,8] despite some studies noting inadequate subject knowledge. Notably, comprehensive studies in this area are lacking in both undergraduate and postgraduate university courses.[9] Favourable prognostic factors include young age (15-25 years); donor tooth with open apex and root length ranging from 2/3rd to fully developed; potential for atraumatic extraction and immediate repositioning of the donor tooth; optimal dental element with suitable root morphology, position and crown size; absence of inflammation; sufficient bone volume and quality; correct management of operation duration, stabilization type, proper follow-up, and appropriate timing for potential endodontic treatment.[10-14]

Contraindications include deciduous dentition, uncooperative patients, and heavily restored or otherwise compromised donor elements. The presence of an infected recipient site is debatable. Some Authors consider it non-contraindicative, while others differ.[15] Immediate autotransplantation into an endodontically infected site, after adequate recipient site treatment involving primary mechanical disinfection followed by irrigant disinfection, can be successful.[16] The success hinges on whether the endodontic or periodontal infection is biofilm-related within the root canal system or on the root surface.[17] Extracting the compromised element under antibiotic cover, followed by adequate site irrigation, seems logically effective in infection control.

Patient selection is critical. Candidates must be in good health, have excellent oral hygiene, and commit to regular follow-up to preserve the transplant prognosis. The transplanted element must align with the recipient site suitability criteria listed above. Effective cooperation and understanding between patient and dentist are essential to ensure successful outcomes.

Success, failure and risk factors

The success of an autotransplantation relies on the periodontal ligament's vitality. Appropriate case selection and correct surgical technique lead to high

success and survival rates. Mejare et al.'s prospective study reported a 4-year survival of 81.4%.[18] Other studies have shown rates of 71-95% over 10 years of follow-up,[19] comparable to or even better than implants.[12] A systematic review with meta-analysis of cases of autotransplanted teeth with completed apices reveals 98% 1-year survival and 90.5% 5-year survival.[20] Similar research indicates 97.4%, 97.8%, and 96.3% survival at 1, 5 and 10 years, respectively.[21]
While the survival percentage rate of the transplanted elements in the arch is very high, success demands the absence of undesirable outcomes like ankylosis, excessive mobility, pulp necrosis or obliteration, and root resorption. These outcomes are influenced by various factors studied extensively,[20,22] including age,[23-26] gender,[27] development stage,[28-30] root anatomy,[31] adequate bone support,[32] atraumatic surgical technique,[33] precise transplanted tooth adaptation in the recipient site,[34] technique and stabilization time,[35] operator expertise,[36] timing of the occlusal loading,[37] and endodontic treatment.[38] Moreover, the presence of infection in the recipient site also plays a role. The factor ensuring maximum survival of a transplanted tooth within the arch, as by a systematic literature review with meta-analysis,[23] is the transplanted tooth's open apex. Teeth with closed apices are more prone to ankylosis, pulp necrosis, and root resorption. Moreover, teeth stabilized using sutures show greater resistance to future extraction compared to those stabilized with orthodontic wire and composite materials. Another meta-analysis[21] identified risk factors, such as lack of antibiotic prophylaxis, rigid fixation and early endodontic treatment within the first 14 days after transplantation. Ankylosis and resorption were more frequent in the anterior, premolar and canine elements.
In conclusion, autotransplantation failure risk is below 10%, dropping to around 3% for teeth with open apices. It is worth noting that, in case of resorption, endodontic treatment with intermediate medications like Ca(OH)2 can potentially halt or even reverse the process.[39,40]

Planning

Prior to autotransplantation, a comprehensive clinical and radiographic examination is essential, followed by careful treatment planning. If the recipient site's mesio-distal dimension does not align with the donor tooth, orthodontic space creation might be necessary before the transplantation. Conversely, the inadequate buccolingual bone volume could warrant the evaluation of regenerative techniques at the recipient site.[4] Pre-operative radiographs also assess apico-coronal recipient site dimensions and donor root length, with possible intraoperative correction of recipient socket depth. Ideally, transplantation is best performed with the donor tooth having the maximal root trunk and potential for pulp regeneration (radiographic apex opening > 1 mm).[7] Root morphology must adapt to the recipient site and ideally converge. Molars exhibit higher failure rates yet fewer post-operative complications (e.g., ankylosis, root resorption). This apparent contradiction might be attributed - pending conclusive data - to the larger root surface, acting as a protective factor against masticatory load, albeit with potential improper surgical socket adaptation.[4]

Technique

Dental autotransplantation involves avulsion followed by a planned reimplantation to minimize trauma. The recipient site is prepared by completely extracting the compromised tooth and curetting the alveolus to remove granulomatous tissues. Here, the donor tooth is gently extracted and placed in the new socket, aiming for minimal mobility. When the fit is satisfactory, immediate tooth placement occurs without further socket preparation. Incongruity necessitates alveolar preparation using drills under saline irrigation until a correct adaptation is achieved. Meantime, the transplant can be stored in a saline solution or temporarily repositioned in the original socket. Once the site preparation has been completed, the element is placed slightly below the occlusal plane (at least 1-2 mm), with adjusted interproximal contact points. Fixation involves crossed mattress sutures on the occlusal surface, possibly retained by composite resin.

Long-term follow-up

At the end of the operation, the patient should receive instructions on correct oral hygiene and be advised to avoid chewing on the operated side. Follow-up appointments are then scheduled: after 7 days to assess suture stability and after 14 days for suture removal. Thereafter, weekly appointments are advised for one month if no complications arise. Finally, check-ups are scheduled at 2/3 months for endodontic treatment, while radiographic follow-up is scheduled at 6-12-24. During the healing process, the transplanted element positioned in infraocclusion emerges. Contact with the opposing arch represents an important sign of periodontal healing for the clinician, while its alarming absence indicates ankylosis. Throughout post-surgery appointments, the tooth must be evaluated clinically and radiographically to exclude the pulp damage noted by intrapulpal calcification, periapical radiolucency or root resorption. Literature data[16] supports that the success of the dental autotransplantation technique hinges on infection-free and inflammation-free recipient sites. However, adequate alveolar bone support in all dimensions and ample keratinized tissue are essential for correctly restoring biological width around the transplanted tooth.

Need for endodontic treatment

In the clinical management of the donor tooth, the approach varies based on whether it has an open or closed apex. The major difference between the two conditions lies in the potential risk of operation failure due to the onset of pulpal pathology. For teeth with fully developed roots and closed apices, several authors recommend prior endodontic treatment before[12,41,42] or within 14 days after transplantation,[4,12] as revascularization and pulpal healing are less likely due to the narrow apical foramen diameter and root length.[43,44] Transplanting a tooth with a completed root does not permit pulp regeneration.[34] Therefore, this successful therapeutic outcome requires prior endodontic treatment.[22] For teeth with a mature apex, the healing process involves substantial pulp necrosis, with revascularization limited to 1-2 mm apically, according to Andreasen. Additionally, the coronal segment is susceptible to ischemic effects, raising the risk of secondary infection.[45] Therefore, through endodontic therapy, inflammatory processes affecting the pulp that could endanger the operation's prognosis are prevented.[4] Chung et al.[20] demonstrated demonstrated a 50% reduction in root resorption rates after autotransplantation when endodontic treatment is performed within 14 days of surgery. Additionally, if the donor tooth is easily accessible, root canal therapy can be performed prior to atraumatic tooth extraction and surgery.[7,34,46] For autotransplanted teeth with complete root formation, endodontic treatment is important, although its optimal timing is still controversial. While various guidelines suggest performing root canal treatment 7-14 days post-autotransplantation,[12,47] recent systematic reviews[48] and meta-analyses[4] have shown comparable failure rates, irrespective of whether the treatment is done within 2 weeks or after it. However, postponing the treatment increases the risk of rhizolysis, as confirmed by previous studies.

Periodontal ligament

One of the critical factors contributing to successful autotransplantation is the presence of periodontal ligament fibres (PDL). It is always advisable to extract a tooth with a sufficient amount of adhering periodontal ligament. This prevents root resorption[4] and supports the formation of the new periodontal attachment.[7]
Healing is rapid, and function is regained almost immediately. The transplanted tooth, with its ligament, maintains osteo-inducing properties, leading to bone defect regeneration around the transplants without graft materials. This reduces time and costs significantly compared to peri-implant regenerative techniques, especially unsuitable for young patients.[7, 27,49]

3D Radiology

Three-dimensional imaging techniques enhanced planning for optimal shape and size, increasing the success and survival rates of transplanted teeth.[8,50,51] A recent study on 100 autotransplanted teeth concluded that a CBCT-guided approach increases the treatment predictability compared to the conventional methods, enabling accurate surgical planning.[52] Some authors[53-55] suggested a alternative use of three-dimensional techniques. Pre-surgical volumetric data can be used to create a stereolithographic print of the maxillary bone and the donor tooth. This removable element allows the operator to prepare the receiving site even before extracting the tooth with a sterilized prototype. This minimizes the extra-alveolar time for the transplanted tooth and reduces associated risks. Furthermore, the anatomical replica allows the surgeon to preview the recipient site, assess volumes and predict any additional preparatory therapies.

Autotransplantation of incompletely formed teeth

Autotransplantation achieves the highest success rates when root development is between half and two-thirds. Transplanting a tooth bud with less than half-formed roots can excessively traumatize and hinder further development.

Teeth with developing roots and open apices show improved prognosis[11] and typically undergo endodontical treatment only upon detecting symptoms of periapical inflammation or its onset.[22]

The transplanted tooth's open apex allows pulp tissue regeneration, which generally negates the need for endodontic intervention.[22,27,56,57] Teeth with immature apices have a particular histological feature, i.e., Hertwig's epithelial sheath, an epithelial-origin membrane that separates the pulp from the dental follicle. Preservation of this sheath is essential for proper root growth, with damage during tooth extraction or repositioning can lead to arrested root formation and periapical invagination of the surrounding bone tissue, usually with maintained periodontal space. Autotransplantation-associated pulp healing occasionally manifests through radiographic indications of pulp obliteration and incomplete apexification.

Post-traumatic pulp healing may involve replacing the pulp organ with bone, periodontal ligament and cementum, leading to tissue metamorphosis or pulp metaplasia.[58,59] Although these phenomena are typically considered pathological after traumatic lesions, they are considered part of a normal post-dental transplant recovery.[60] Despite inflammation following pulp necrosis, Hertwig's epithelial sheath continues to function, demonstrating that root development alone is not a criterion for diagnosing pulp vitality.

Pulp healing of the transplanted teeth with immature apices follows well-defined stages. Microangiography and contrast medium reveal blood vessels in the apical half of canals after ten days post-surgery, extending throughout the pulp after 30 days. Consequently, the coronal half of the pulp survives without vascular supply for weeks. The revascularization of pulpal horns and the entire endodontium occurs over more than 30 days. The coronal area may experience aseptic necrosis. Regardless, 6 months post-surgery, pulpal blood vessels generally decrease, favouring partial or complete obliteration by dentinal tissue.[61]

Even with necrosis, well-vascularized connective tissue initiates repair, reaching the pulpal horn around 30 days post-operation. If the pulp tissue survives post-operation, it has a normal radiographic appearance and histological odontoblastic survival signs. Andreasen[45] also noted immediate coronal necrosis due to ischemic damage during extraction, with revascularization beginning at 4 days from the apical foramen, where the damaged pulp tissue is gradually replaced by proliferating and capillary mesenchymal cells. Revascularization completes within 4-5 weeks post-operation, where some cases with anastomosis between newly formed vessels and those of the transplanted element, achieving early revascularization, even one week post-surgery.

The healing process first forms osteo-dentine, a hard tissue lacking dentinal tubules and occasionally incorporating cells. In some cases, canal wall cells subsequently begin transforming into odontoblasts, resulting in a layer of tubular dentin.

Based on both animal and human studies, nerve fibre regeneration usually occurs around 1 to 2 months post-operation.[62] However, the best time for an autotransplantation surgery aligns with the radiographic evidence of an apical foramen (2 mm) and 50-75% root development.[63] Transplanting a tooth with an open apex is normally indicated in 12-year-old (using premolar elements) or 18-year-old (using third molars) patients. This approach is recommended in these patients due to ongoing maxillofacial growth and contraindications for titanium dental implant placement.

Prognosis of autotransplantation of incompletely formed teeth

Upon reviewing the literature, it becomes evident that autotransplanting teeth with immature apices has a very favourable prognosis. Many authors have measured the survival rates of premolars and molars with immature apices undergoing autotransplantation, reporting short-term survival rates ranging from 88.4% to 100%.[8,22,23,33,64-67]

Likewise, the success rates appear high, meeting the essential criteria for defining method success: absence of endodontic pathologies, suppuration, bone defects, periodontal pockets and post-surgery resumption of root development.[7,57]

Regarding the long-term prognosis, several reviews reported similar data. Andreasen et al. followed 370 autotransplanted premolars for 1-13 years and reported a 95% long-term survival for teeth with incomplete root formation.[14] Czochrowska et al. reported a 90% survival rate for 33 teeth after 17-41 years.[60] Jonsson and Sigurdsson's 2-22-year follow-up of 40 premolars resulted in a 97.5% survival rate.[68] Additionally, Watanabe et al., based on extended data with a mean follow-up of 9.2 years, recommended performing tooth transplantation before complete root development. They also highlighted the vital importance of high-quality root canal obturation for the long-term prognosis, as inadequate endodontic treatment has been linked to failure or pathology in most failed transplants.[69] Finally, Rohof's meta-analysis, incorporating 32 studies on immature teeth, reported survival rates of 97.4%, 97.8%, and 96.3% at 1, 5 and 10 years, respectively, with a complication rate of < 5%.[70] Similarly, Van Westerveld reported an overall cumulative survival rate of 95.4% for all transplanted teeth, varying slightly by tooth used.[71]

Additional authors corroborated this conclusion, hypothesizing that root morphology and extraction-related challenges can cause iatrogenic periodontal damage.[27,72,73]

Chung et al.'s[20] meta-analysis showed a 2% failure rate for self-transplanted mature apex teeth, with 1-year and 5-year survival rates at approximately 98% and 90.5%, respectively. These findings were consistent with those from a long-term observational study by Andreasen.[12]

Autotransplantation of impacted or malpositioned teeth

The complex series of events from dental germ emergence to the tooth eruption in its correct position can be disrupted by various events leading to dental impaction.

Predominantly, third molars are impacted, with canines (the upper ones more often than the lower ones) also experiencing partial or complete impaction.

Infrequently, other elements may encounter failed eruption incidents.

When feasible space is available, a common treatment involves surgical exposure followed by the application of orthodontic forces to align the tooth functionally. In cases of insufficient arch space, orthodontic treatment is required first to create sufficient space to accommodate the tooth.

For impacted teeth in an unfavourable position—deviating significantly from the norm or distant from their intended location—complex orthodontic correction may necessitate avulsion and reimplantation at the appropriate site.

The presence of supernumerary elements is a factor causing dental impaction, can hinder proper permanent tooth eruption and needs surgical removal.

In some instances, considering simultaneous extraction and reimplantation of the impacted tooth to its definitive site during surgery may be warranted.

In the clinical cases of this chapter, a 12-year-old boy presented a rare partial inclusion of an upper premolar fused to a supernumerary, which prevented its eruption. Extracting and reimplanting the premolar, post-separation of the twin teeth, and extraoral endodontic treatment ensured tooth persistence in the arch, thereby yielding predictable positive functional and bone development outcomes.

Given the absence of a periodontal ligament on the complete sectioned root due to supernumerary coalescence suggests a potential future root resorption. However, the clinical consequences of any resorption will occur when bone development nears completion, leaving an optimal implant placement site.

Conclusions

In conclusion, the autotransplantation technique offers numerous periodontal ligament preservation-related advantages.

The proprioceptive function is maintained and alveolar bone volume is preserved. The dentofacial development and the jaw growth remain uncompromised, allowing for orthodontic treatment. Furthermore, when using a donor tooth with incomplete root development, it is feasible to maintain pulp vitality and support ongoing root development.[74,75]

Some exemplary clinical cases of the autotransplantation technique are illustrated below, performed with different indications and described in the captions.

CLINICAL CASES

Autotransplantation of 48 in site 46 with follow-up at 19 years

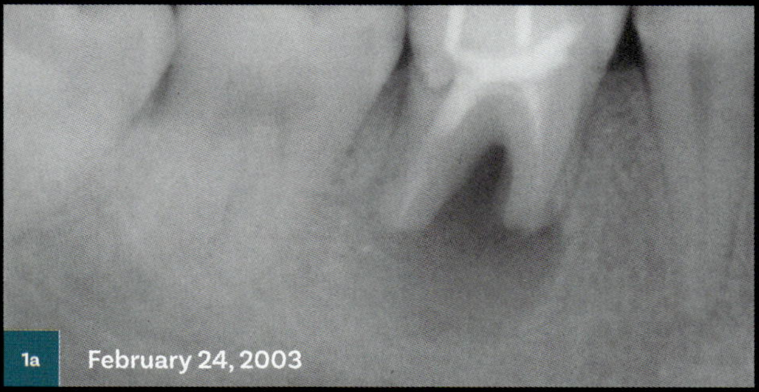

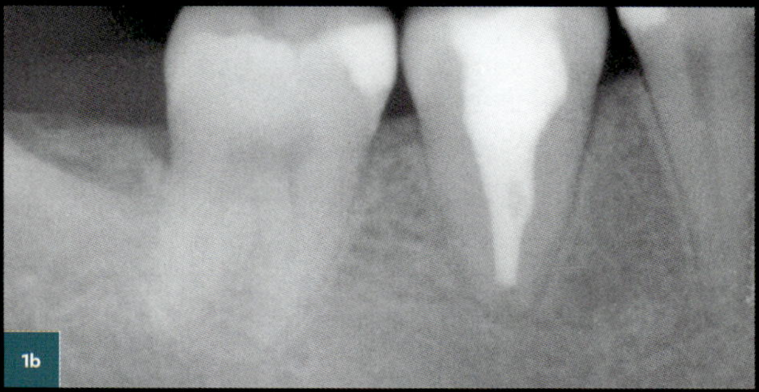

Fig. 1a ■ The patient, A.V.M., aged 16, presents with the 46 which is not suitable for further conservative procedures. The 48 has the requisites to be a good candidate for autotransplantation.

Fig. 1b ■ Periapical Rx after 6 months.

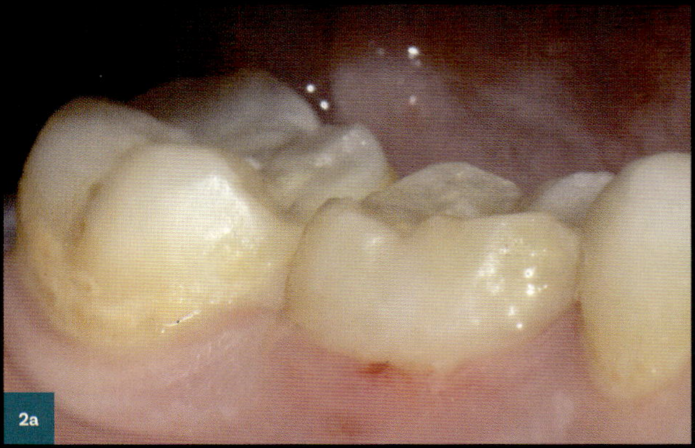

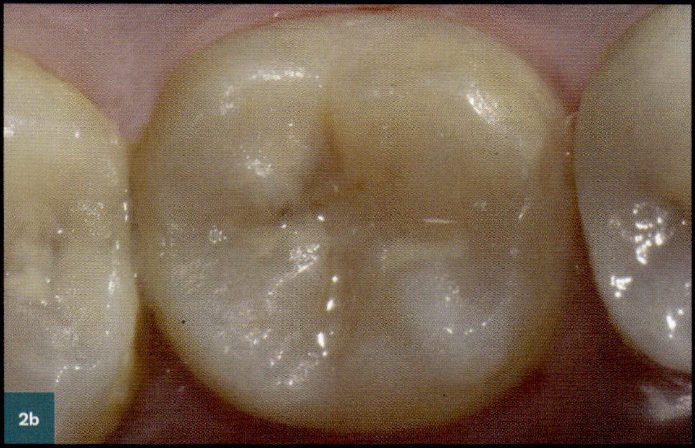

Figs. 2a,b ■ Clinical images at 6 months.

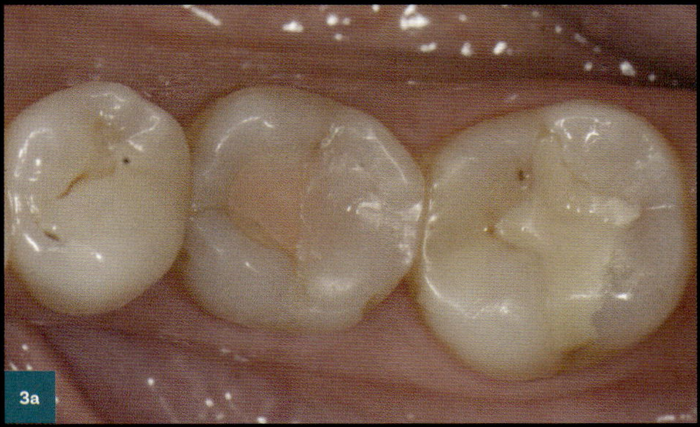

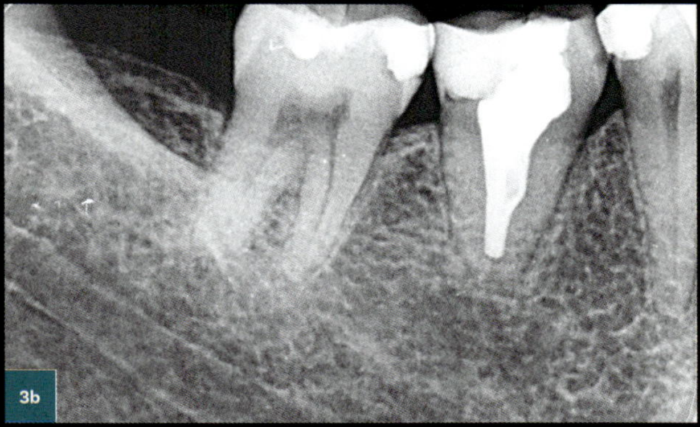

Figs. 3a,b ■ Clinical and radiographic check-up 19 years following autotransplantation.

Autotransplantation of 18 in position 17

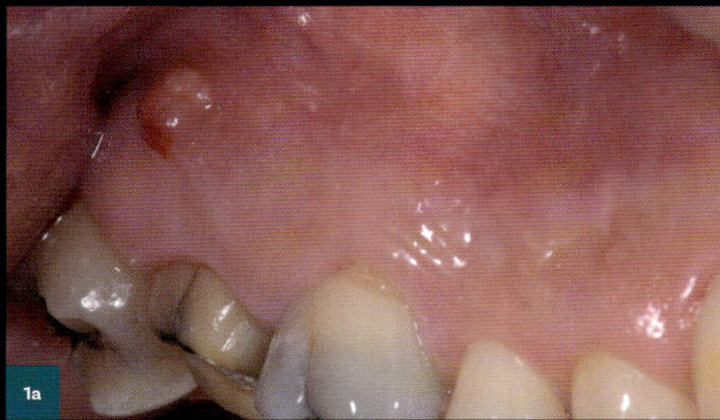

Fig. 1a ■ The 33-year-old patient, M.C., was referred to evaluate the possibility of retreating tooth 17. The tooth has already been subjected to two attempts at endodontic treatment, without resolution of the symptoms, and indeed with the appearance of a fistula. Clinical examination with intraoral X-ray and CBCT is carried out. a: buccal view, with fistula.

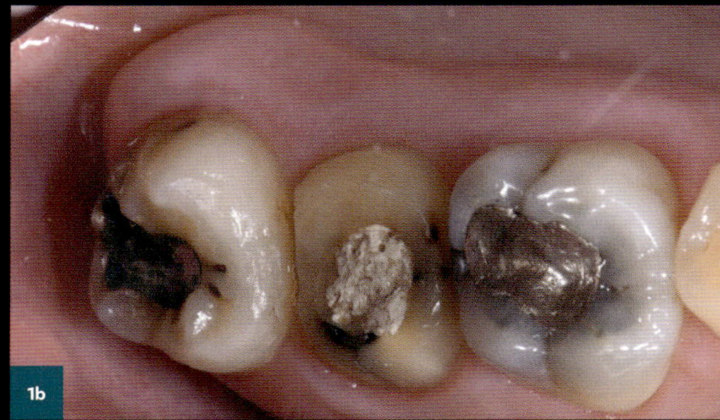

Fig. 1b ■ Occlusal view.

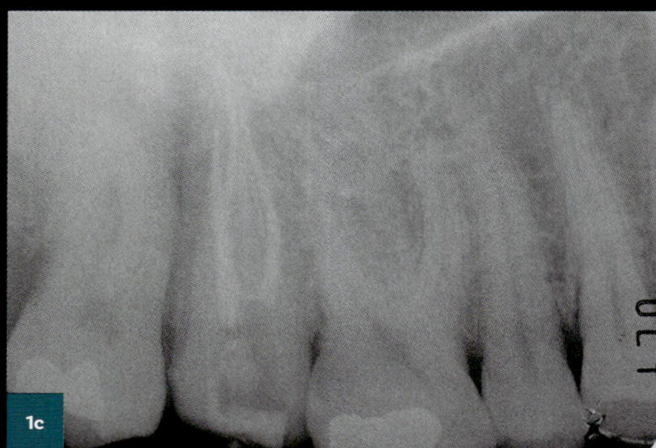

Fig. 1c ■ Periapical Rx.

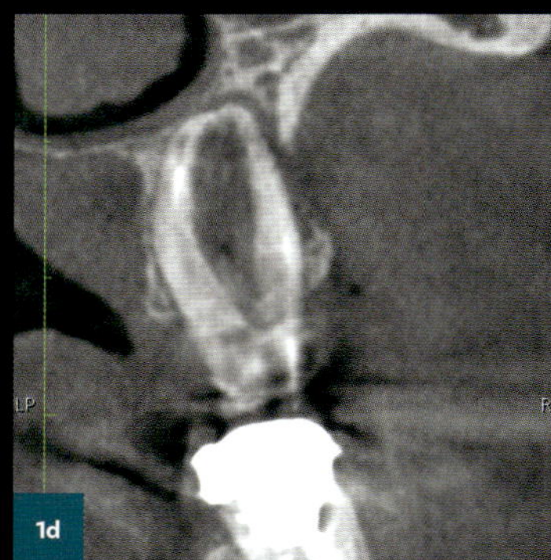

Fig. 1d ■ Bucco-lingual section of CBCT.

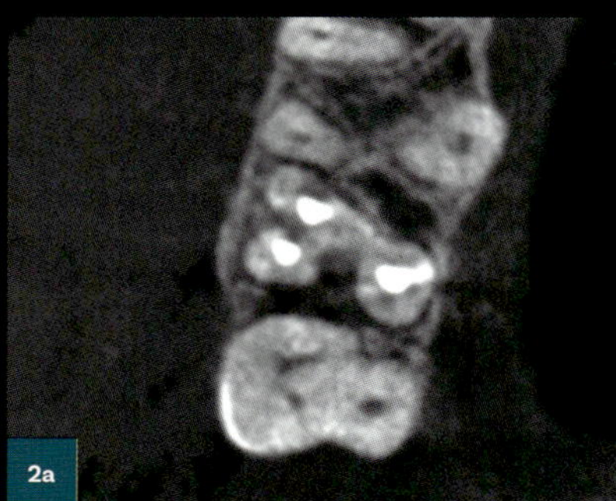

Fig. 2a ■ Horizontal section that shows perforation of pulp chamber floor.

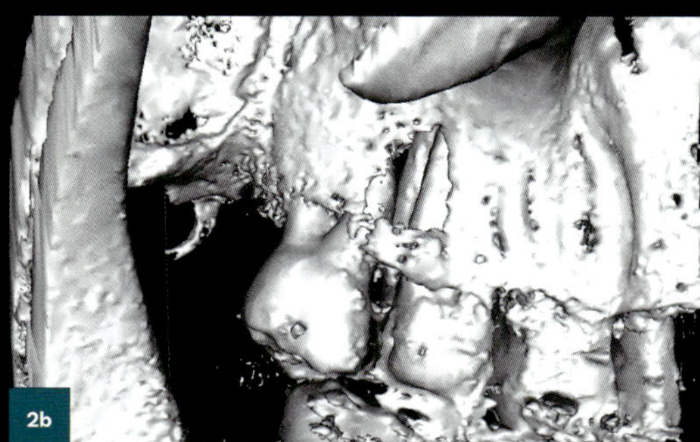

Fig. 2b ■ 3 D reconstruction that shows the bone defect between 17 and 18.

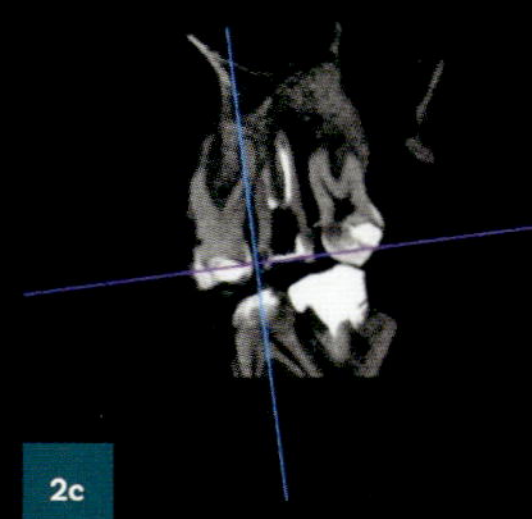

Fig. 2c ■ Sagittal section.

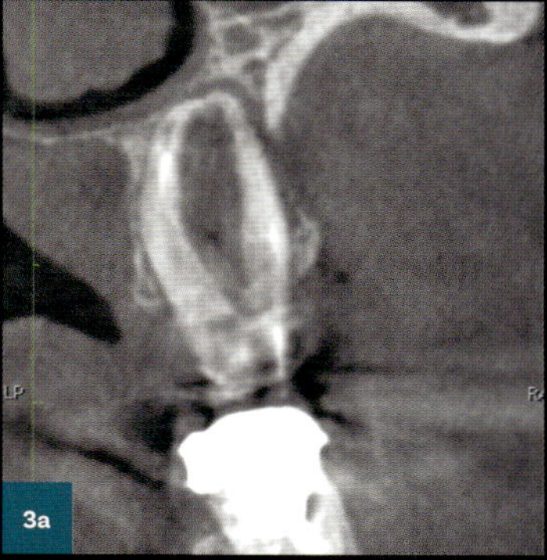

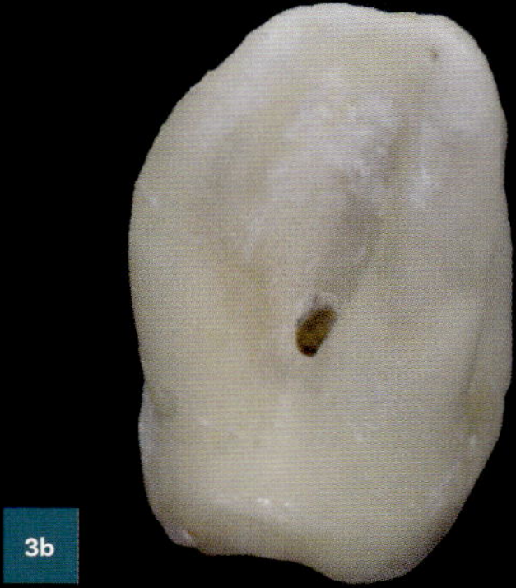

Fig. 3a ▪ The presence of a long-standing floor perforation (existing for three years) suggests that the result of another orthograde retreatment is highly unpredictable. The large size of the lesion is another negative prognostic factor. After discussing with the patient, it was decided to proceed with the extraction of tooth 17 and the contextual autotransplantation of tooth 18. **a**: coronal section.

Fig. 3b ▪ Extracted tooth with perforation.

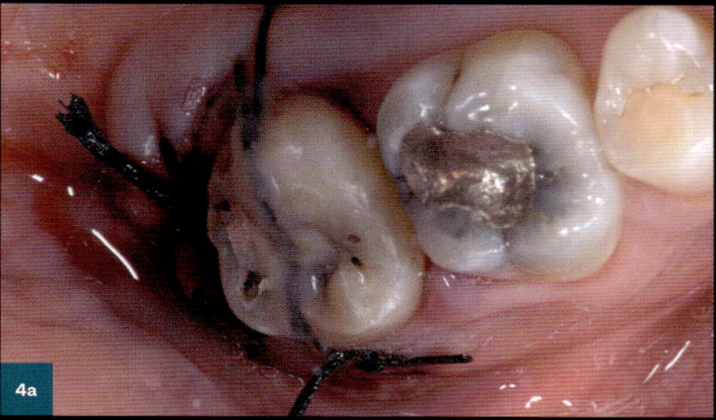

Fig. 4a ▪ Autotransplantation was just performed. Tooth 18 is secured in the alveolus of the tooth 17 using suture, and then fixed with flow composite on the occlusal surface.

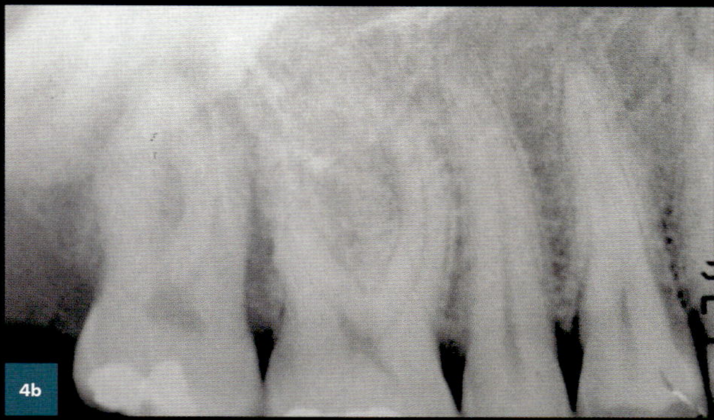

Fig. 4b ▪ Periapical Rx.

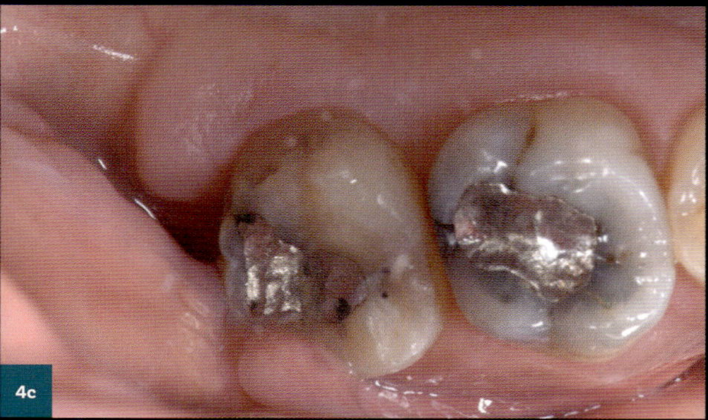

Fig. 4c ▪ Check-up after 2 weeks, following removal of the sutures.

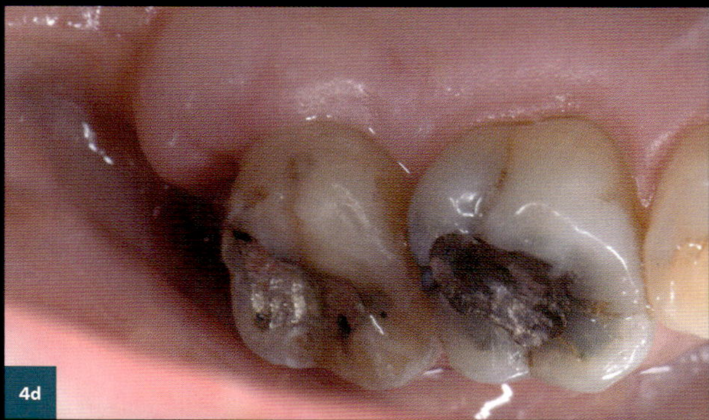

Fig. 4d ▪ Check-up after 2 months.

CONT'D >

> CONT'D

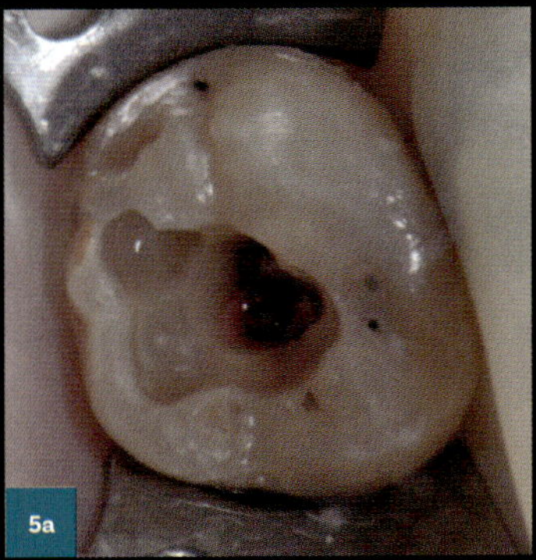

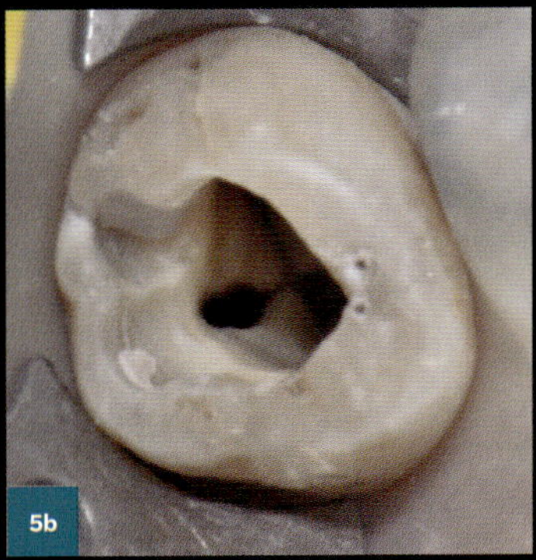

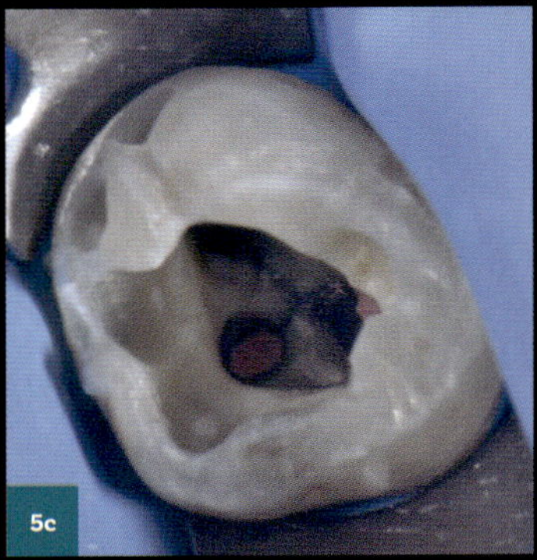

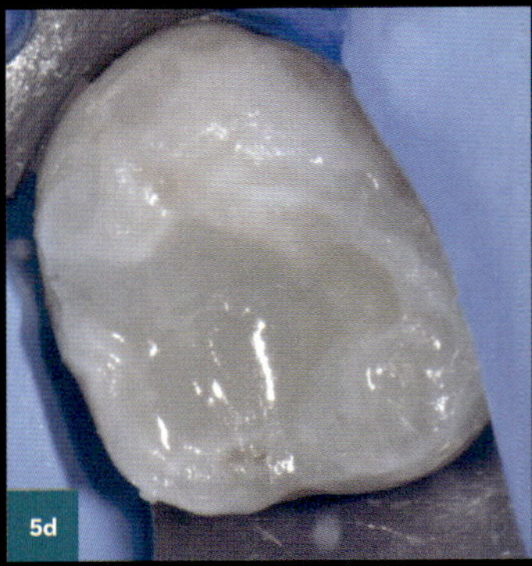

Fig. 5a ■ Endodontic treatment 2 months following transplantation. **a**: access cavity.

Fig. 5b ■ Instrumented canals.

Fig. 5c ■ Canal obturation.

Fig. 5d ■ Closure of access cavity.

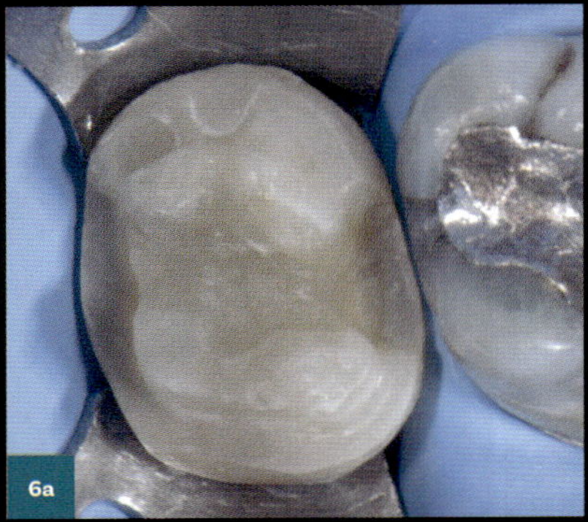

Fig. 6a ■ Onlay preparation.

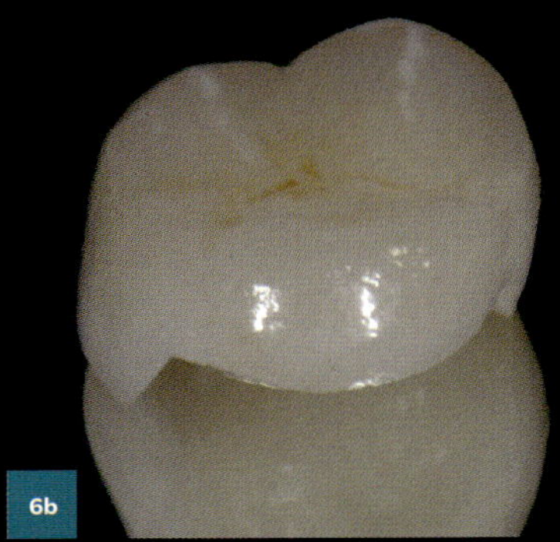

Fig. 6b ■ Onlay in lithium disilicate.

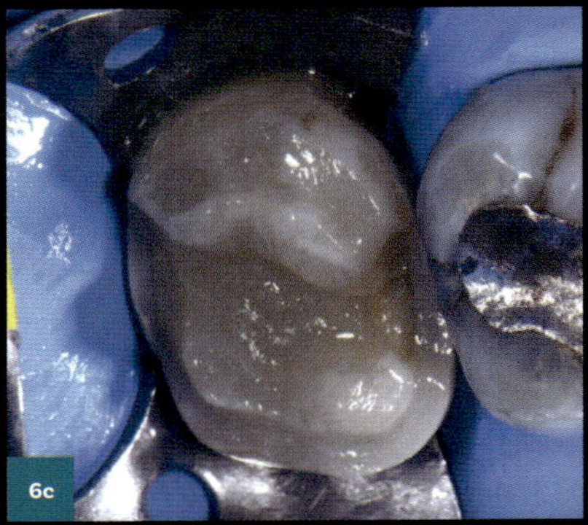

Fig. 6c ■ Adhesion.

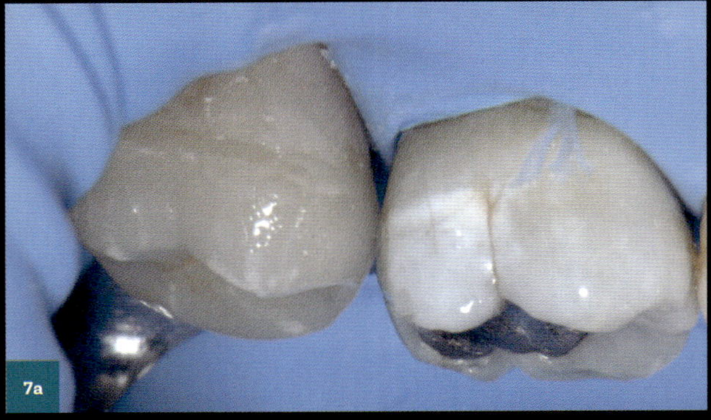

Fig. 7a ■ Buccal view of cemented onlay.

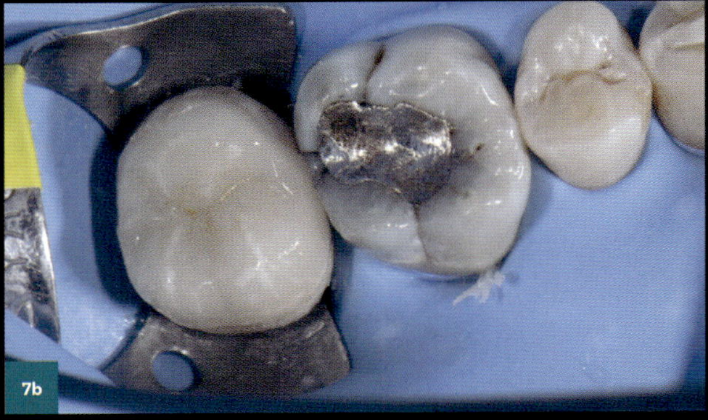

Fig. 7b ■ Occlusal view of cemented onlay.

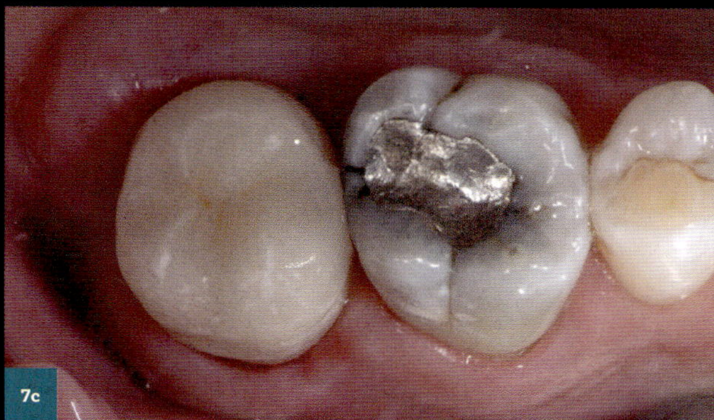

Fig. 7c ■ After rubber dam removal.

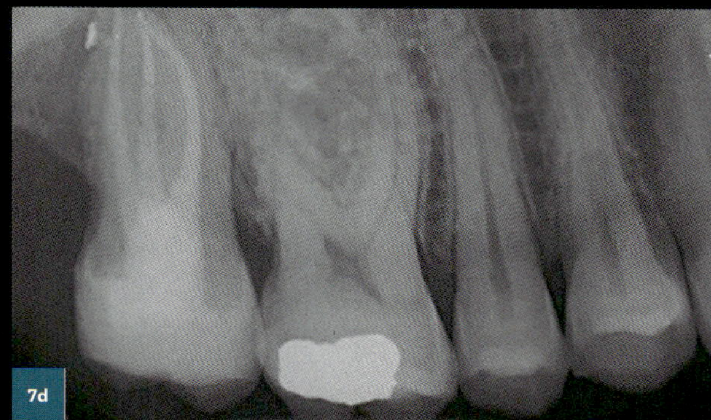

Fig. 7d ■ Check-up with periapical radiograph.

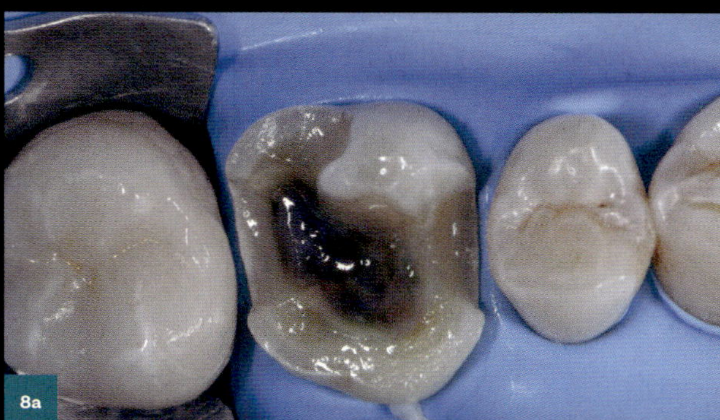

Fig. 8a ■ The treatment of the sextant is concluded by carrying out an overlay on tooth 16, which presented a deteriorated amalgam and various discontinuities and cracks. At one year, the remarkable stability of the hard and soft tissues can be noted. **a**: preparation.

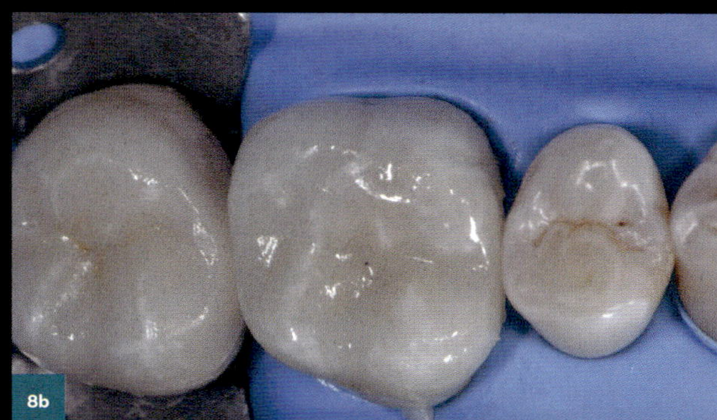

Fig. 8b ■ Cementation.

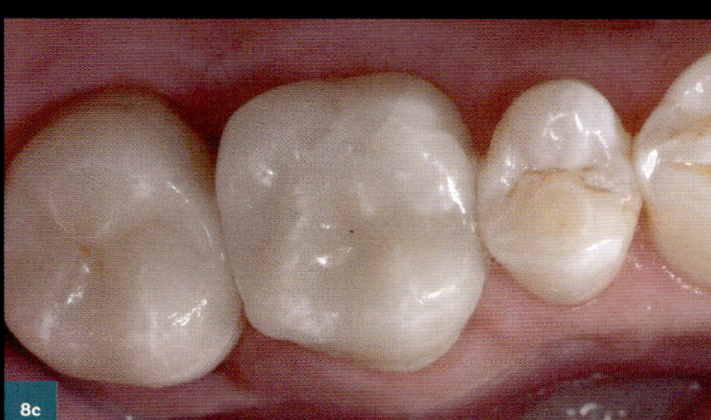

Fig. 8c ■ Following rubber dam removal.

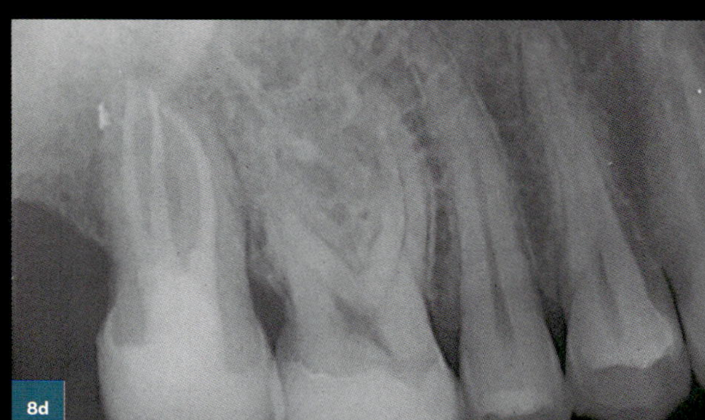

Fig. 8d ■ Check-up with periapical radiograph.

CLINICAL CASES

Incompletely formed teeth

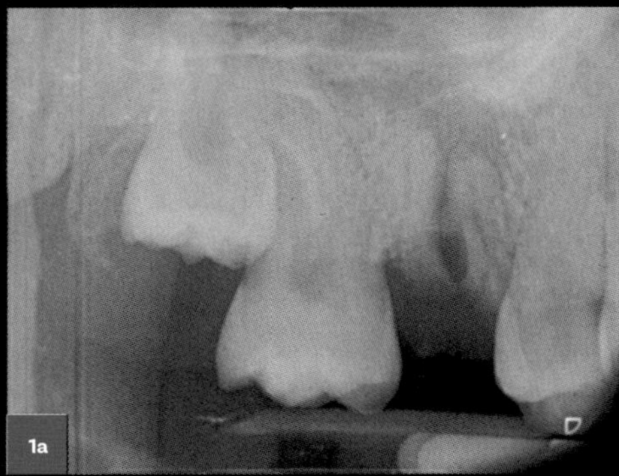

Fig. 1a ■ Patient, S.S., 16 years old. Upper right first molar for extraction. Third molars are not erupted, with root formation between 1/2 and 2/3.

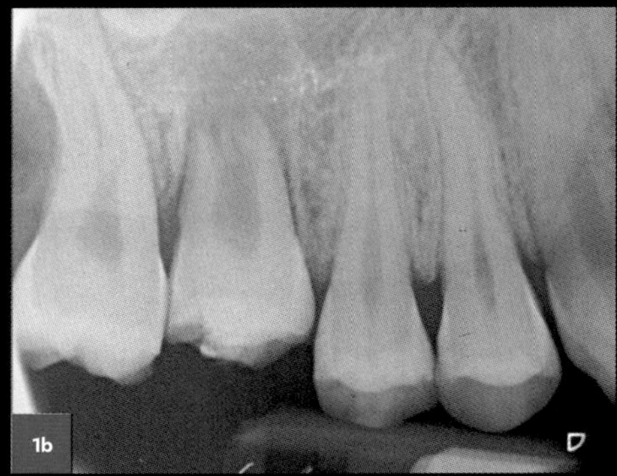

Fig. 1b ■ Completed autotransplantation.

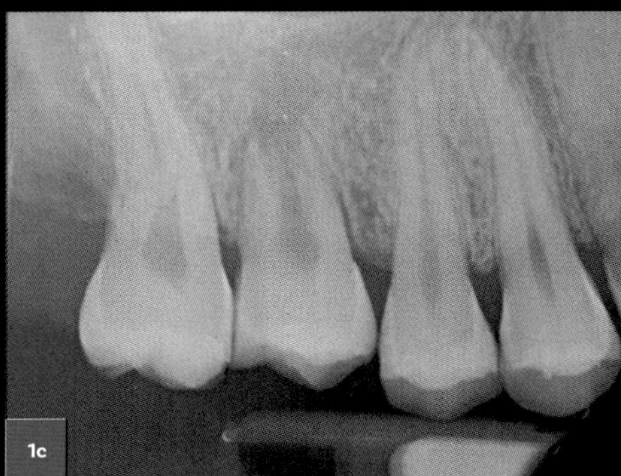

Fig. 1c ■ Check-up after 3 months.

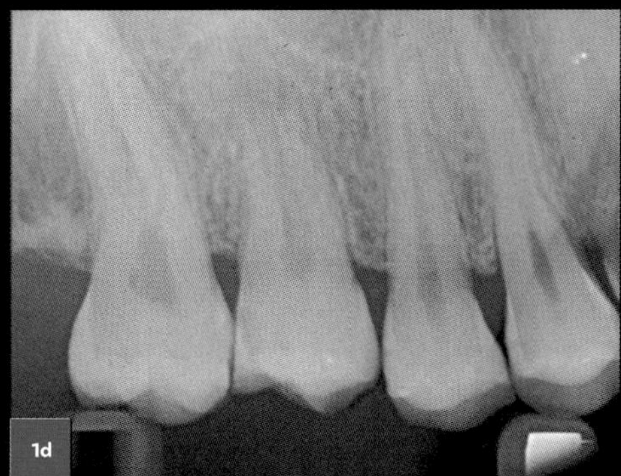

Fig. 1d ■ Check-up at 18 months. Root development continues. In these cases, endodontic treatment is not indicated.

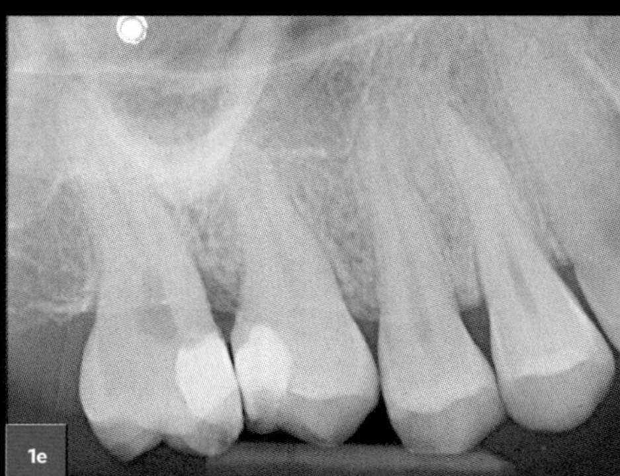

Fig. 1e ■ Check-up at 8 years with the root of the transplanted tooth having completed its formation.

Autotransplantation using a 3D printed guide, thanks to the integration of CBCT data and an intraoral scan

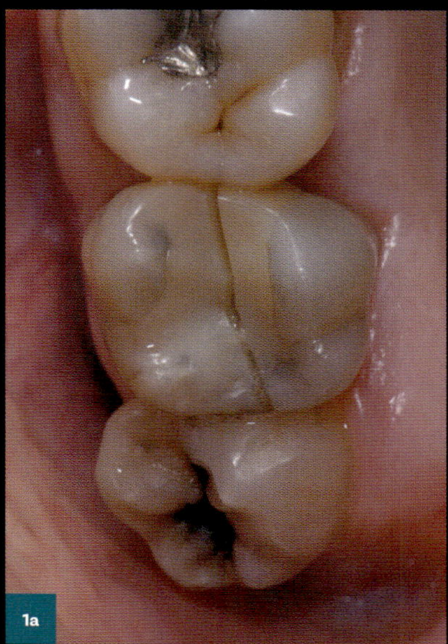

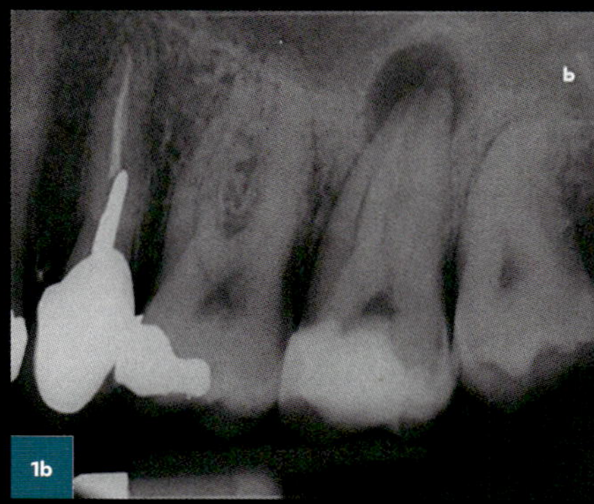

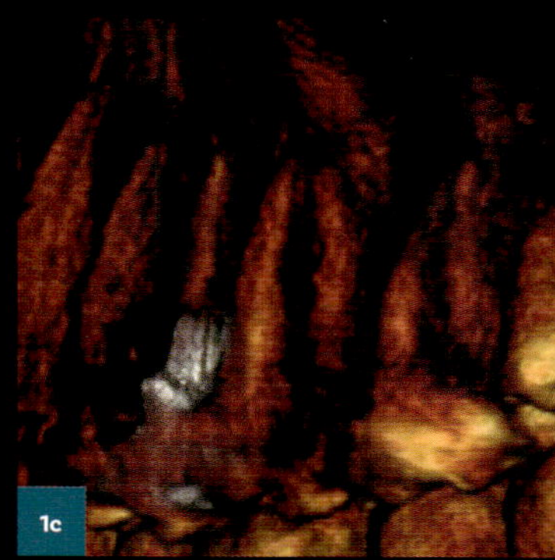

Figs. 1a-c ■ This 56-year-old male patient presents with a complaint of pain while chewing on tooth 27. Physical and radiological examinations show a vertical root fracture. The presence of a third molar in good condition suggests the possibility of performing an autotransplantation. Given the significant difference in shape between the roots of the two teeth—the one that needs to be extracted and the one that will be transplanted—a CBCT scan is performed in order to construct aids capable of facilitating the transplant.

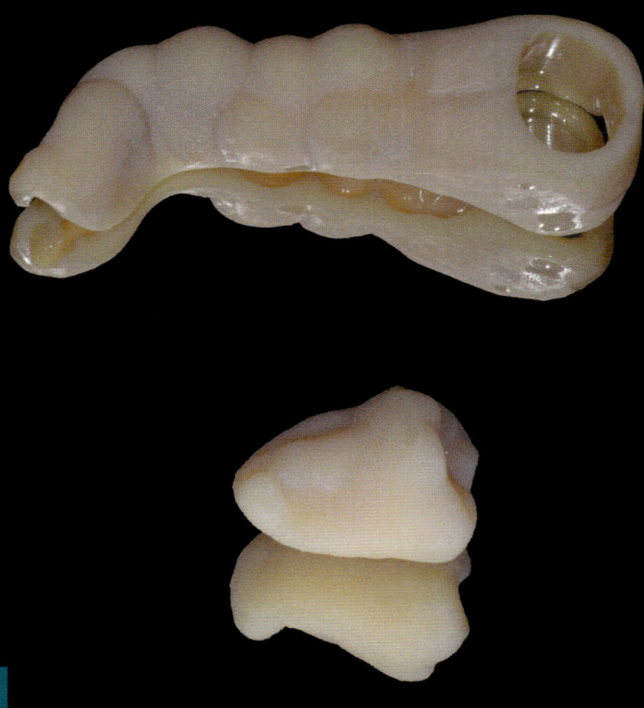

Fig. 2 ■ Thanks to the CBCT, a replica of the tooth to be transplanted and a surgical guide are constructed to facilitate correct positioning.

CONT'D >

CONT'D

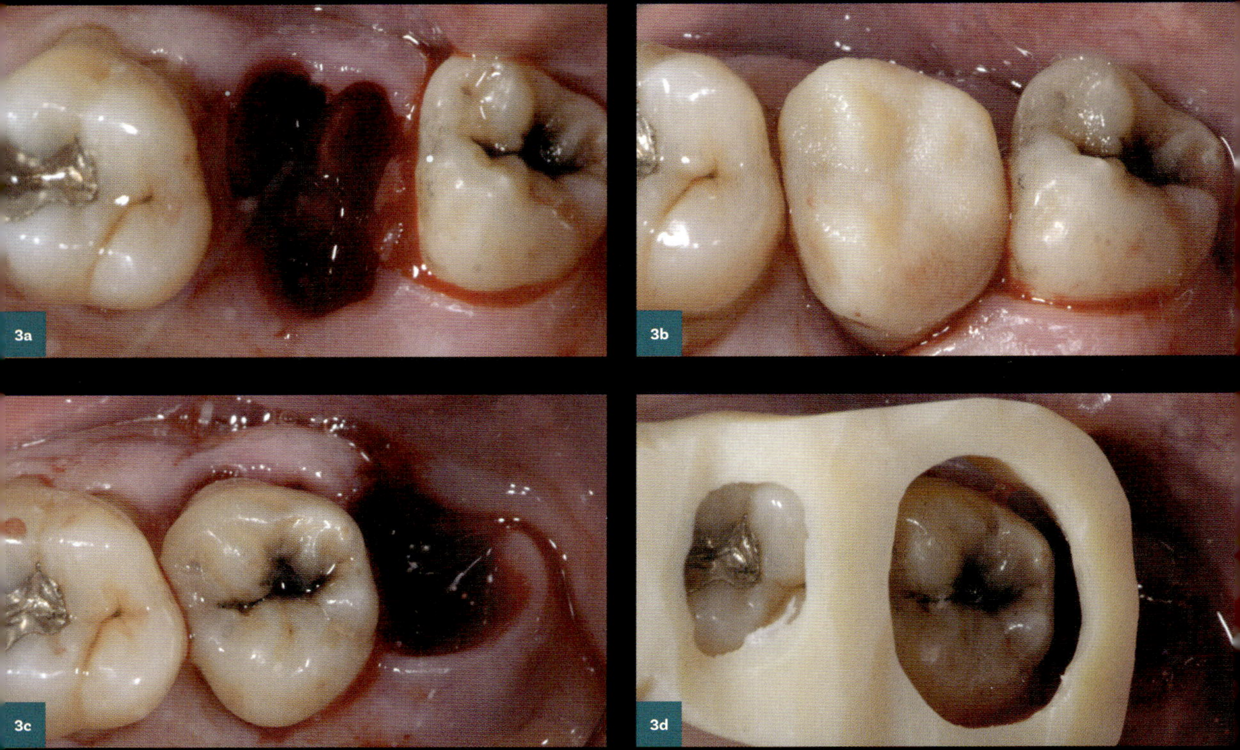

Figs. 3a-d ■ After the extraction of the fractured tooth, the replica is used to verify the possibility of inserting the third molar to be transplanted. Once the correct positioning of the replica has been obtained, the third molar is extracted and positioned in the alveolus with the help of the surgical guide.

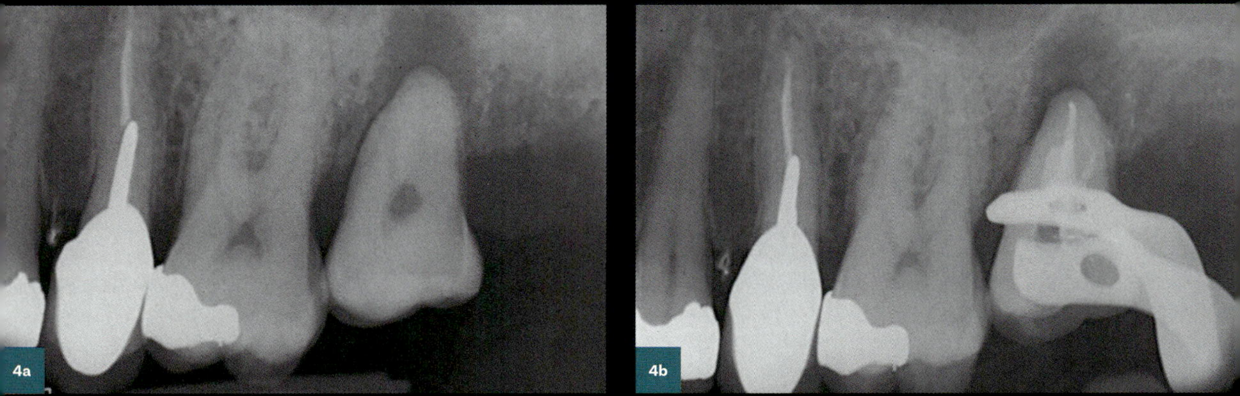

Figs. 4a,b ■ Despite the significant difference in shape and size, good stability is achieved. At 30 days endodontic treatment is per-

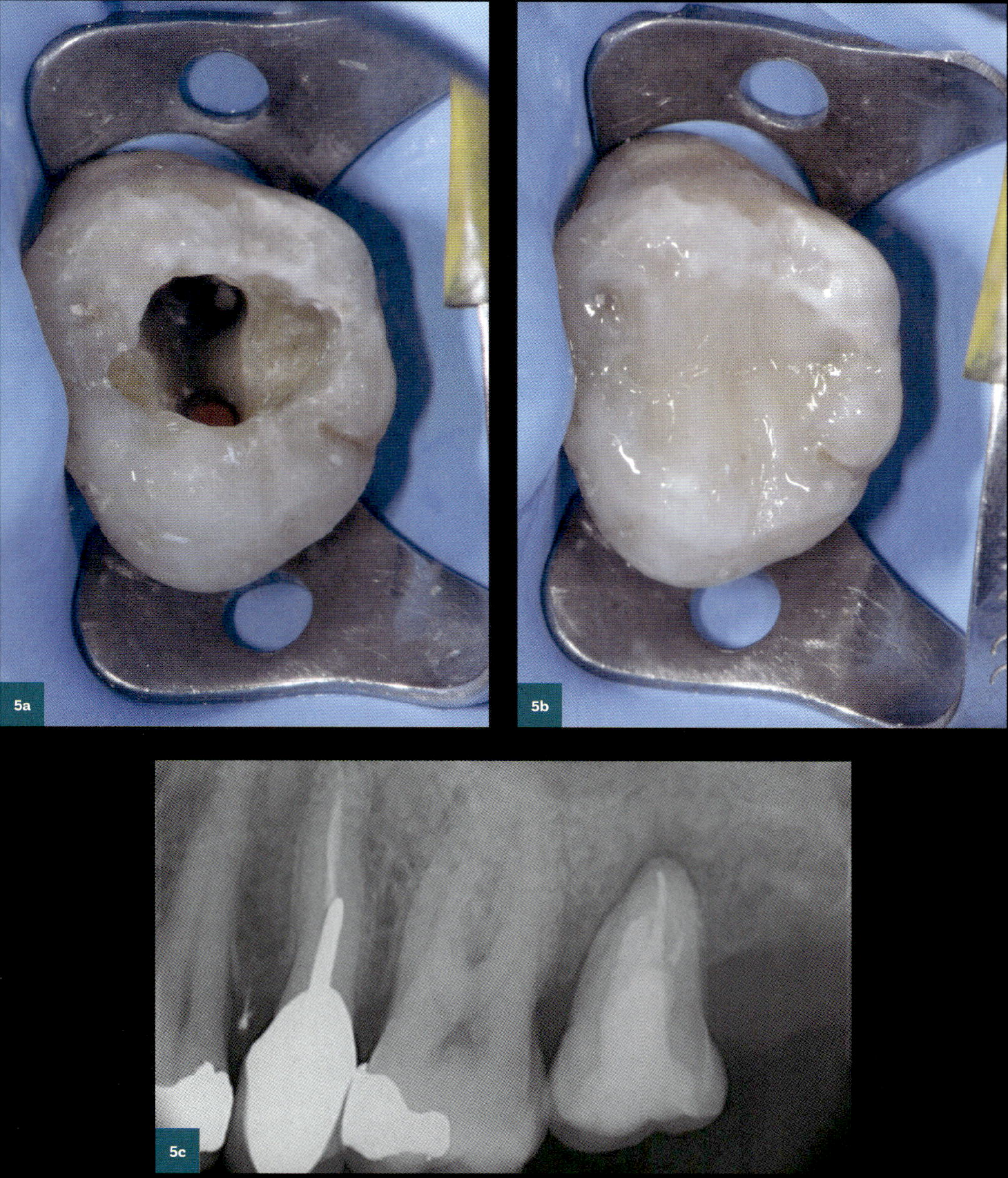

Figs. 5a-c ■ The restoration of the tooth is done. The Rx shows an advanced stage of healing.

Autotransplantation of impacted 18 in position 36

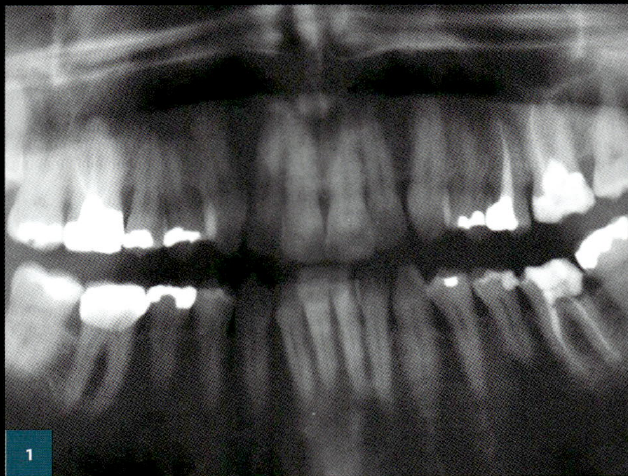

Fig. 1 ■ Orthopantomography. Patient T.P., 35 years old, presents with pain in the lower left first molar. The tooth is affected by root caries, extending to the floor of the pulp chamber, which contraindicates any conservative treatment and requires extraction. Note the presence of an impacted upper right eight. In agreement with the patient, it was decided to perform an autotransplantion of the 18 into position 36.

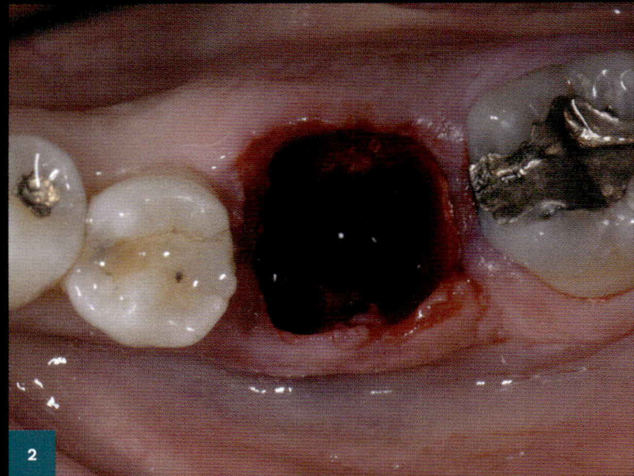

Fig. 2 ■ Once the extraction has been carried out, osteotomy of the interradicular septum is performed using a rongeur, keeping the fragment in physiological solution, to make the socket compatible with the shape of the root of 18.

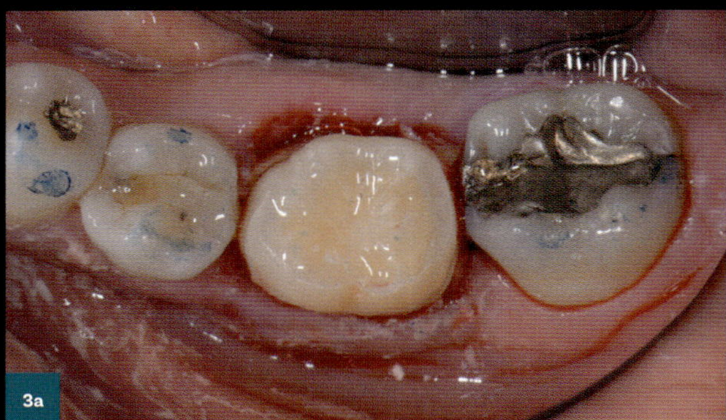

Fig. 3a ■ The 18 is positioned in the alveolus.

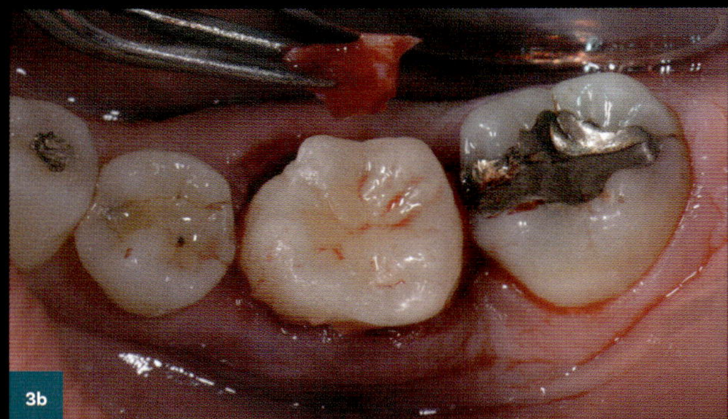

Fig. 3b ■ The bone fragment taken from the septum is wedged between the lingual cortex and root trunk of the transplanted tooth to compensate for the volumetric discrepancy.

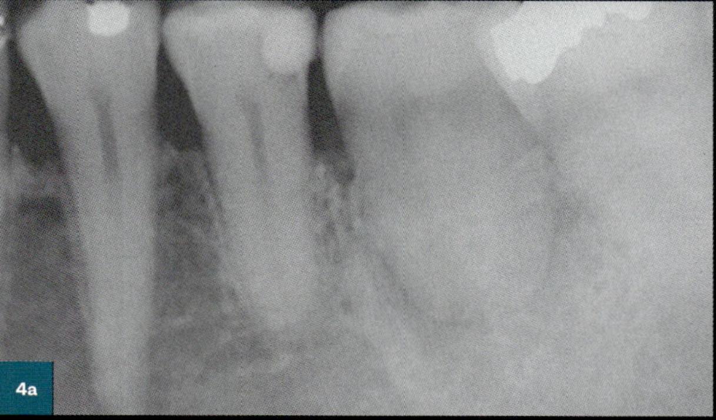

Fig. 4a ■ Periapical Rx after the procedure.

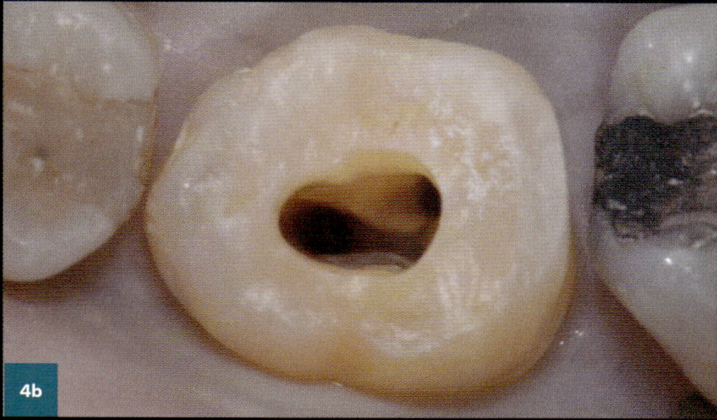

Fig. 4b ■ Access cavity for endodontic treatment 2 months following the procedure.

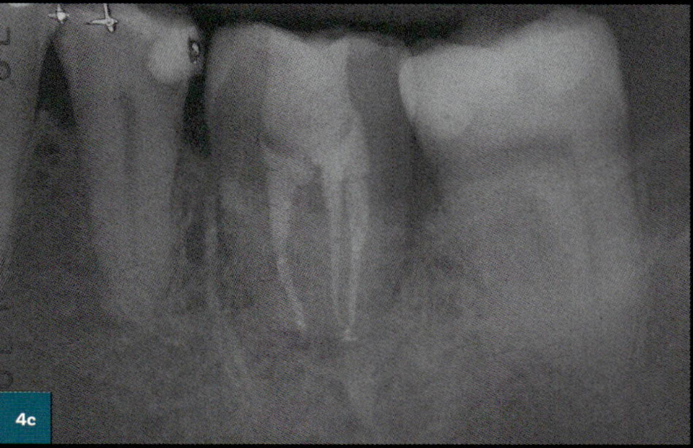

Fig. 4c ■ Periapical Rx after endodontic treatment and closure of the access cavity.

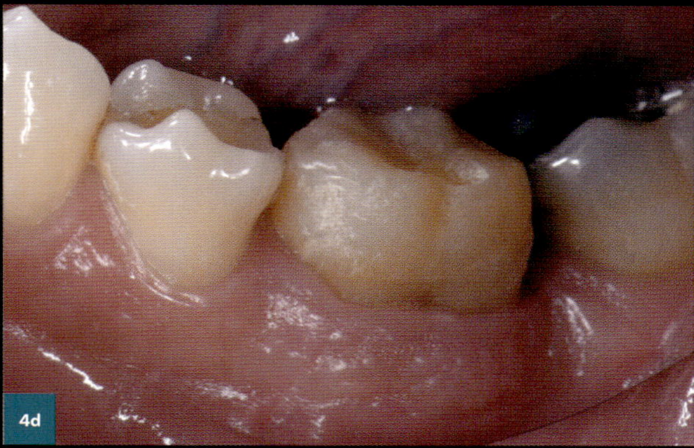

Fig. 4d ■ Buccal view showing the good soft tissue adaptation.

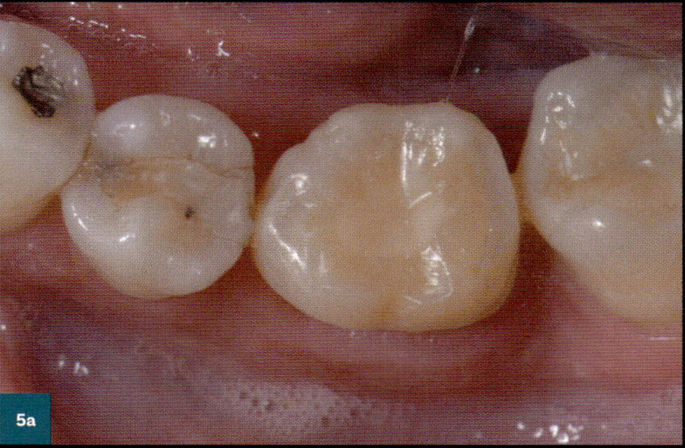

Fig. 5a ■ Check-up at 3 months. It is decided to do an all-ceramic crown to adapt the morphology of the upper molar to the new position.

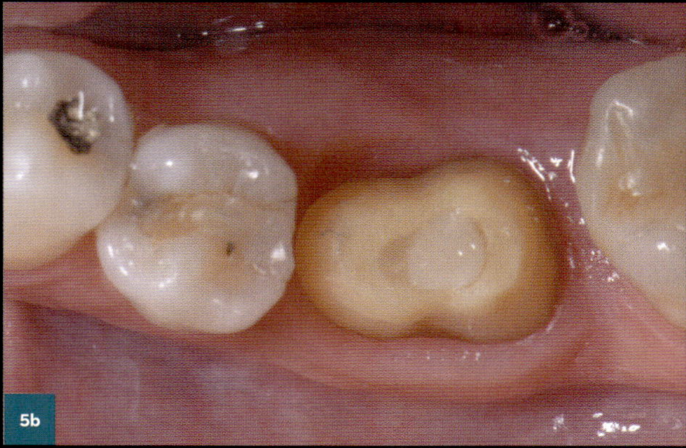

Fig. 5b ■ Crown preparation keeping the margins supragingival.

> CONT'D

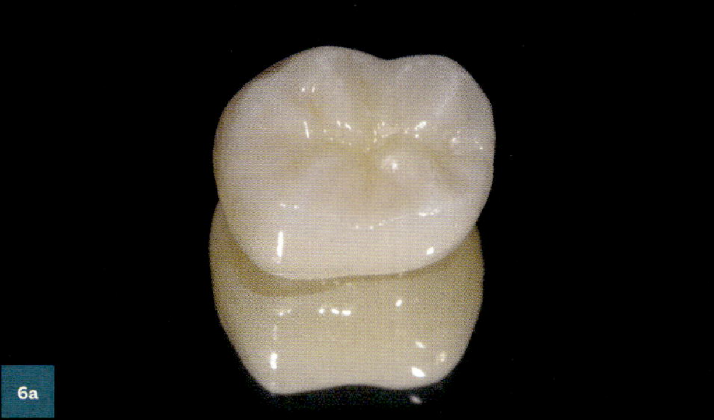

6a

Fig. 6a ■ Prosthetic crown.

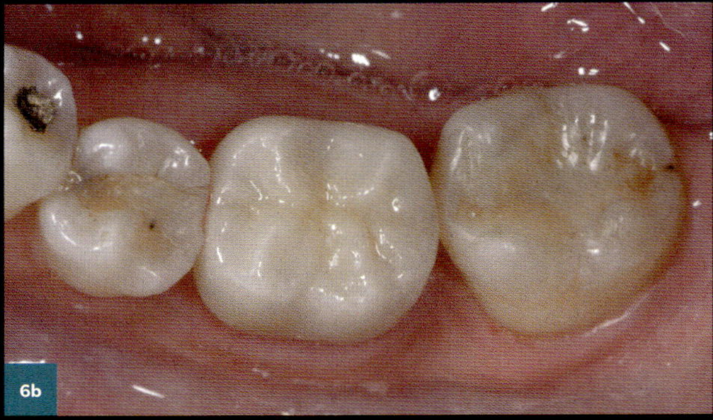

6b

Fig. 6b ■ Occlusal view.

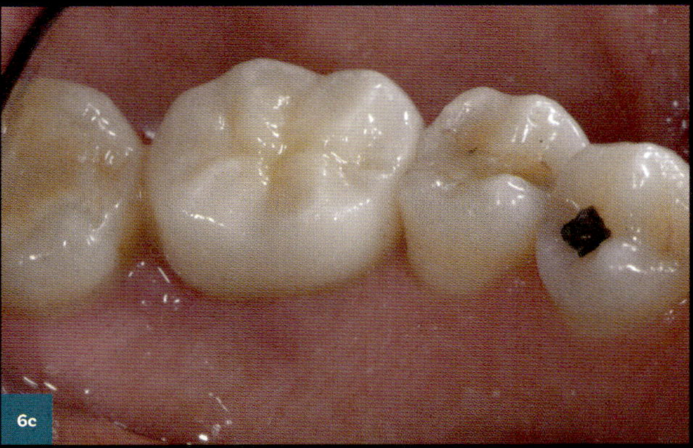

6c

Fig. 6c ■ Lingual view.

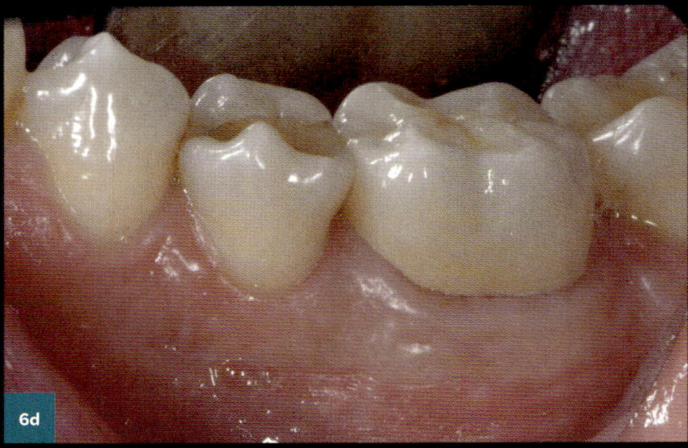

6d

Fig. 6d ■ Buccal view. Note the good adaptation of the soft tissue, attained thanks to the precocious stability guaranteed by the small bone graft.

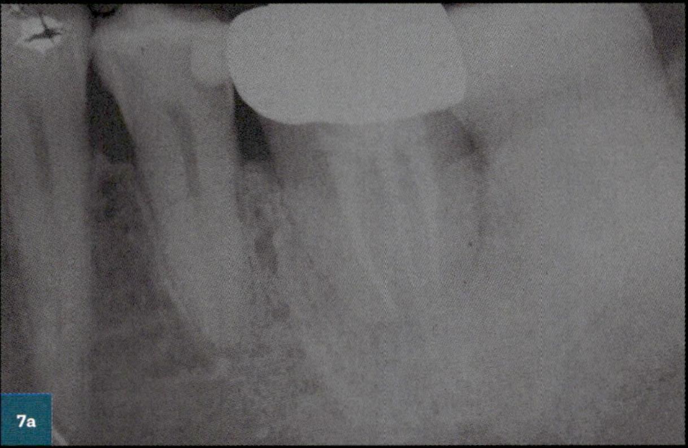

7a

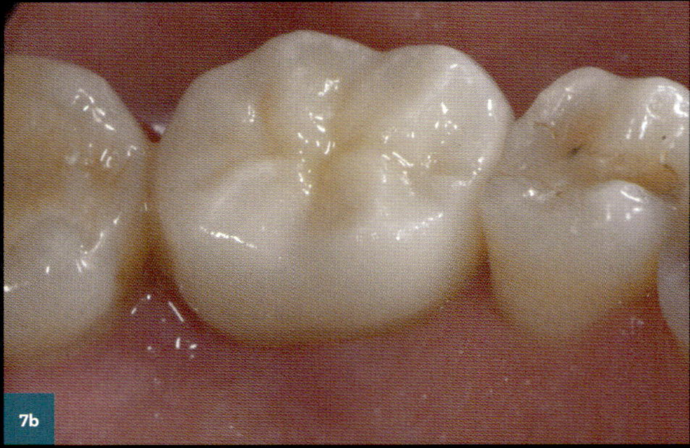

7b

Figs. 7a,b ■ Radiographic and clinical check-up at 3 years showing the stability of the result.

Autotransplantation of 18 into position 26, in the presence of a large cystic lesion

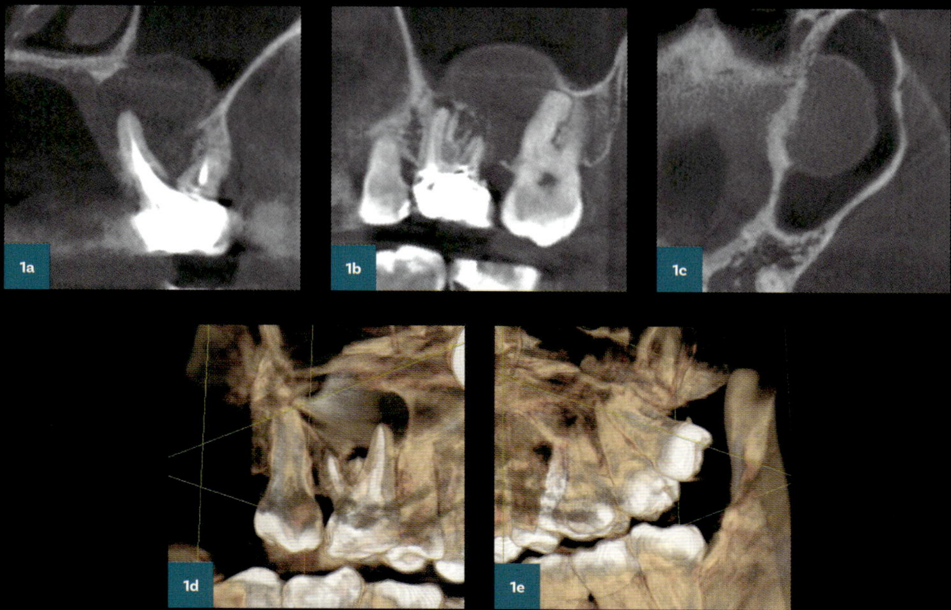

Figs. 1a-e ■ The 24-year-old patient, C.C., was referred by a colleague due to the presence of a cystic lesion in the left upper arch. This area frequently experiences flare-ups and is located near a previously treated upper sixth tooth that has been endodontically treated and restored with a cast post and ceramic fused to metal crown. Clinically, vestibular and palatal fracture lines are visible, with deep punctiform probing. Radiographic evaluation with CBCT confirms the presence of a cystic lesion, which also invades the maxillary sinus (**a-d**). The presence of a contralateral upper eight is noted, malpositioned and a good candidate as a donor for autotransplantation (**e**).

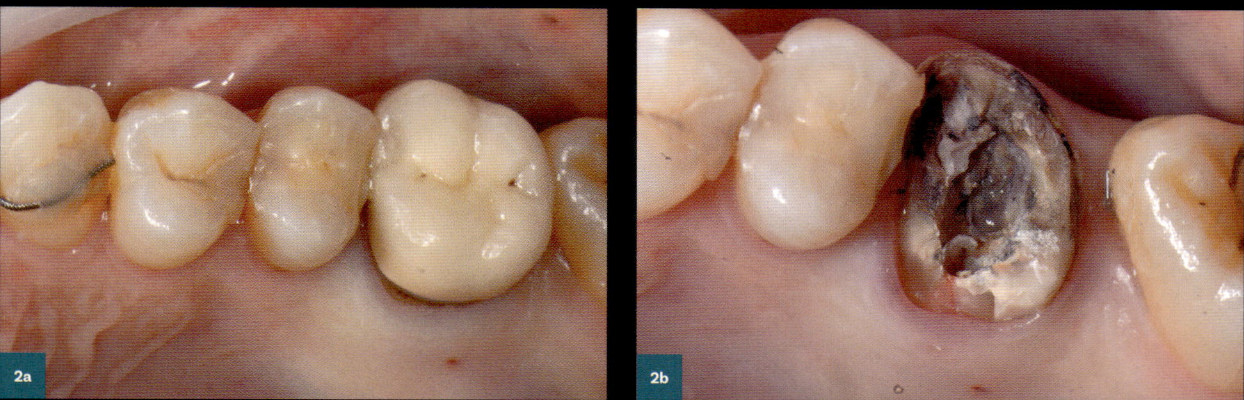

Figs. 2a,b ■ The initial clinical situation (**a**) and after (**b**) removal of the crown. The presence of a fracture is confirmed.

> CONT'D

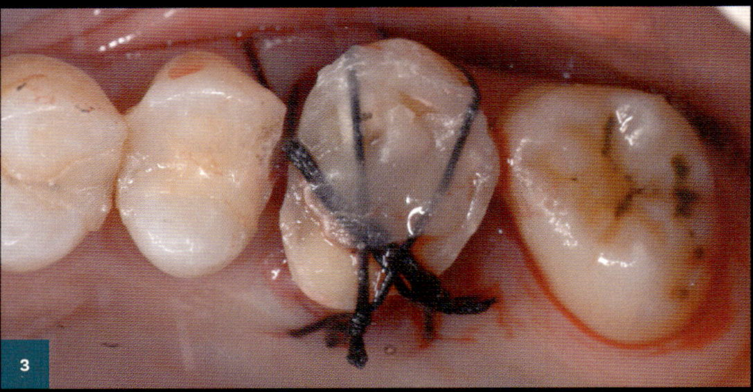

Fig. 3 ■ The contralateral eight positioned in the alveolus and stabilized with sutures.

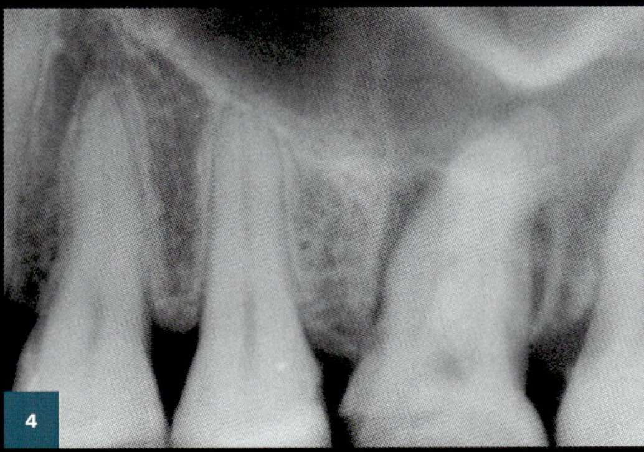

Fig. 4 ■ Periapical radiograph of the autotransplanted eight.

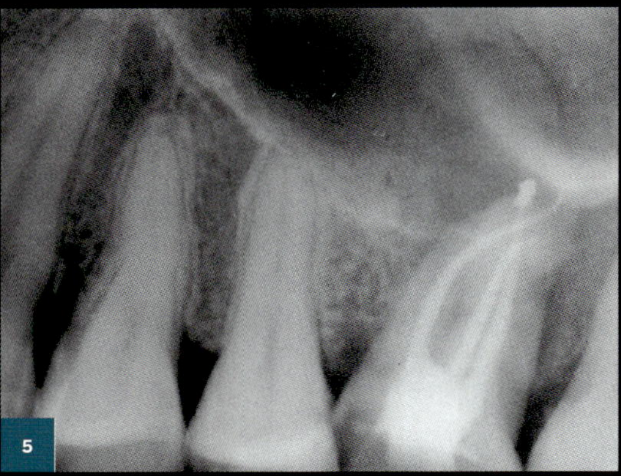

Fig. 5 ■ Endodontic treatment is done two months after autotransplantation.

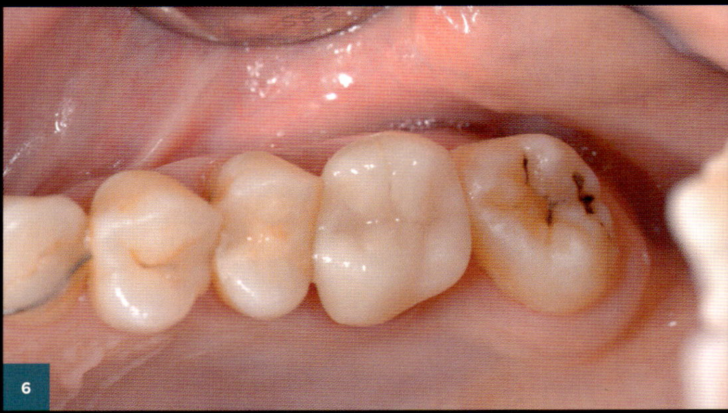

Fig. 6 ■ The case completed with the placement of a ceramic overlay.

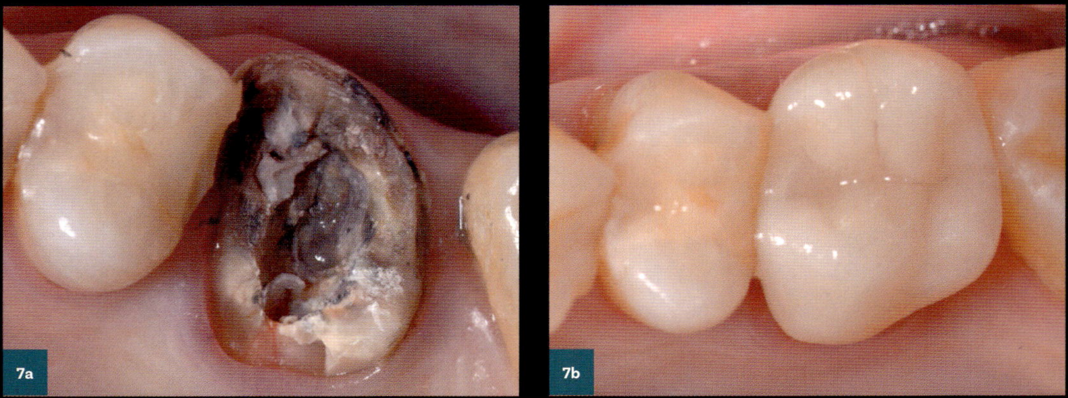

Figs. 7a,b ■ The case before and after the autotransplantation.

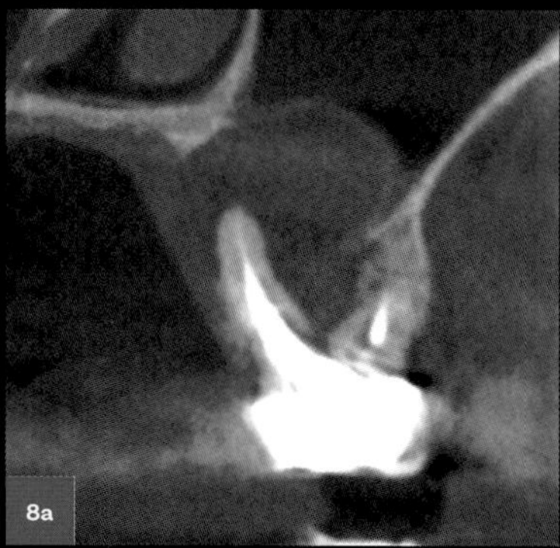

Fig. 8a ■ Diagnostic CBCT.

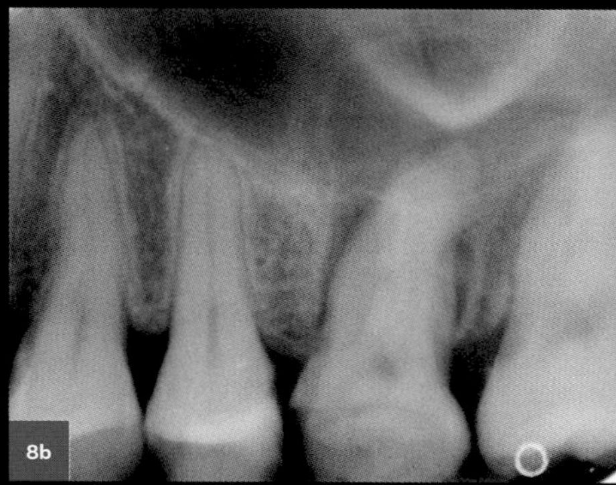

Fig. 8b ■ Periapical radiograph done immediately after the procedure.

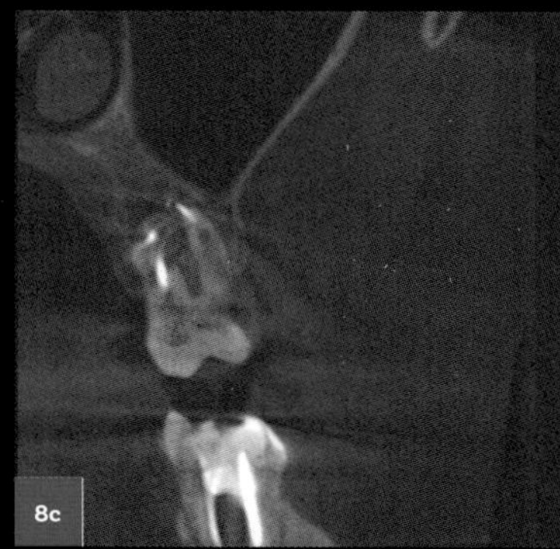

Fig. 8c ■ CBCT check-up 6 months after the procedure.

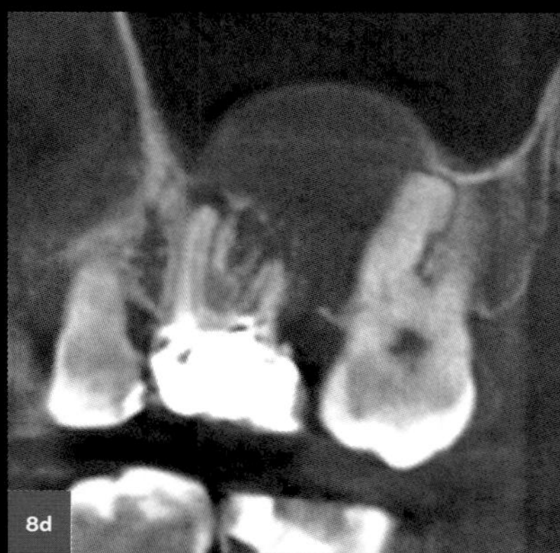

Fig. 8d ■ Parasagittal CBCT images. **d**: diagnostic.

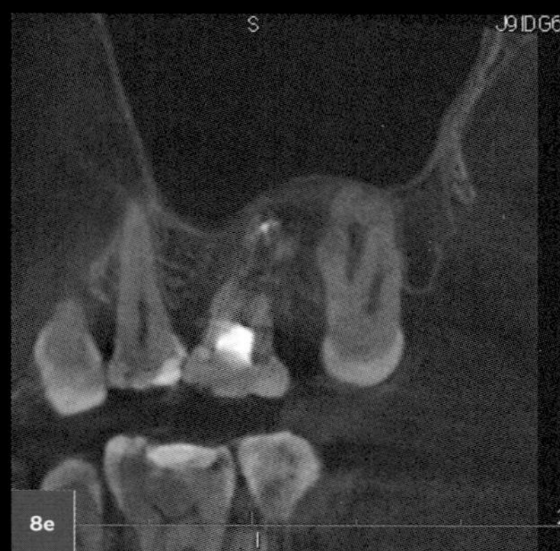

Fig. 8e ■ Check-up after 6 months.

Supernumerary fused with premolar, which prevents its eruption. The supernumerary is removed, the premolar extracted, treated extraorally and reimplanted

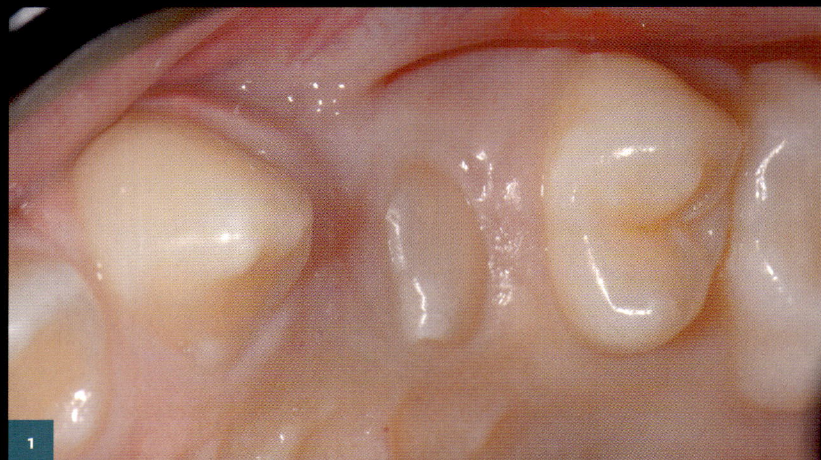

Fig. 1 ■ Patient, G.P., 12 years old, complains that the left upper first premolar has failed to erupt.

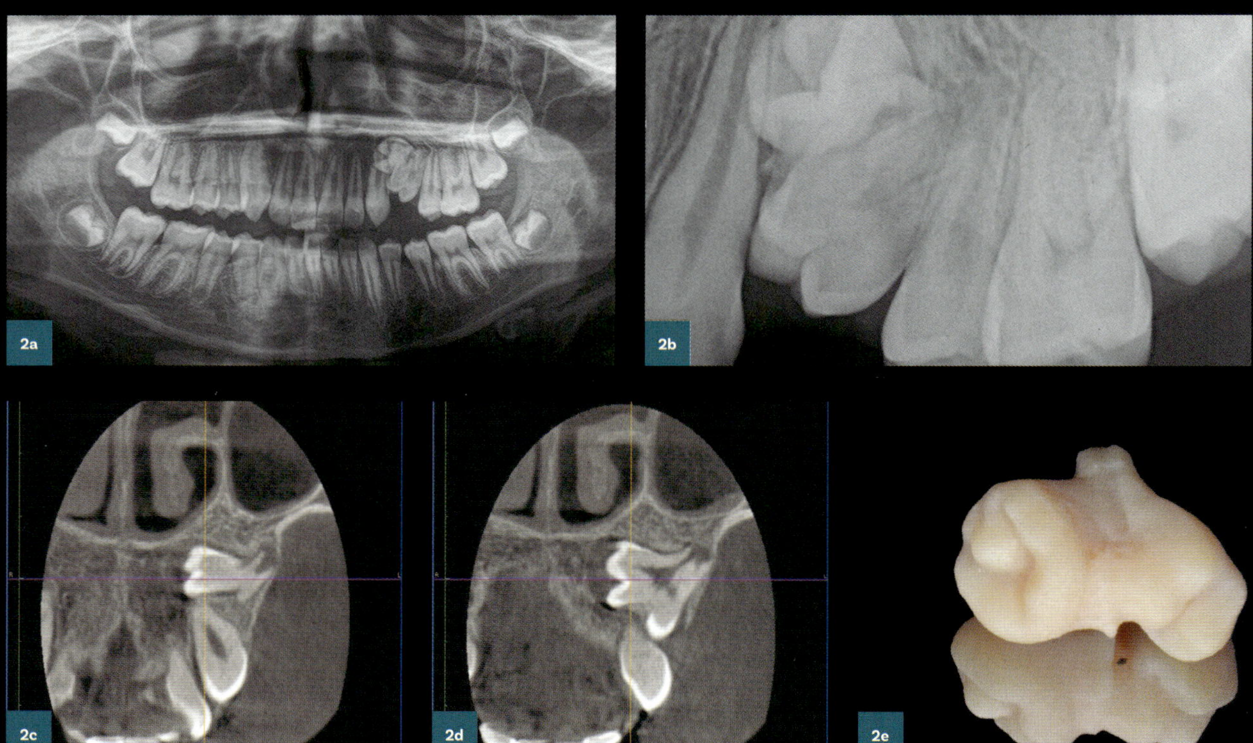

Figs. 2a-e ■ Radiological findings: **a**: orthopantomography; **b**: periapical X-ray; **c**, **d**: CBCT sections; **e**: stereolithographic model. After extensive discussion and orthodontic advice, the decision was made for the extraction of the supernumerary and the extraction and reimplantation of the premolar.

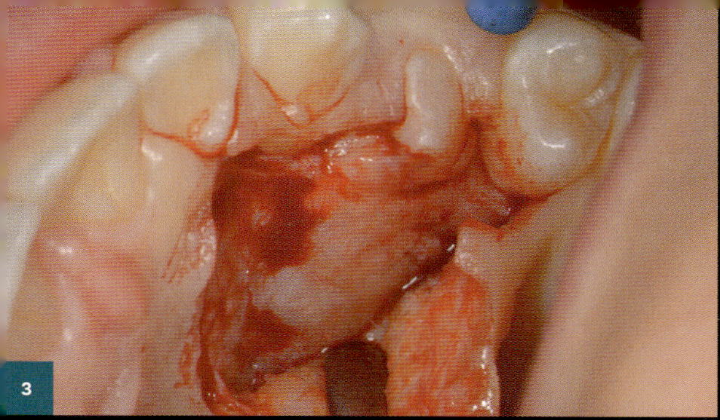

Fig. 3 ■ Access flap.

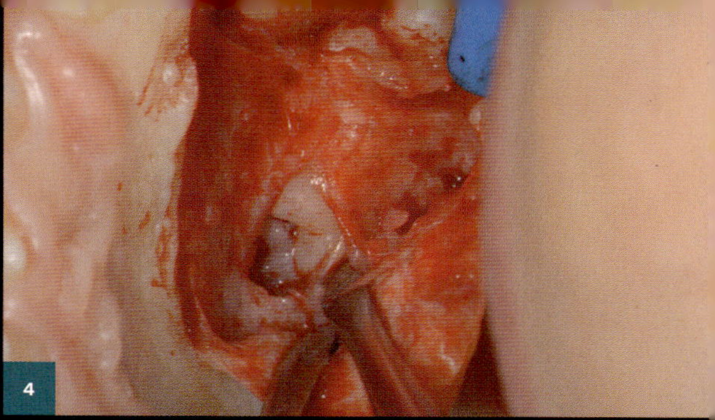

Fig. 4 ■ Ostectomy that exposes the crown of the supernumerary

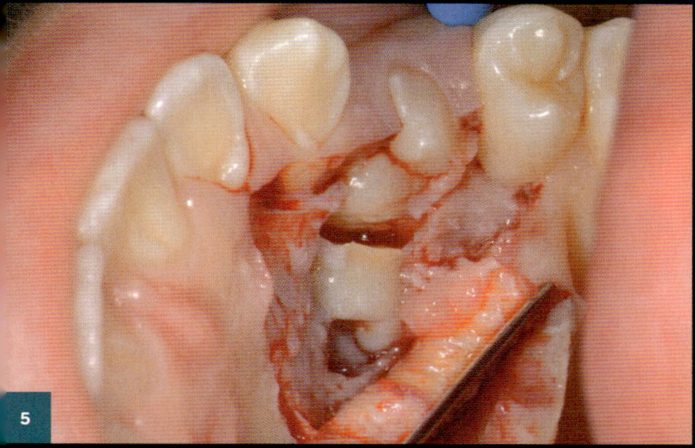

Fig. 5 ■ Odontotomy of the supernumerary.

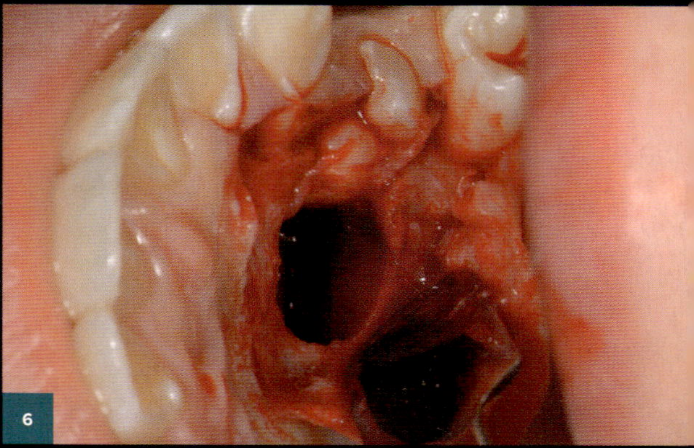

Fig. 6 ■ Post-extraction alveolus of the supernumerary.

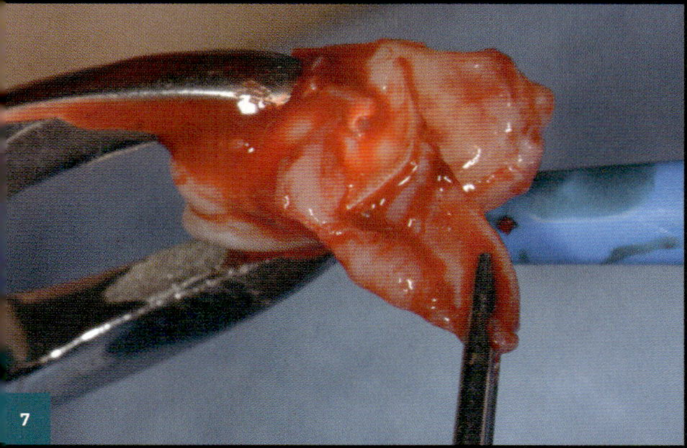

Fig. 7 ■ The premolar is extracted. The pulp tissue is removed

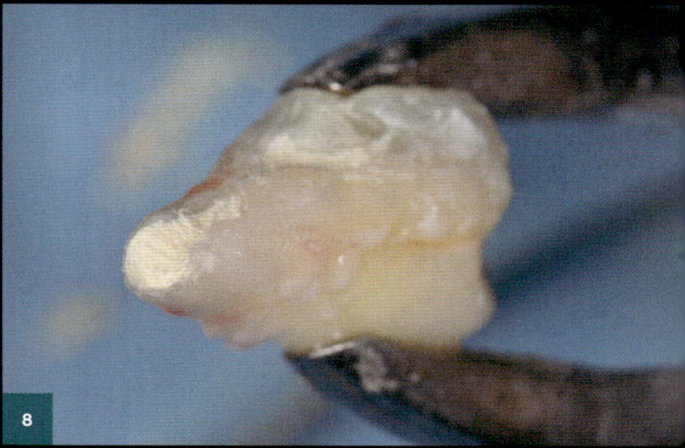

Fig. 8 ■ The apex and the odontotomy gap are filled with bioce-

> CONT'D

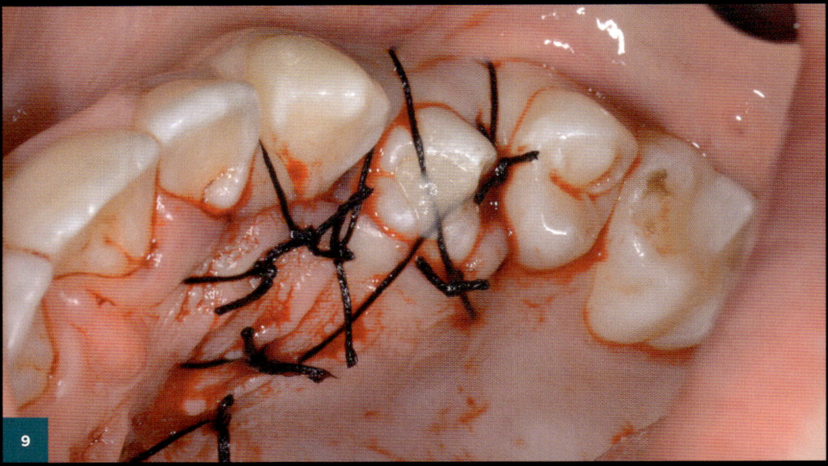

9

Fig. 9 ■ The premolar is repositioned in the socket and stabilized with a suture. The flap is sutured.

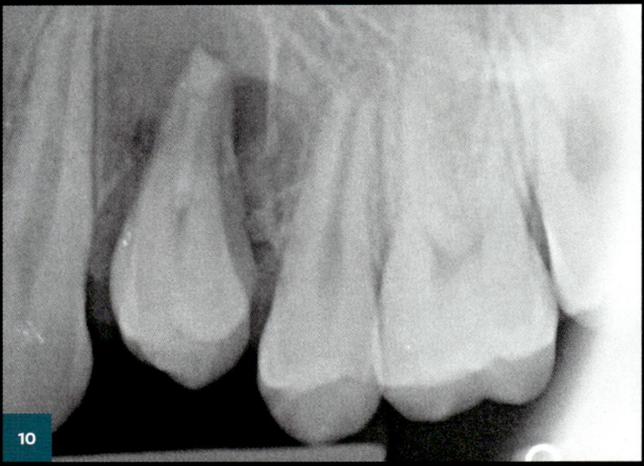

10

Fig. 10 ■ Post-operative periapical radiograph.

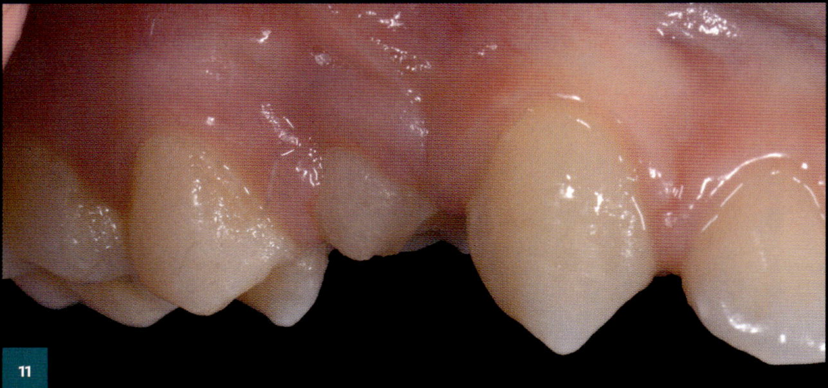

11

Fig. 11 ■ Check-up 15 days after the procedure.

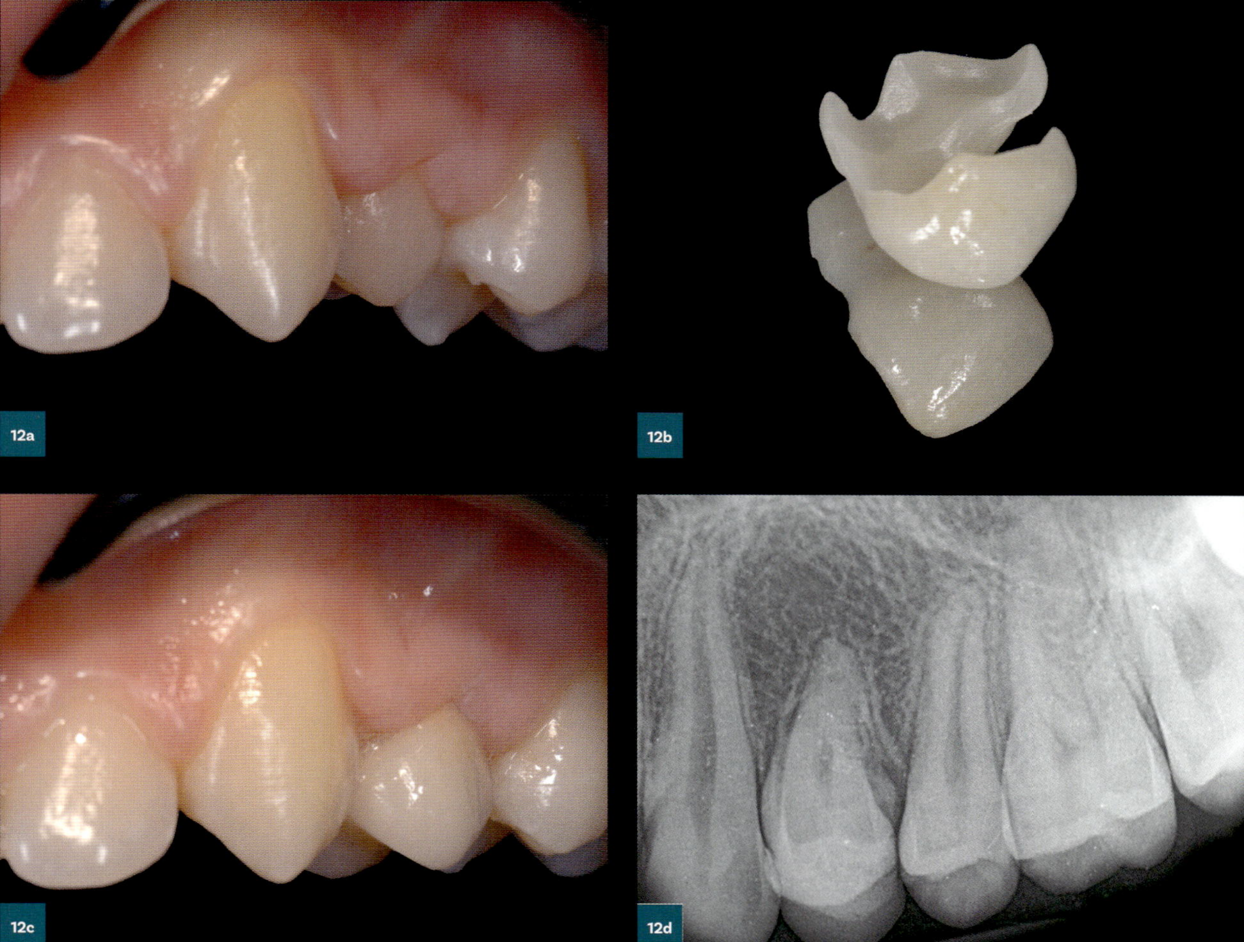

Figs. 12a-d ■ **a:** control at 1 year. The premolar is partially erupted, but is not perfectly functional or aligned in the arch. It is considered appropriate to avoid orthodontic movements. After scanning, an additional ceramic inlay is produced (**b**) which is then cemented (**c**). **d**: Periapical X-ray check-up.

Placement of impacted canine not suitable for orthodontic therapy in the appropriate site

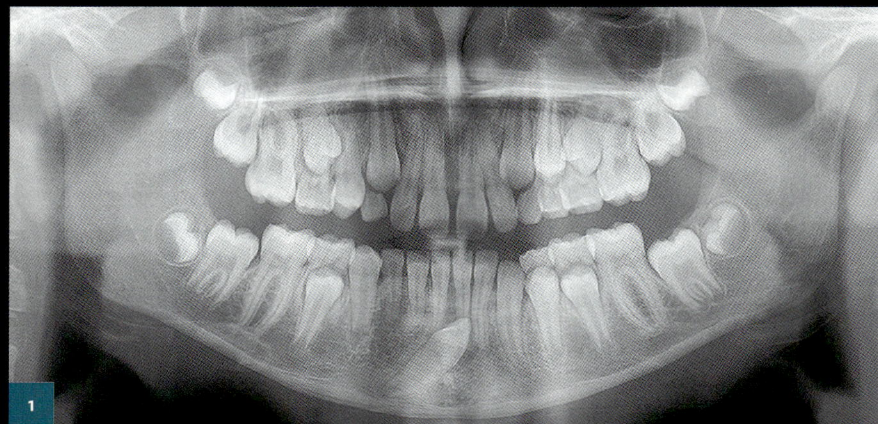

Fig. 1 ■ Patient, A.V., aged 13. Orthopantomography. Referred by the orthodontist for impaction of the lower right canine in a situation such as to make orthodontic repositioning inadvisable, both due to the peculiarities of the mandibular bone and the position of the tooth. It is decided, in agreement with the patient, the parents and the colleague, to proceed with an autotransplantation.

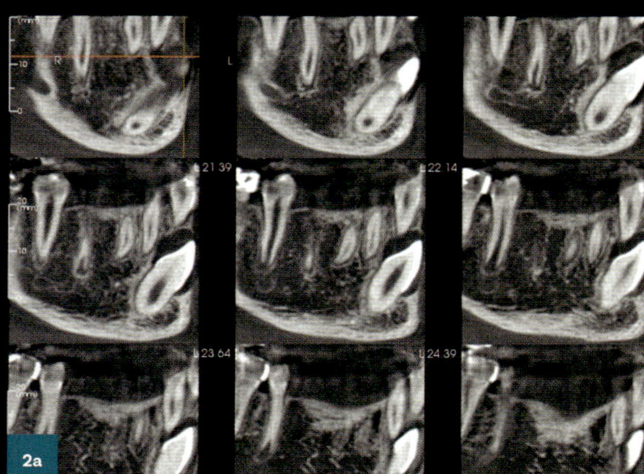

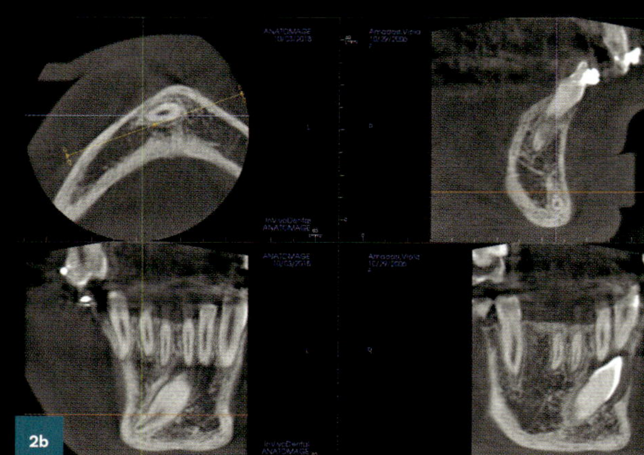

Figs. 2a,b ■ 3D evaluation using a CBCT. In agreement with the orthodontist, given the size of the tooth to be transplanted and the root shape, orthodontics is done to obtain a space in the arch greater than strictly necessary.

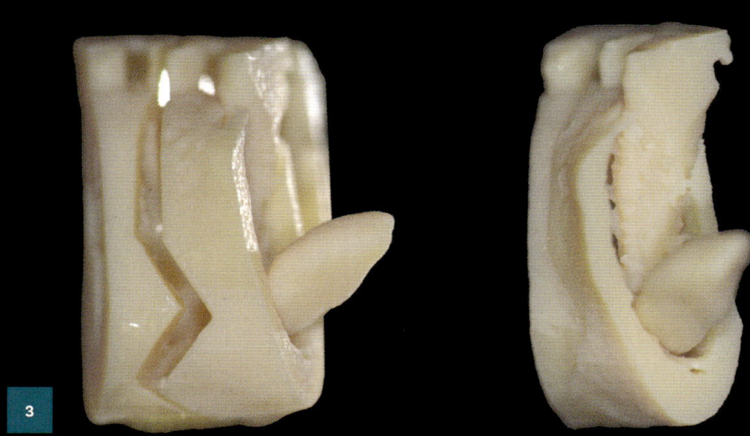

Fig. 3 ■ Stereolithographic model with removable canine to simulate repositioning.

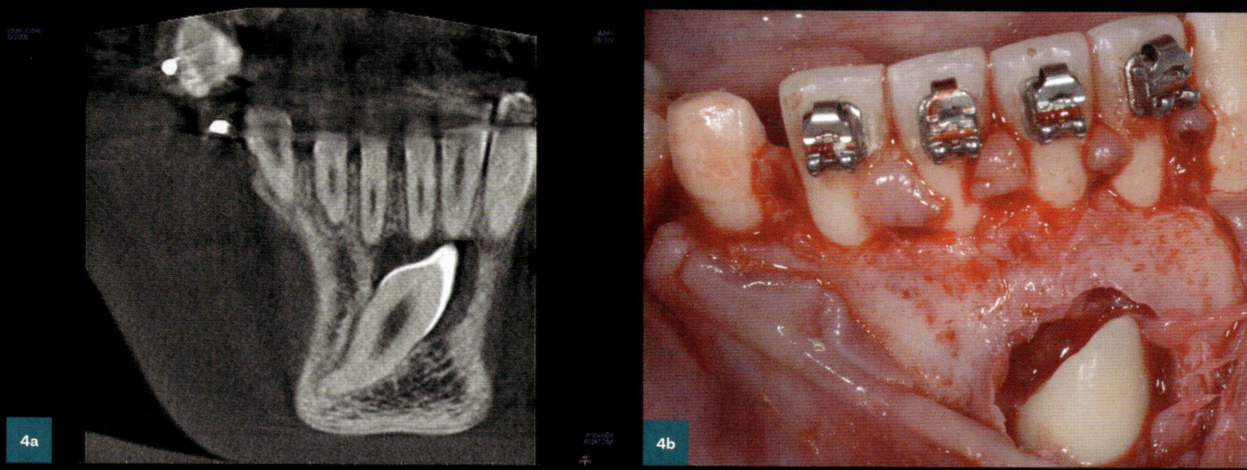

Figs. 4a,b ■ Correspondence between the CBCT findings and the surgical situation after incision with preservation of the papillae, flap elevation and exposure of the crown of the canine.

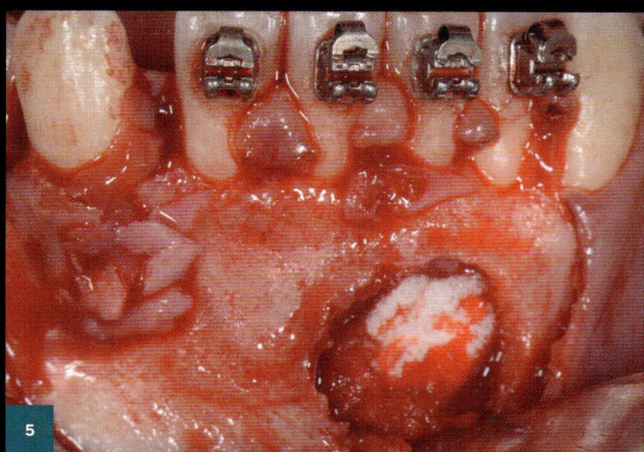

Fig. 5 ■ The canine is extracted and repositioned in its site. The bone chips resulting from the exposure of the impacted canine are grafted buccally. A haemostatic sponge is placed in the ectopic socket.

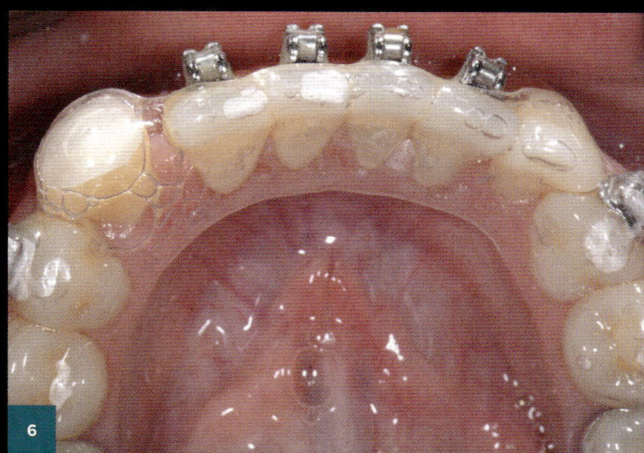

Fig. 6 ■ During healing, stabilization is ensured with a mask.

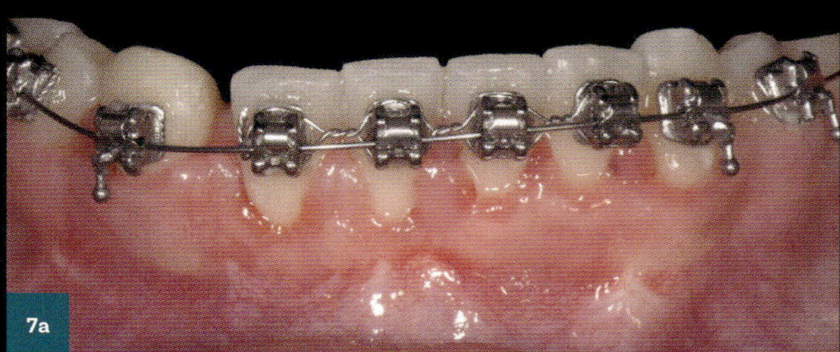

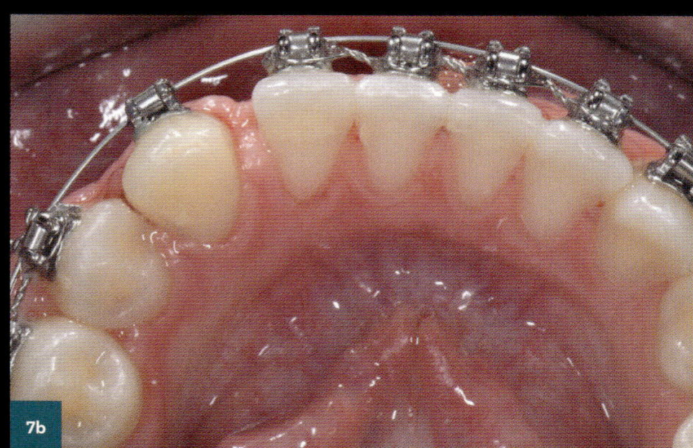

Figs. 7a,b ■ Once healing is complete, the orthodontic treatment is resumed to close the spaces.

CONT'D >

> CONT'D

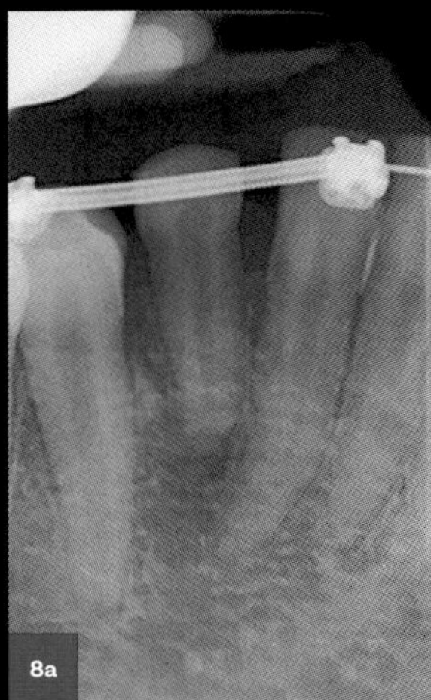

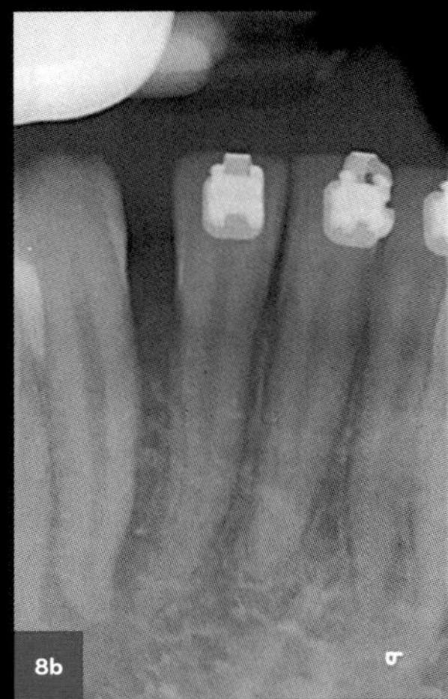

Fig. 8a ■ Pre-operative periapical radiograph, with deciduous canine in place.

Fig. 8b ■ Post-operative periapical Rx, with transplanted canine. Particular care has been applied to the precise positioning of the root in relation to the roots of the contiguous elements.

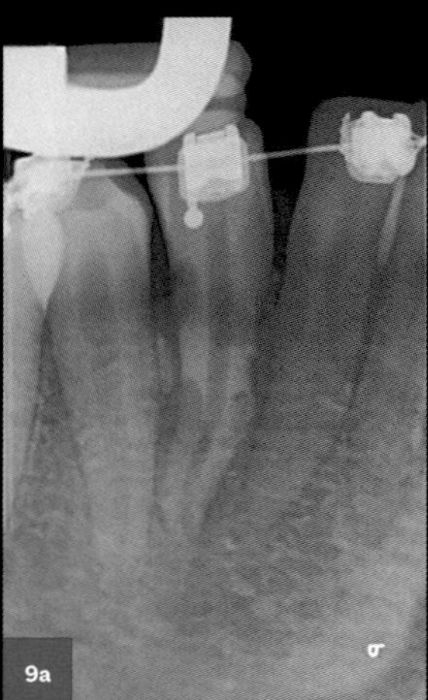

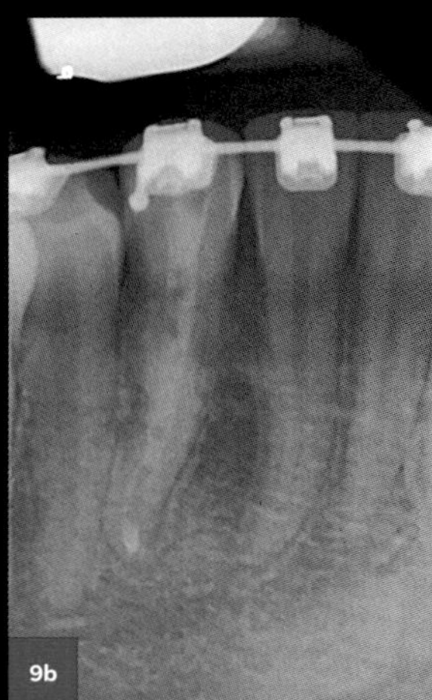

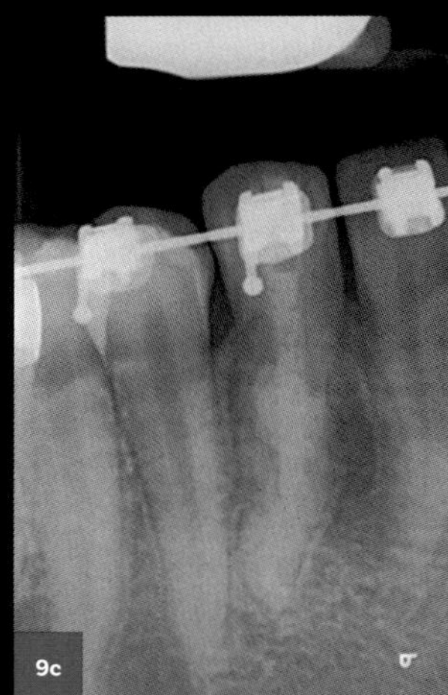

Fig. 9a ■ On the X-ray check-up before endodontic treatment, the radiological signs of root resorption are evident in the absence of any symptoms.

Fig. 9b ■ We then proceed with the placement of calcium hydroxide with 2% chlorhexidine, to be renewed every 21 days for a period of 6 months while the endodontic treatment continued.

Fig. 9c ■ Check-up at six months. The resorption appears arrested.

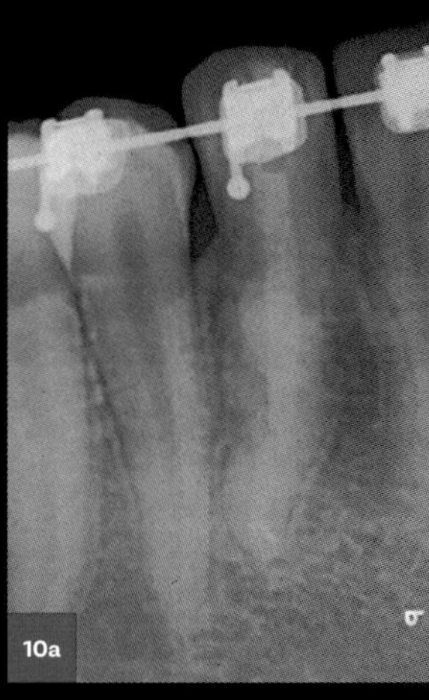

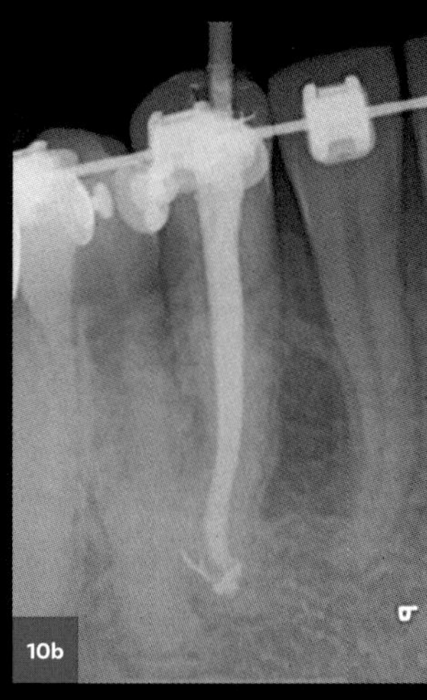

Fig. 10a ■ Radiograph at seven months confirms remission of the resorption.

Fig. 10b ■ Closure of the root canal with carrier-based gutta-percha.

Autotransplantation of premolar in position 21 following trauma

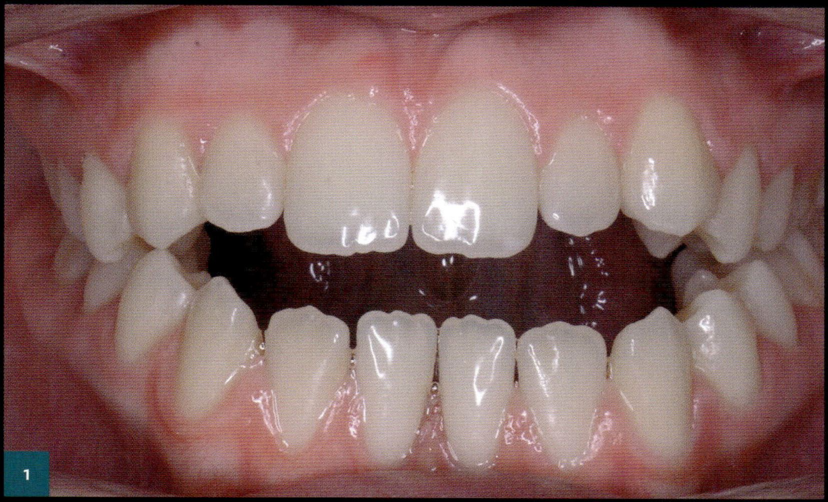

Fig. 1 ■ Patient, M.P., aged 13. Archive image from the orthodontist, who was studying an orthodontic and possible surgical treatment plan.

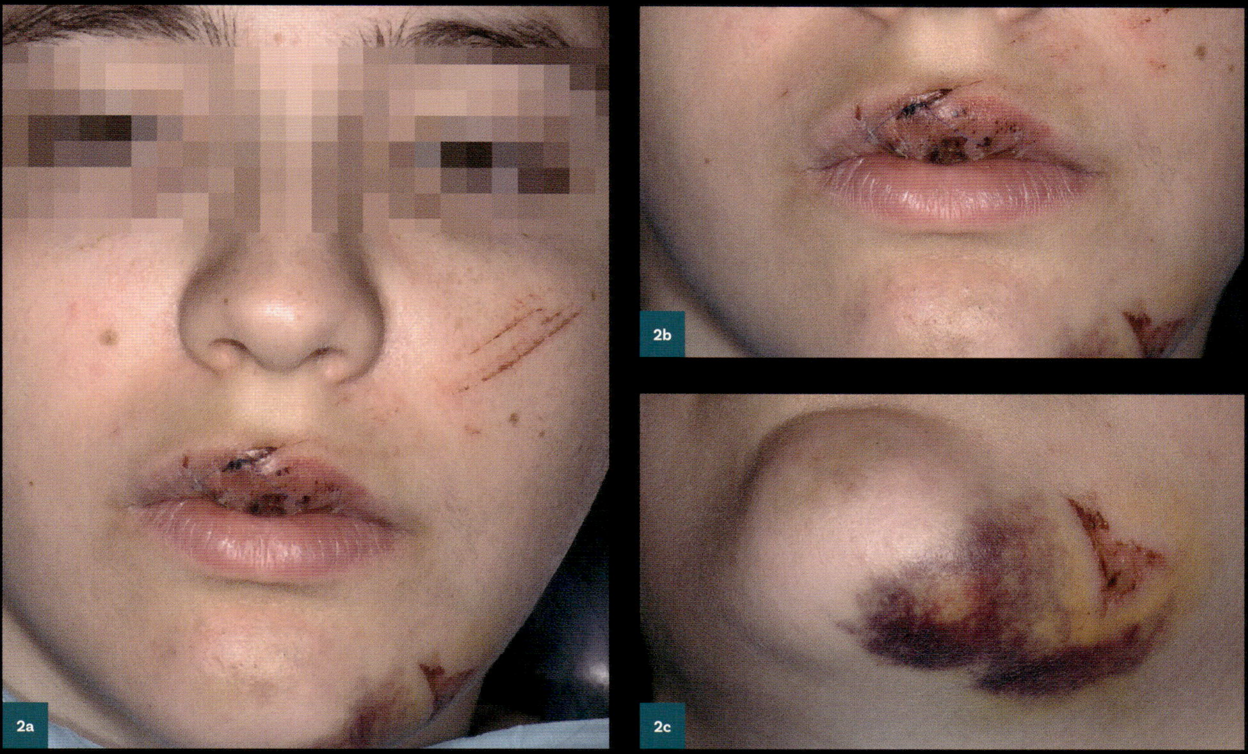

Figs. 2a-c ■ Unfortunately, the patient suffered a trauma while skiing, being run over by another skier. From the visible signs on the face, it is evident that one of the patient's skis crossed the middle and lower third of the facial mass transversely, from top left to bottom right. The trauma involves the upper dental arch, with the traumatic avulsion of teeth 21, 23 and 24 and the coronal fracture of 22. The 23 is recovered from the scene of the accident, while 21 and 24 are not. The 23 recovered was promptly reimplanted, and the wounds sutured.

> CONT'D

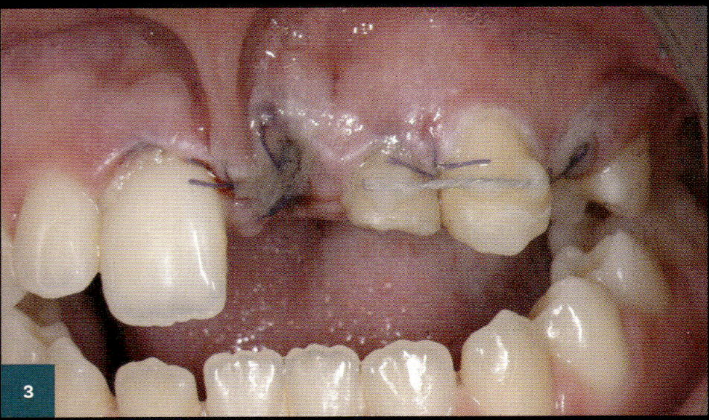

Fig. 3 ■ The patient attended a consultation with the avulsion of teeth 21 and 24, and the 23 reimplanted and splinted with metal wire to the stump of 22.

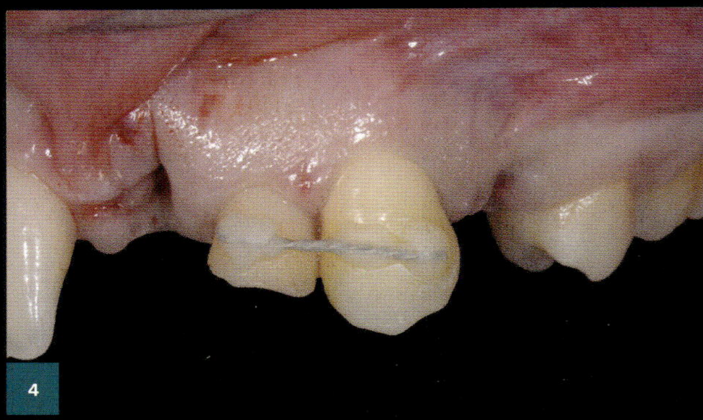

Fig. 4 ■ Suture removal ten days after the incident.

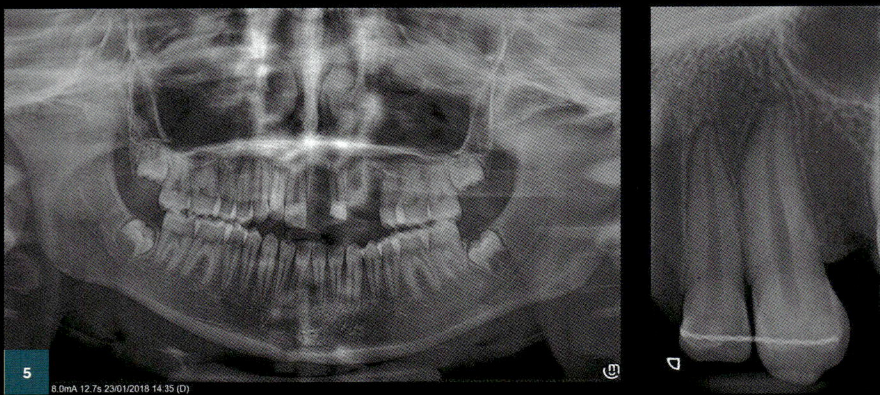

Fig. 5 ■ Two-dimensional radiological evaluations, orthopantomography and periapical of 22 and 23. Widening of the periodontal space is noted in teeth 22 and 23, which respond negatively to thermal and electrical tests.

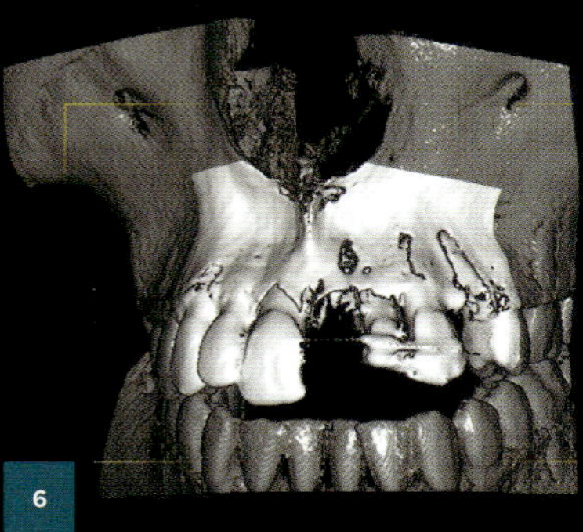

Fig. 6 ■ CBCT: 3D reconstruction frontal view.

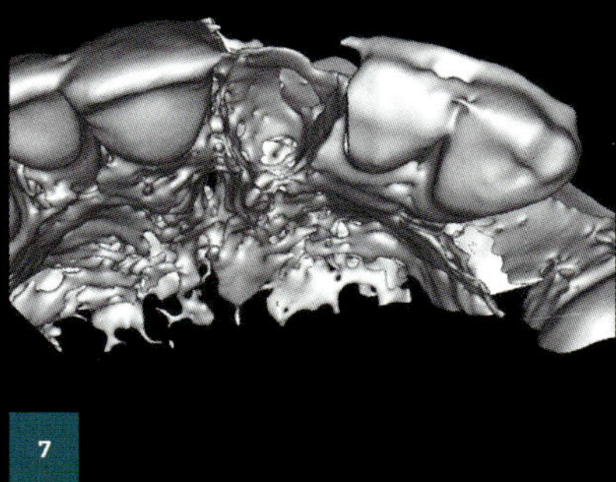

Fig. 7 ■ CBCT: 3D reconstruction occlusal view.

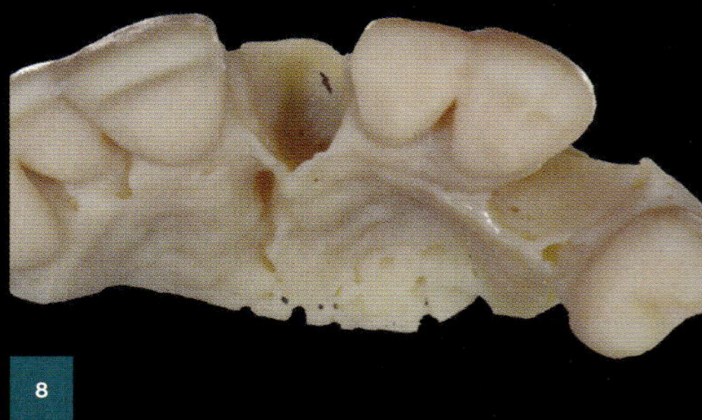

Fig. 8 ■ Stereolithography.

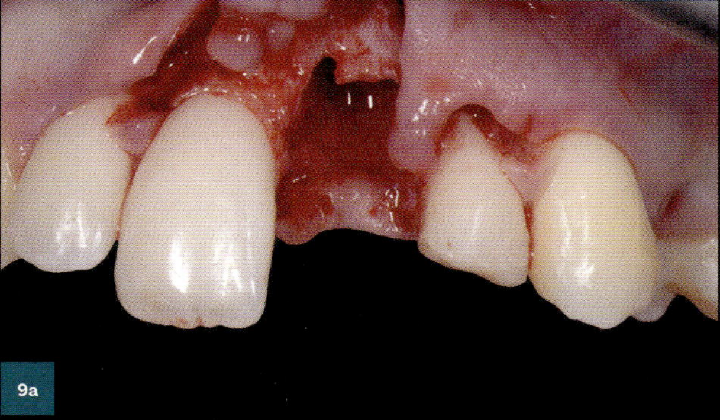

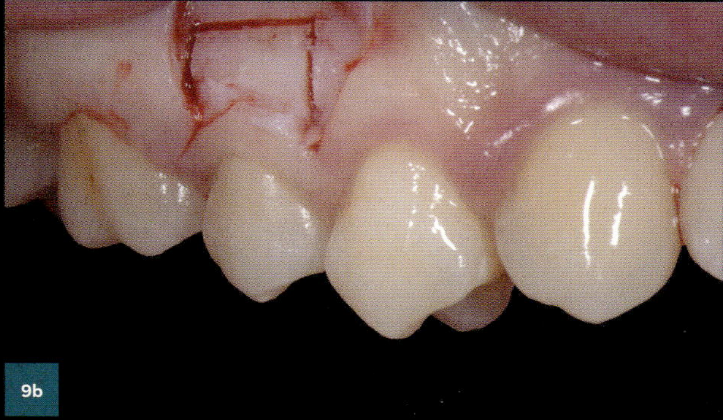

Fig. 9a ■ After extensive discussion with the patient, the parents and the orthodontist, the following treatment plan was agreed upon: autotransplantation of 15 in site 21, after endodontic treatment of 15, 22 and 23. Coronal reconstructions and adaptations as per aesthetic and functional needs. The orthodontist will then be responsible for closing the edentulous spaces in locations 15 and 24. In this way, symmetry and the possibility of development of the maxilla will be restored as far as possible. a: after the elevation of the mucoperiosteal flap.

Fig. 9b ■ Removal of the upper second premolar, with attached keratinized gingiva and cortical bone fragment, to compensate for the buccal bone dehiscence.

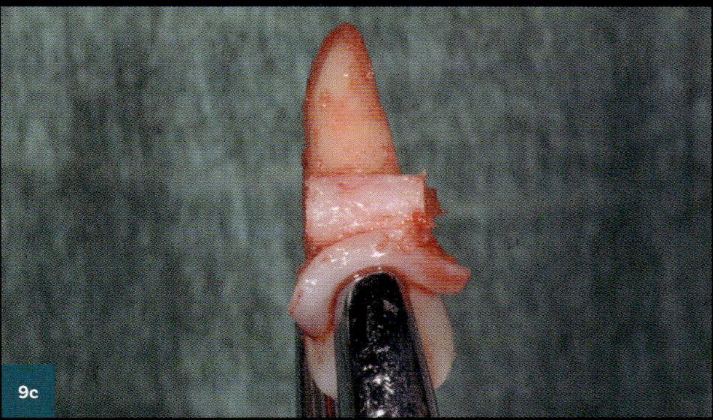

Fig. 9c ■ Removed premolar.

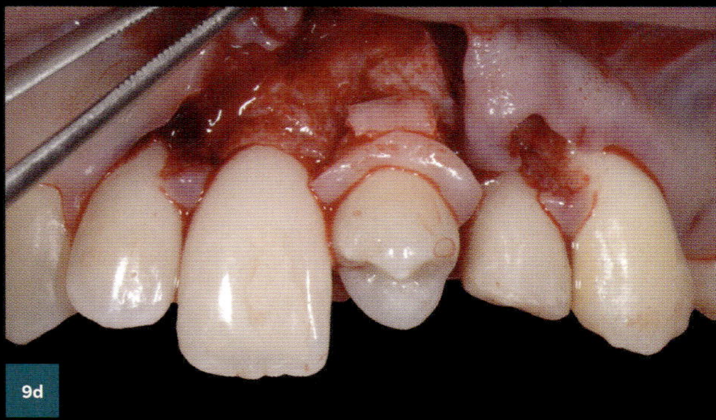

Fig. 9d ■ Premolar positioned in the 21 alveolus.

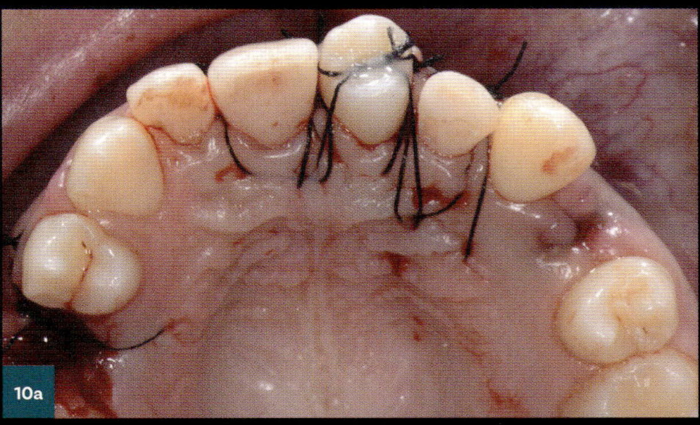

Fig. 10a ■ Premolar stabilized with sutures, 22 partially reconstructed, flaps and socket of 15 sutured.

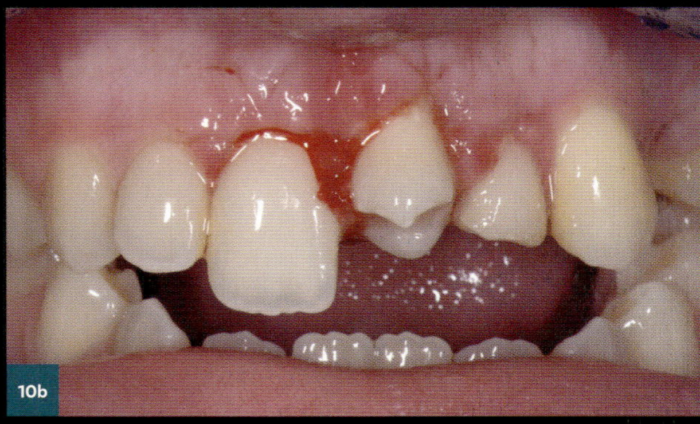

Fig. 10b ■ Suture removal at one week. Normally, the stabilizing sutures of the transposed element are removed after 15 days, but in this case, it was possible to anticipate their removal.

CONT'D >

CONT'D

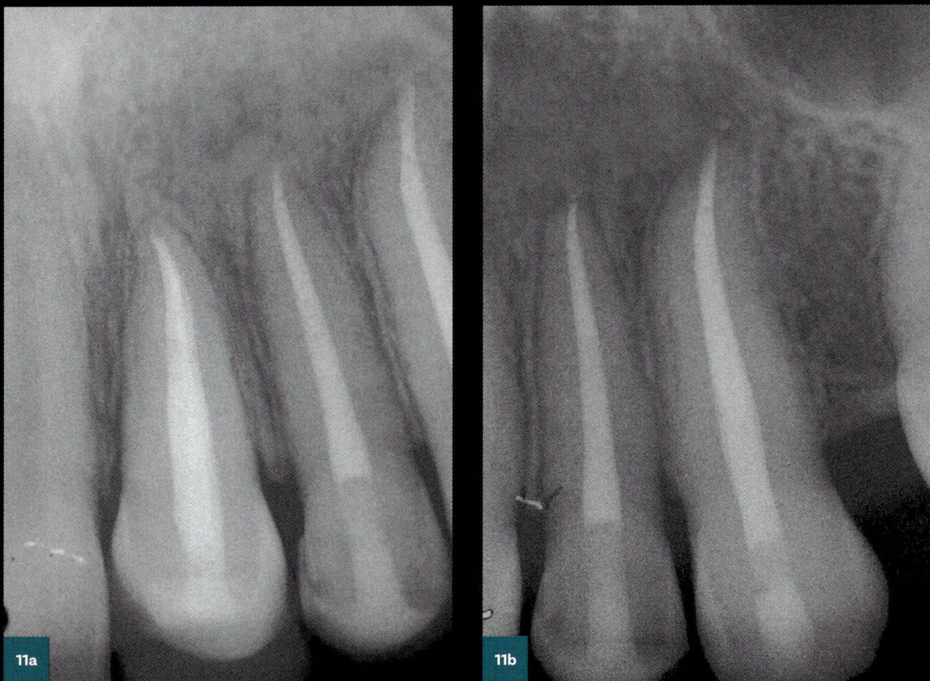

Figs. 11a,b ■ Post-operative periapical radiograph. Endodontic treatments were performed before surgery.

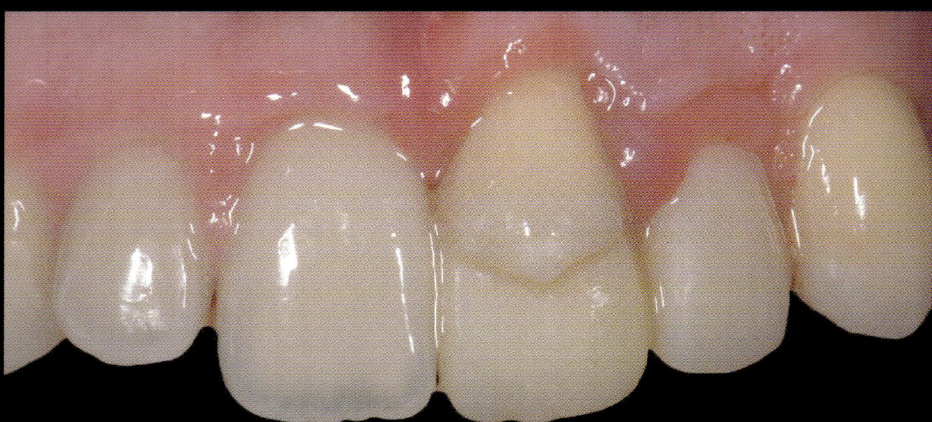

12

Fig. 12 ■ Check-up 1 month after surgery. Provisional direct reconstruction of the 21 and 22 is performed.

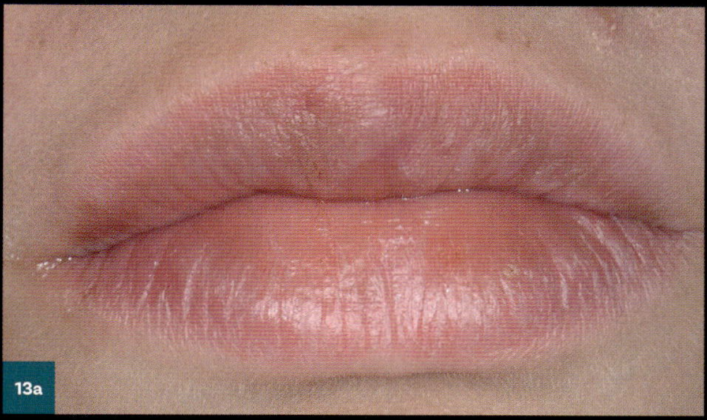

13a

Fig. 13a ■ View with closed lips, the good aesthetic result of the smooth skin is appreciated.

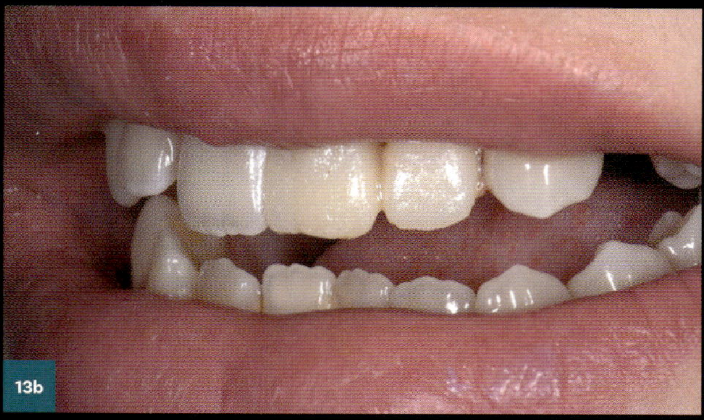

13b

Fig. 13b ■ View with lips apart.

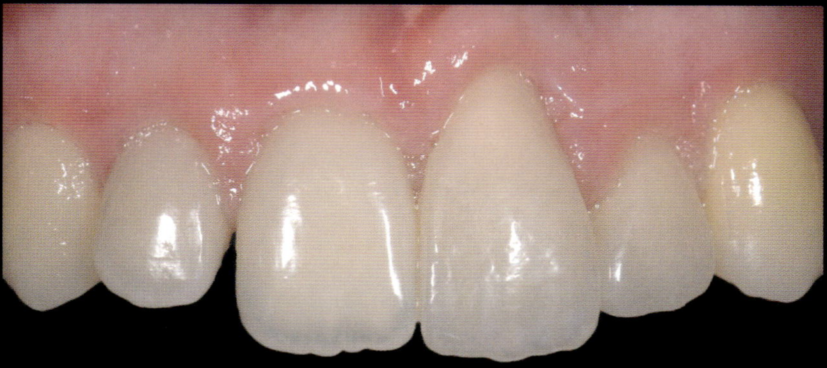

14

Fig. 14 ■ Indirect composite restorations, which will be re-evaluated after the orthognathic treatment for correction of the open bite and at the end of growth.

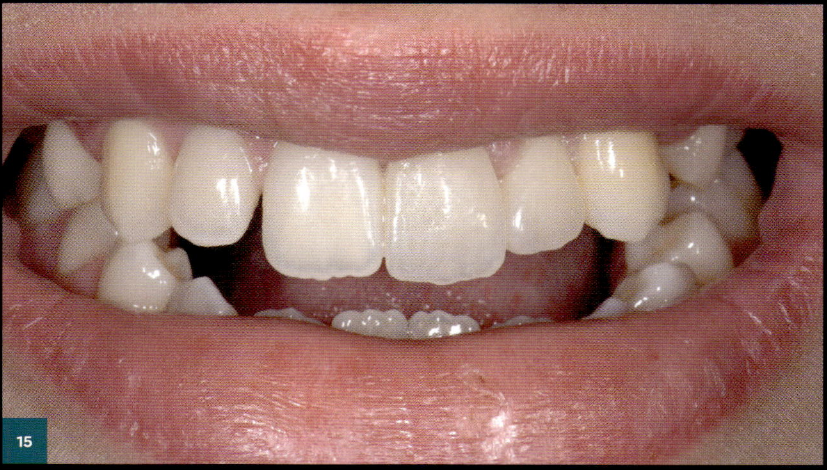

15

Fig. 15 ■ Smile showing the well-preserved papillae, while the slight recession does not require treatment for the moment, as it is not visible.

Bibliography

1. Northway WM, Konigsberg S. Autogenic Tooth Transplantation the "State of the Art". *Am J Orthodont.* 1980;77(2):146-162.
2. Nimčenko T, Omerca G, Varinauskas V, et al. Tooth auto-transplantation as an alternative treatment option: A literature review. *Dent Res J* (Isfahan). 2013;10(1):1-6.
3. Clokie CM, Yau DM, Chano L. Autogenous tooth transplantation: an alternative to dental implant placement? *J Can Dent Assoc.* 2001;67(2):92-96.
4. Cohen AS, Shen TC, Pogrel MA. Transplanting teeth successfully: autografts and allografts that work. *JADA.* 1995;126(4):481-500.
5. Hale ML. Autogenous transplants. *Oral Surg Oral Med Oral Pathol.* 1956;9(1):76-83.
6. Bertani P, Generali P. Third molar autotransplantation: A undervalued therapeutic alternative. *Dental Cadmos.* 2019;87(1):50-55.
7. Tsukiboshi M. Autotransplantation of Teeth: Requirements for Predictable Success. *Dent Traumatol.* 2002;18(4):157-180.
8. Cross D, El-Angbawi A, McLaughlin P, et al. Developments in autotransplantation of teeth. *Surgeon.* 2013;11(1):49-55.
9. Nagori SA, Jose A, Arora A, et al. Misconceptions Regarding Autogenous Tooth Transplantations: A Survey. *J Maxillofac Oral Surg.* 2016;15(2):173-178.
10. Rohof EC, Kerdijk W, Jansma J, Livas C, Ren Y. Autotransplantation of Teeth with Incomplete Root Formation: A Systematic Review and Meta-Analysis. *Clin Oral Invest.* 2018;22(4):1613-1624.
11. Andreasen JO, Paulsen HU, Yu Z, Ahlquist R, Bayer T, Schwartz O. A Long-Term Study of 370 Autotransplanted Premolars. Part I. Surgical Procedures and Standardized Techniques for Monitoring Healing. *Eur J Orthod.* 1990;12(1):3-13.
12. Andreasen JO, Paulsen HU, Yu ZZ, Bayer T, Schwartz O. A Long-Term Study of 370 Autotransplanted Premolars. Part II. Tooth Survival and Pulp Healing Subsequent to Transplantation. *Eur J Orthod.* 1990;12(1):14-24.
13. Andreasen JO, Paulsen HU, Yu Z, Schwartz O. A Long-Term Study of 370 Autotransplanted Premolars. Part III. Periodontal Healing Subsequent to Transplantation. *Eur J Orthod.* 1990;12(1):25-37.
14. Andreasen JO, Paulsen HU, Yu Z, Bayer T. A Long-Term Study of 370 Autotransplanted Premolars. Part IV. Root Development Subsequent to Transplantation. *Eur J Orthod.* 1990;12(1):38-50.
15. Martin K, Nathwani S, Bunyan R. Autotransplantation of teeth: An evidence-based approach. *Br Dent J.* 2018;224(11):861-864.
16. Al-Khanati NM. Immediate autotransplantation of immature maxillary third molar: A case report with 4-year clinical and radiographic follow-up. *Saudi Endod J.* 2019;9(3):226-230.
17. Rusu D, Stratul S, Calniceanu H, et al. A qualitative and semiquantitative SEM study of the morphology of the biofilm on root surfaces of human teeth with endodontic-periodontal lesions. *Exp Ther Med.* 2020;20(6):201.
18. Mejare B, Wannfors K, Jansson L. A study on transplantation of third molars with complete root formation. *Oral Surg Oral Med Oral Pathol Oral Radiol Endod.* 2004;97(2):231-238.
19. Sugai T, Yoshizawa M, Kobayashi T, et al. Clinical study on prognostic factors for autotransplantation of teeth with complete root formation. *Int J Oral Maxillofac Surg.* 2010;39(12):1193-1203.
20. Chung WC, Tu YK, Lin YH, Lu HK. Outcomes of autotransplanted teeth with complete root formation: a systematic review and meta-analysis. *J Clin Periodontol.* 2014;41(4):412-423.
21. Rohof ECM, Kerdijk W, Jansma J, et al. Autotransplantation of teeth with incomplete root formation: a systematic review and meta-analysis. *Clin Oral Investig.* 2018;22(4):1613-1624.
22. Almpani K, Papageorgiou SN, Papadopoulos MA. Autotransplantation of teeth in humans: a systematic review and meta-analysis. *Clin Oral Investig.* 2015;19(6):1157-1179.
23. Lundberg T, Isaksson S. A clinical follow-up study of 278 autotransplanted teeth. *Br J Oral Maxillofac Surg.* 1996;34(2):181-185.
24. Schwartz O, Bergmann P, Klausen B. Autotransplantation of human teeth. *Int J Oral Surg.* 1985;14(3):245-258.
25. Hernandez SL, Cuestas-Carnero R. Autogenic tooth transplantation: a report of ten cases. *J Oral Maxillofac Surg.* 1988;46(12):1051-1055.
26. Altonen M, Haavikko K, Malmström M. Evaluation of autotransplantations of completely developed maxillary canines. *Int J Oral Surg.* 1978;7(5):434-441.
27. Yoshino K, Ishizuka Y, Sugihara N, et al. Gender difference in tooth autotransplantation with complete root formation: a retrospective survey. *J Oral Rehabil.* 2013;40(5):363-374.
28. Kristerson L. Autotransplantation of human premolars. A clinical and radiographic study of 100 teeth. *Int J Oral Surg.* 1985;14(2):200-213.
29. Andreasen JO, Hjorting-Hansen E, Jolst O. A clinical and radiographic study of 76 autotransplanted third molars. *Scand J Dent Res.* 1970;78(6):512-523.
30. Bauss O, Zonios I, Rahman A. Root development of immature third molars transplanted to surgically created sockets. *J Oral Maxillofac Surg.* 2008;66(6):1200-1211.
31. Hasselgren G, Larsson Å, Rundquist L. Pulpal status after autogenous transplantation of fully developed maxillary canines. *Oral Surg Oral Med Oral Pathol.* 1977;44(1):106-112.
32. Hürzeler MB, Quiñones CR. Autotransplantation of a tooth using guided tissue regeneration. *J Clin Periodontol.* 1993;20(7):545-548.
33. Reich PP. Autogenous transplantation of maxillary and mandibular molars. *J Oral Maxillofac Surg.* 2008;66(11):2314-2317.
34. Kim E, Jung JY, Cha IH, Kum KY, Lee SJ. Evaluation of the prognosis and causes of failure in 182 cases of autogenous tooth transplantation. *Oral Surg Oral Med Oral Pathol Oral Radiol Endod.* 2005;100(1):112-119.
35. Kristerson L, Lagerström L. Autotransplantation of teeth in cases with agenesis or traumatic loss of maxillary incisors. *Eur J Orthod.* 1991;13(6):486-492.

36. Sobhi MB, Rana MJ, Manzoor MA, Ibrahim M, Tasleem-ul-Hudda. Autotransplantation of endodontically treated third molars. *J Coll Physicians Surg Pak.* 2003;13(7):372-374.

37. Yan Q, Li B, Long X. Immediate autotransplantation of mandibular third molar in China. *Oral Surg Oral Med Oral Pathol Oral Radiol Endod.* 2010;110(4):436-440.

38. Paulsen HU, Andreasen JO, Schwartz O. Pulp and periodontal healing, root development and root resorption subsequent to transplantation and orthodontic rotation: a long-term study of autotransplanted premolars. *Am J Orthod Dentofacial Orthop.* 1995;108(6):630-640.

39. Herrera H, Leonardo MR, da Silva LA. Treatment of external inflammatory root resorption after autogenous tooth transplantation: case report. *Oral Surg Oral Med Oral Pathol Oral Radiol Endod.* 2006;102(6):e51-e54.

40. Trope M, Moshonov J, Nissan R, et al. Short vs. long-term calcium hydroxide treatment of established inflammatory root resorption in replanted dog teeth. *Endod Dent Traumatol.* 1995;11(3):124-128.

41. Eliasson S, Låftman AC, Strindberg L. Autotransplanted teeth with early-stage endodontic treatment: a radiographic evaluation. *Oral Surg Oral Med Oral Pathol.* 1988;65(5):598-603.

42. Akiyama Y, Fukuda H, Hashimoto K. A clinical and radiographic study of 25 autotransplanted third molars. *J Oral Rehabil.* 1998;25(8):640-644.

43. Gault PC, Warocquier-Clerout R. Tooth auto-transplantation with double periodontal ligament stimulation to replace periodontally compromised teeth. *J Periodontol.* 2002;73(5):575-583.

44. Marques-Ferreira M, Rabaça-Botelho MF, Carvalho L, Oliveiros B, Palmeirão-Carrilho EV. Autogenous tooth transplantation: evaluation of pulp tissue regeneration. *Med Oral Patol Oral Cir Bucal.* 2011;16(7):e984-e989.

45. Andreasen JO. Relationship between Surface and Inflammatory Resorption and Changes in the Pulp after Replantation of Permanent Incisors in Monkeys. *J Endod.* 1981;7(7):294-301.

46. Bae JH, Choi YH, Cho BH, Kim YK, Kim SG. Autotransplantation of teeth with complete root formation: a case series. *J Endod.* 2010;36(8):1422-1426.

47. Flores MT, Andreasen JO, Bakland LK, et al. Guidelines for the Evaluation and Management of Traumatic Dental Injuries. *Dent Traumatol.* 2001;17(5):193-198.

48. Hinckfuss SE, Messer LB. An evidence-based assessment of the clinical guidelines for replanted avulsed teeth. Part I: Timing of pulp extirpation. *Dent Traumatol.* 2009;25(1):32-42.

49. Herrera-Gimbernat D, Recio-Lora C, Torres-Lagares D, Romero-Ruiz MM, Gutiérrez-Pérez JL. Current State of Dental Autotransplantation. *Med Oral Patol Oral Cir Bucal.* 2011;16(7):e948-e952.

50. Armstrong L, O'Reilly C, Ahmed B. Autotransplantation of Third Molars: A Literature Review and Preliminary Protocols. *Br Dent J.* 2020;228(4):247-251.

51. Juslin J, Jääsaari P, Teerijoki-Oksa T, Suominen A, Thorén H. Survival of Autotransplanted Teeth With Open Apices: A Retrospective Cohort Study. *J Oral Maxillofac Surg.* 2020;78(6):902.e1-902.e9.

52. EzEldeen M, Wyatt J, Al-Rimawi A, et al. Use of CBCT Guidance for Tooth Autotransplantation in Children. *J Dent Res.* 2019;98(4):406-413.

53. Lee SJ, Jung IY, Lee CY, Choi SY, Kum KY. Clinical Application of Computer-Aided Rapid Prototyping for Tooth Transplantation. *Dent Traumatol.* 2001;17(3):114-119.

54. Honda M, Uehara H, Uehara T, et al. Use of a Replica Graft Tooth for Evaluation before Autotransplantation of a Tooth. A CAD/CAM Model Produced Using Dental-Cone-Beam Computed Tomography. *Int J Oral Maxillofac Surg.* 2010;39(10):1016-1019.

55. Anssari Moin D, Derksen W, Verweij JP, van Merkesteyn R, Wismeijer D. A Novel Approach for Computer-Assisted Template-Guided Autotransplantation of Teeth with Custom 3D Designed/Printed Surgical Tooling. An Ex Vivo Proof of Concept. *J Oral Maxillofac Surg.* 2016;74(5):895-902.

56. Waikakul A, Punwutikorn J, Kasetsuwan J, Korsuwannawong S. Alveolar bone changes in autogenous tooth transplantation. *Oral Surg Oral Med Oral Pathol Oral Radiol Endod.* 2011;111(3):e1-7.

57. Waldon K, Barber SK, Spencer RJ, Duggal MS. Indications for the use of auto-transplantation of teeth in the child and adolescent. *Eur Arch Paediatr Dent.* 2012;13(4):210-216.

58. Andreasen JO, Kristerson L, Andreasen FM. Damage of the Hertwig's epithelial root sheath: effect upon root growth after autotransplantation of teeth in monkeys. *Endod Dent Traumatol.* 1988;4(4):145-151.

59. Andreasen JO. Pulp and Periodontal Tissue Repair - Regeneration or Tissue Metaplasia after Dental Trauma. A Review. *Dent Traumatol.* 2012;28(1):19-24.

60. Czochrowska EM, Plakwicz P. Autotransplantation and healing. *Am J Orthod Dentofacial Orthop.* 2019;156(3):299-300.

61. Skoglund A, Tronstad L. Pulpal changes in replanted and autotransplanted immature teeth of dogs. *J Endod.* 1981;7(7):309-316.

62. Schendel KU, Schwartz O, Andreasen JO, Hoffmeister B. Reinnervation of autotransplanted teeth. A histological investigation in monkeys. *Int J Oral Maxillofac Surg.* 1990;19(4):247-249.

63. Cronin RJ Jr, Oesterle LJ. Implant use in growing patients. Treatment planning concerns. *Dent Clin North Am.* 1998;42(1):1-34.

64. Verweij JP, Anssari Moin D, Mensink G, Wismeijer D, van Merkesteyn JP. Autotransplantatie 2.0. Overwegingen, uitkomsten en nieuwste technieken [Autotransplantation 2.0. Considerations, results and the latest techniques]. *Ned Tijdschr Tandheelkd.* 2016;123(7-8):348-353.

65. Mensink G, van Merkesteyn R. Autotransplantation of premolars. *Br Dent J.* 2010;208(3):109-111.

66. Kvint S, Lindsten R, Magnusson A, Nilsson P, Bjerklin K. Autotransplantation of teeth in 215 patients. A follow-up study. *Angle Orthod.* 2010;80(3):446-451.

67. Josefsson E, Brattström V, Tegsjö U, Valerius-Olsson H. Treatment of lower second premolar agenesis by autotransplantation: four-year evaluation of eighty patients. *Acta Odontol Scand.* 1999;57(2):111-115.

68. Jonsson T, Sigurdsson TJ. Autotransplantation of premolars to premolar sites. A long-term follow-up study of 40 consecutive patients. Am *J Orthod*

Dentofacial Orthop. 2004;125(6):668-675.

69. Watanabe Y, Mohri T, Takeyama M, et al. Long-Term Observation of Autotransplanted Teeth with Complete Root Formation in Orthodontic Patients. *Am J Orthod Dentofacial Orthop.* 2010;138(6):720-726.

70. Rohof ECM, Kerdijk W, Jansma J, Livas C, Ren Y. Autotransplantation of teeth with incomplete root formation: a systematic review and meta-analysis. *Clin Oral Investig.* 2018;22(4):1613-1624.

71. van Westerveld KJH, Verweij JP, Toxopeus EE, Fiocco M, Mensink G, van Merkesteyn JPR. Long-term outcomes 1-20 years after autotransplantation of teeth: clinical and radiographic evaluation of 66 premolars and 8 molars. *Br J Oral Maxillofac Surg.* 2019;57(7):666-671.

72. Mendoza-Mendoza A, Solano-Reina E, Iglesias-Linares A, Garcia-Godoy F, Abalos C. Retrospective Long-Term Evaluation of Autotransplantation of Premolars to the Central Incisor Region. *Int Endod J.* 2012;45(1):88-97.

73. Gonnissen H, Politis C, Schepers S, et al. Long-Term Success and Survival Rates of Autogenously Transplanted Canines. *Oral Surg Oral Med Oral Pathol Oral Radiol Endod.* 2010;110(5):570-578.

74. Generali P, Bertani P. How to Give a Second Life to Third Molars: A Case Series with Follow-Up. 2019. https://www.dental-tribune.com/clinical/how-to-give-a-second-life-to-third-molars-a-caseseries-with-follow-up/.

75. Milani S, Generali P. Tooth Autotransplantation. What's the Limit of Our Possibilities in Conservative Treatments? *G Ital Endod.* 2018;32(2):86-91.

17

Orthodontic-restorative solutions with dental agenesis and traumatic extractions

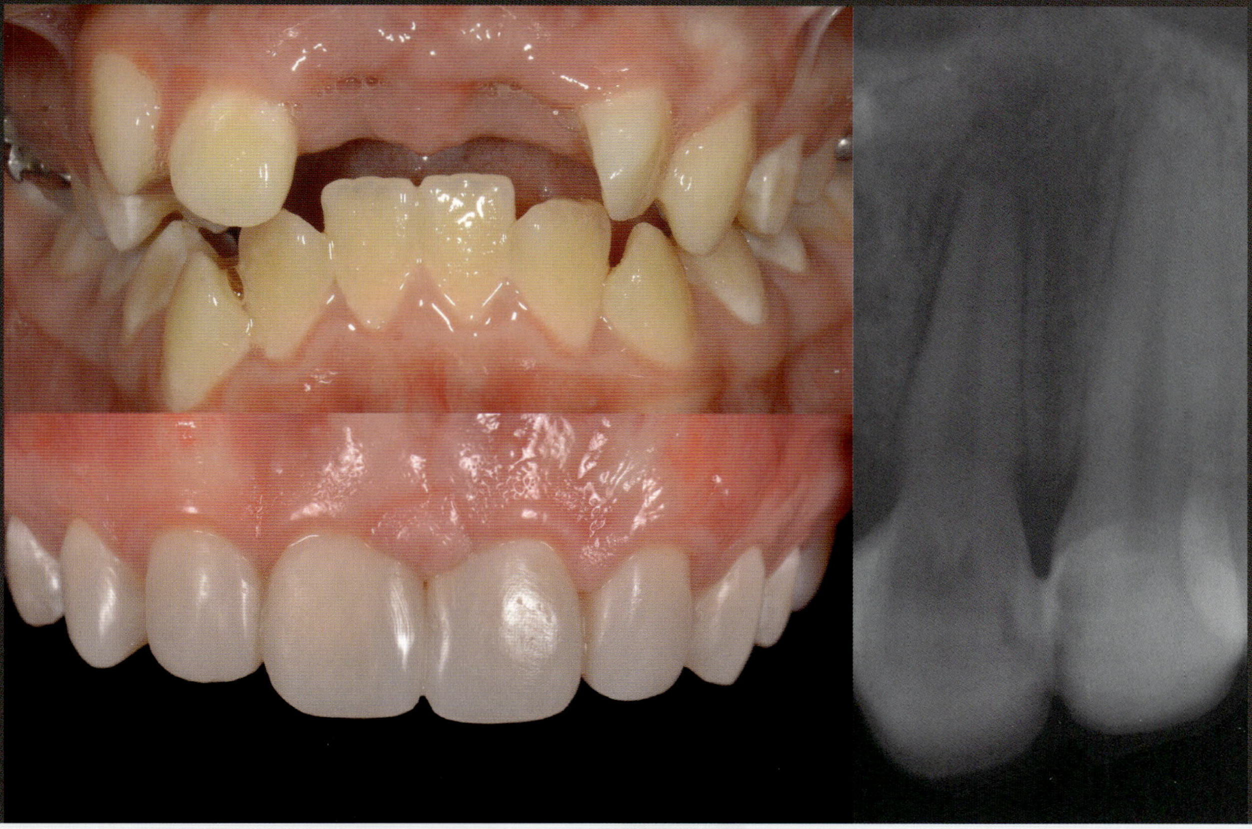

Agenesis

The absence of teeth prompts consideration for suitable replacements within the dental arch. The synergy between adhesive dentistry and orthodontics is often the optimal choice. However, in a minority of cases, implants could also be significant.[1]

Agenesis occurs in approximately 9% of the Caucasian population. Notably, attention is particularly warranted for cases involving the front teeth, especially the lateral incisors, which are absent in about 1% of the population. Although this prevalence is consistent between genders, agenesis is more commonly unilateral, often with a contralateral malformed tooth.[2] The relevance of agenesis in this context is substantial. Until recently, diverse solutions existed without consensus on the optimal therapeutic approach. Proposed remedies frequently included osseointegrated implants or invasive prosthetic procedures. However, when these approaches are applied to young patients, they could jeopardize the long-term integrity of the masticatory system.[3-5]

Fortunately, both orthodontic and prosthetic clinical experiences have led to significant improvements, offering highly effective solutions.[6-8]

Within orthodontics, a significant amount of literature supports the choice of closing spaces resulting from agenesis.[9,10] Similarly, in restorative dentistry, the increasing use of adhesive techniques enables aesthetic adjustments for improperly relocated dental elements, ensuring both a pleasing appearance and functionally validity.[11] Based on these principles, we have explored additional options for utilizing the auto-transplantation technique to relocate non-functional or redundant teeth from their original sites to replace missing teeth in more critical areas.

In this short chapter, we address the aforementioned challenges and offer practical guidance for both the diagnostic and clinical phases. It's crucial to highlight that successful outcomes depend on seamless collaboration among diverse specialists, each contributing their unique expertise. These disciplines include orthodontics, periodontics, restorative dentistry, and, in specific instances, oral surgery.

In many cases, patients present with the sole absence of an upper lateral incisor, often accompanied by a small or conical-shaped contralateral tooth. This scenario adds to therapeutic uncertainties. The decision to retain the conical tooth and address aesthetics using adhesive techniques, rather than extracting it and treating the case as a dual agenesis, remains a recurrent topic of discussions.

In such cases, the initial observation period may reveal dental malpositioning in the anterior sector due to migrating teeth that are not in contact. Additionally, concomitant skeletal dysgnathia of skeletal origin should be considered.

Consequently, orthodontic intervention is crucial to address these issues, with the understanding that the restoration of missing dental structure is within the scope of restorative dentistry. It is evident that the shared goal is to preserve hard tissue, leading both disciplines to prioritize tooth preservation. Therefore, any aesthetic enhancement procedure should prioritize minimal invasiveness.

Given these considerations, it is clear that achieving an optimal aesthetic outcome might necessitate the adhesive reconstruction of the six upper front teeth over time.

Literature underscores that composite restorations and veneers, whether using CADCAM techniques or traditional ceramics, yield excellent long-term outcomes when employing appropriate methods and materials.[12,13]

Orthodontic-restorative solutions

A relevant literature analysis helps refine therapeutic approaches, offering insights into the need for unilateral space closure or the possible avoidance of contralateral malformed superior lateral extraction. Furthermore, for patients with concurrent malocclusion on the same side as maxillary agenesis, the preferred approach is upper space closure.

During the extended transition from adolescence to

adulthood,[14] "Maryland" adhesive bridges serve as a viable solution, often eliminating the requirement for a single dental implant, especially in cases with a prominent smile line.

The dynamic interplay between orthodontics and modern adhesive dentistry necessitates a well-considered decision tree for optimal patient-specific treatment selection.

A robust 95% success rate has been reported for cantilevered bonded bridges with extensions, and a mere 5% rate of veneer decementation after 10 years, establishing their reliability.[15] Biologically, aesthetically and periodontally, a natural tooth or root consistently outweighs an implant due to minimal side effects.[16] This is particularly important in the aesthetic area, where achieving enduring tissue stability presents a challenge.

Finally, it must be reiterated that, in most instances, orthodontic treatment is essential to counteract adjacent tooth migration. This approach offers a shorter treatment duration and a superior cost-benefit ratio compared to available alternatives (**Table 17.1**).

This consideration holds significant importance when treating pediatric and young adult patients. Among numerous studies, the oldest study, conducted by Nordquist and McNeil,[17] compared 39 cases of space closure and 19 cases of space opening using prosthetic replacements (13 bridges, 6 removable partial dentures) over a 10-year period after treatment.

Their findings concluded that:

- Patients undergoing space closure exhibit better periodontal health compared to those with prosthetic devices.
- There is no disparity in terms of occlusal function.
- The presence or absence of bonded restorations to enlarge the canine does not correlate with periodontal status.
- No evidence supports the notion that the Class I canine relationship is the preferred treatment method.

The most compelling conclusion is that "space closure" represents the most effective long-term approach to completing cases involving the absence of one or more upper lateral incisors due to agenesis or trauma. These teeth can be transformed using minimally invasive adhesive techniques, supported by an aesthetic analysis after suitable repositioning. Such techniques are applicable to single teeth and teeth with extensions like "Maryland type" bridges featuring a single anchoring wing.[18-21]

Below, we present a concise review of clinical cases illustrating the achievement of functionally robust and aesthetically optimal outcomes through a multidisciplinary approach. These outcomes are sustainable for extended periods, negating the necessity for highly invasive techniques required by implants or specific prosthetic devices.

Table 17.1 ■ Why close agenesis spaces orthodontically.

Produces satisfactory aesthetic results for patients
Does not impair the function of the temporomandibular joint (TMJ)
Preserves periodontal health

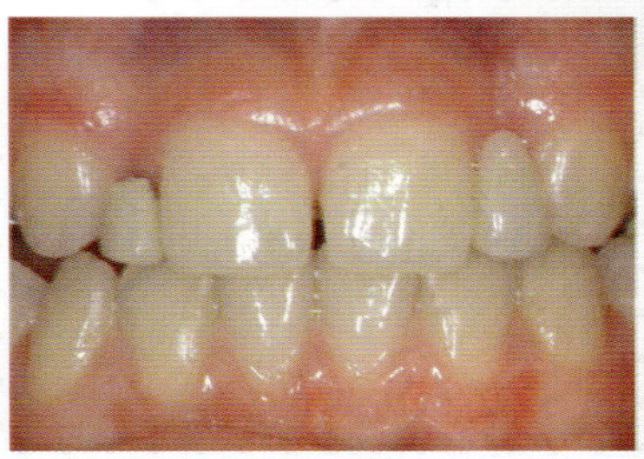

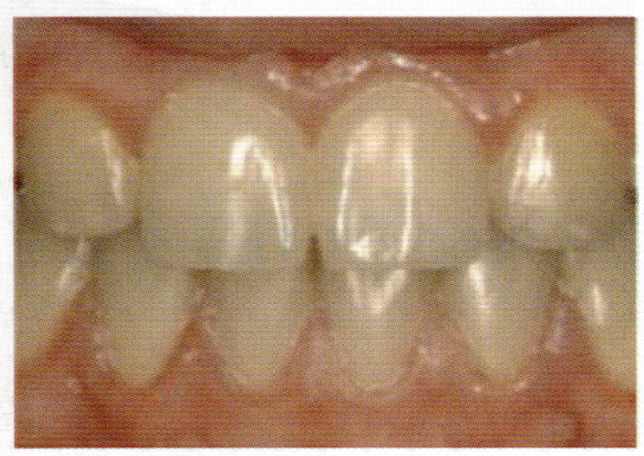

Orthodontic retreatment in a 14-year-old female patient with bilateral agenesis of the upper lateral incisors

The featured case is emblematic. The patient, now fourteen, underwent orthodontic treatment to create space for two osseointegrated implants once they have finished growing, which is expected to be around the age of twenty. A temporary solution involved a removable metallic appliance supporting the missing teeth (12 and 22). Seeking an alternative, the patient consulted a specialist.

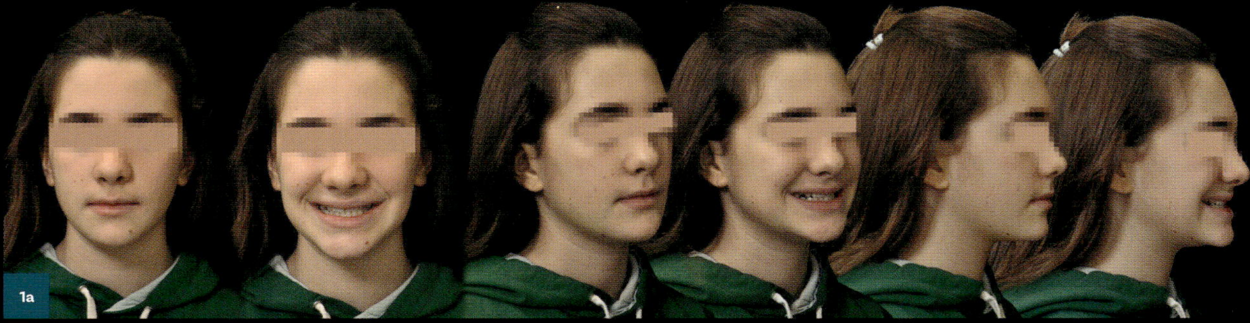

1a

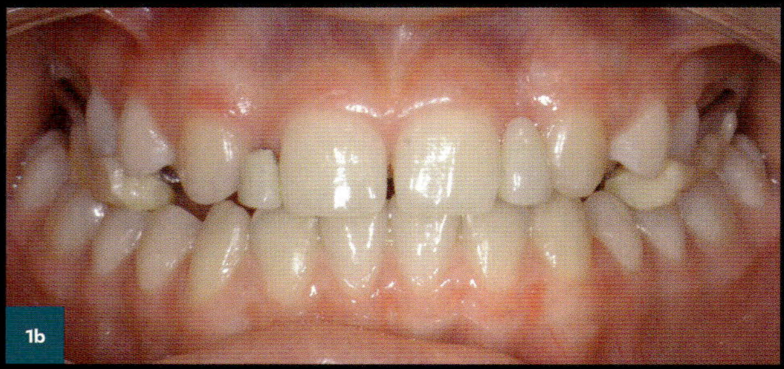

1b

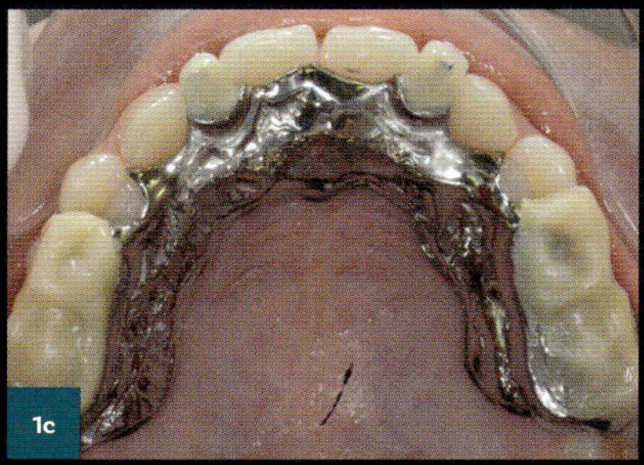

1c

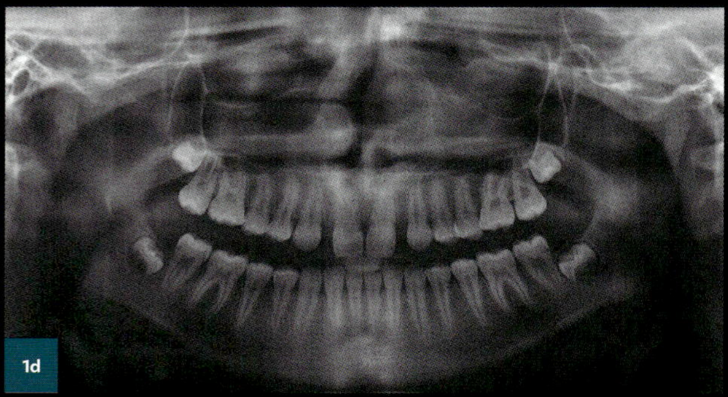

1d

Figs. 1a-d ■ **(a)** The young patient's facial photographs show mild maxillary retrusion associated with a slight mandibular prominence. **(b)** The frontal intraoral view shows the agenesis of both upper lateral incisors, which have been replaced with a removable prosthetic device **(c)** to maintain the aesthetics. However, the experience was not particularly pleasant or comfortable for the patient. **(d)** The panoramic radiographic view confirms the presence of bilateral agenesis of teeth 12 and 22.

The analysis of the case highlighted a clear tendency towards skeletal Class III. Due to the patient's late advanced stage, observation for about a year was necessary. Once skeletal relationships stabilized, orthodontic treatment was implemented. This aimed to close residual spaces, enhance aesthetics using adhesive techniques, and address emerging issues.

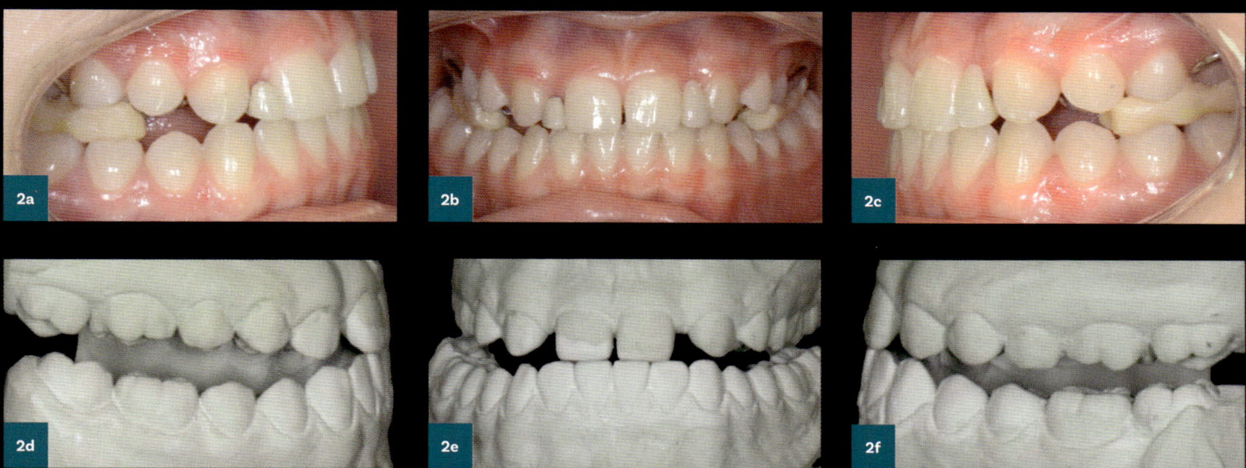

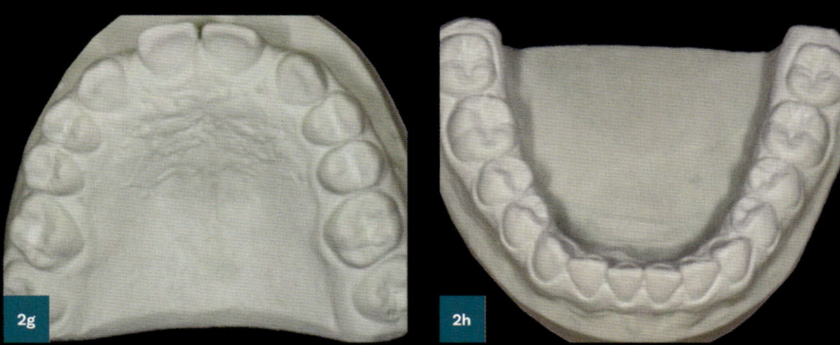

Figs. 2a-h ■ Mounting in the articulator allows for the evaluation of the incisor relationship in edge-to-edge position and the potential for orthodontic correction by closing the spaces caused by agenesis. This is necessary because reopening these spaces accurately is not possible.

CONT'D >

CONT'D

n particular, special attention should be given to the unique orthodontic treatment phase (see Figs. 6a-i) Here, canine extrusion and simultaneous intrusion of the corresponding first premolar are executed. This simplifies subsequent aesthetic transformations and aligns with the teeth's new roles. Five years (see Figs. 6a-i post-orthodontic and restorative treatment, the case's review affirms the validity of the chosen approach Medium-term stability confirms that the implant-free solution was indeed the wisest approach.

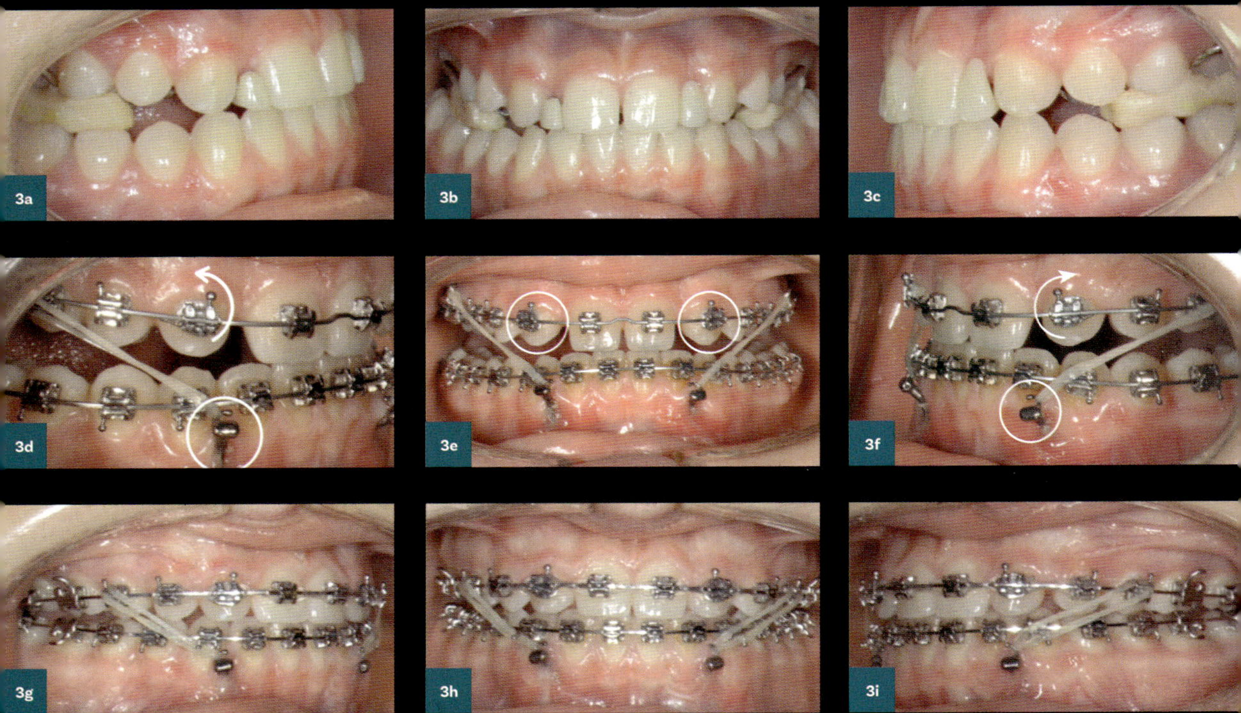

Figs. 3a-i ■ The orthodontic treatment, using mandibular TADs and Class III elastics, successfully corrected the overjet and overbite while also establishing a stable posterior occlusion.

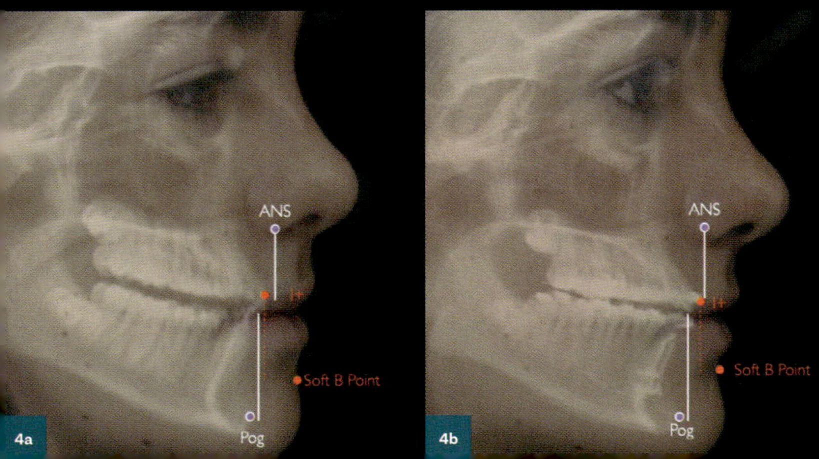

Figs. 4a,b ■ The cephalometric examination shows that the orthodontic correction has not produced significant dento-alveolar compensation. This allows for a possible surgical solution in case of unfavourable late growth of the mandible

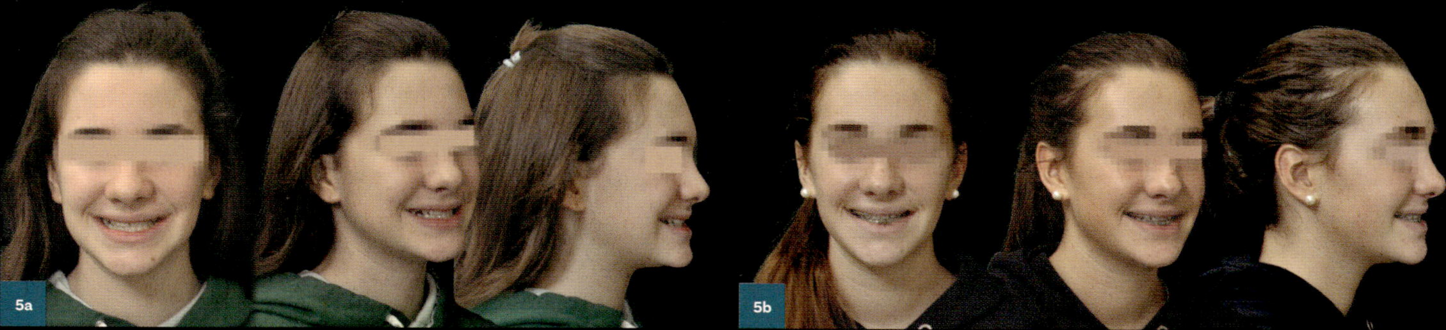

Figs. 5a,b ■ During the treatment, verifying the good clinical outcome of the dento-maxillary repositioning was possible, which improved the patient's aesthetic appearance, refining her profile.

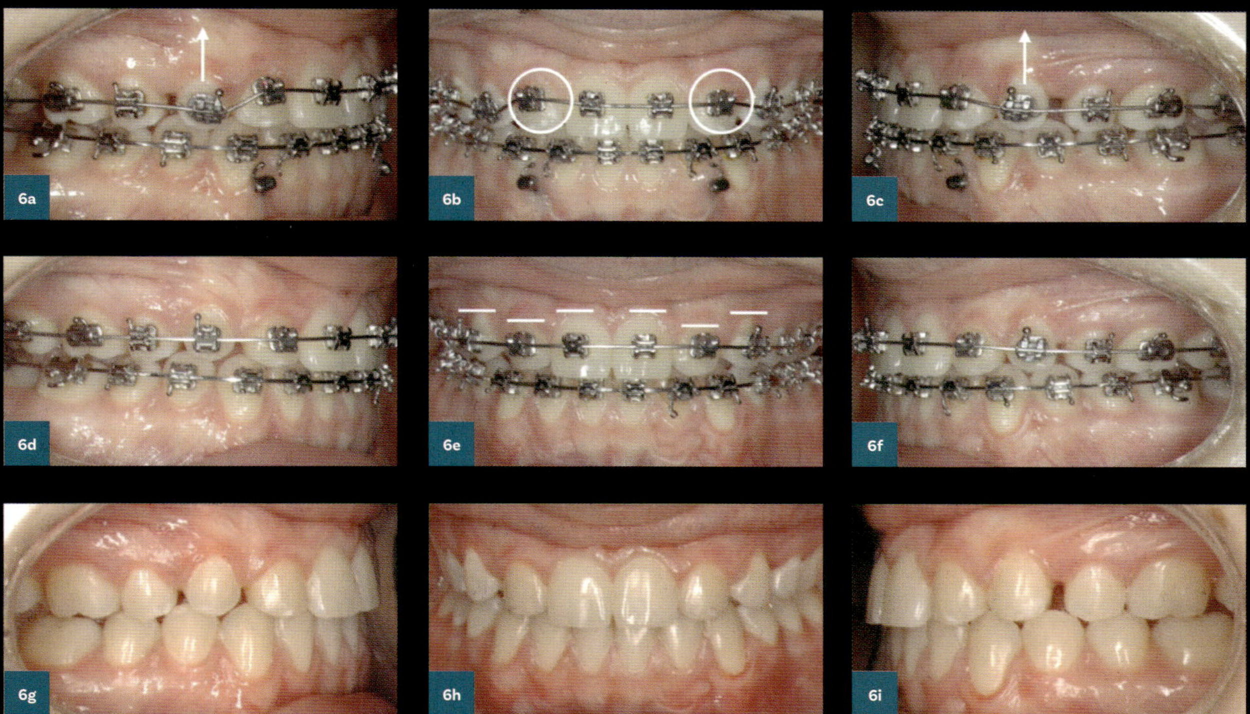

Figs. 6a-i ■ A peculiar feature of these cases, from an orthodontic point of view, is the relocation of the canines to replace the missing laterals and successively reviewing the position of the first premolars. The former must be slightly extruded to make the transformation process into laterals easier; likewise, the upper first premolars must be intruded since their role will be to replace the canines during the normal operations of aesthetic-functional transformation.

> CONT'D

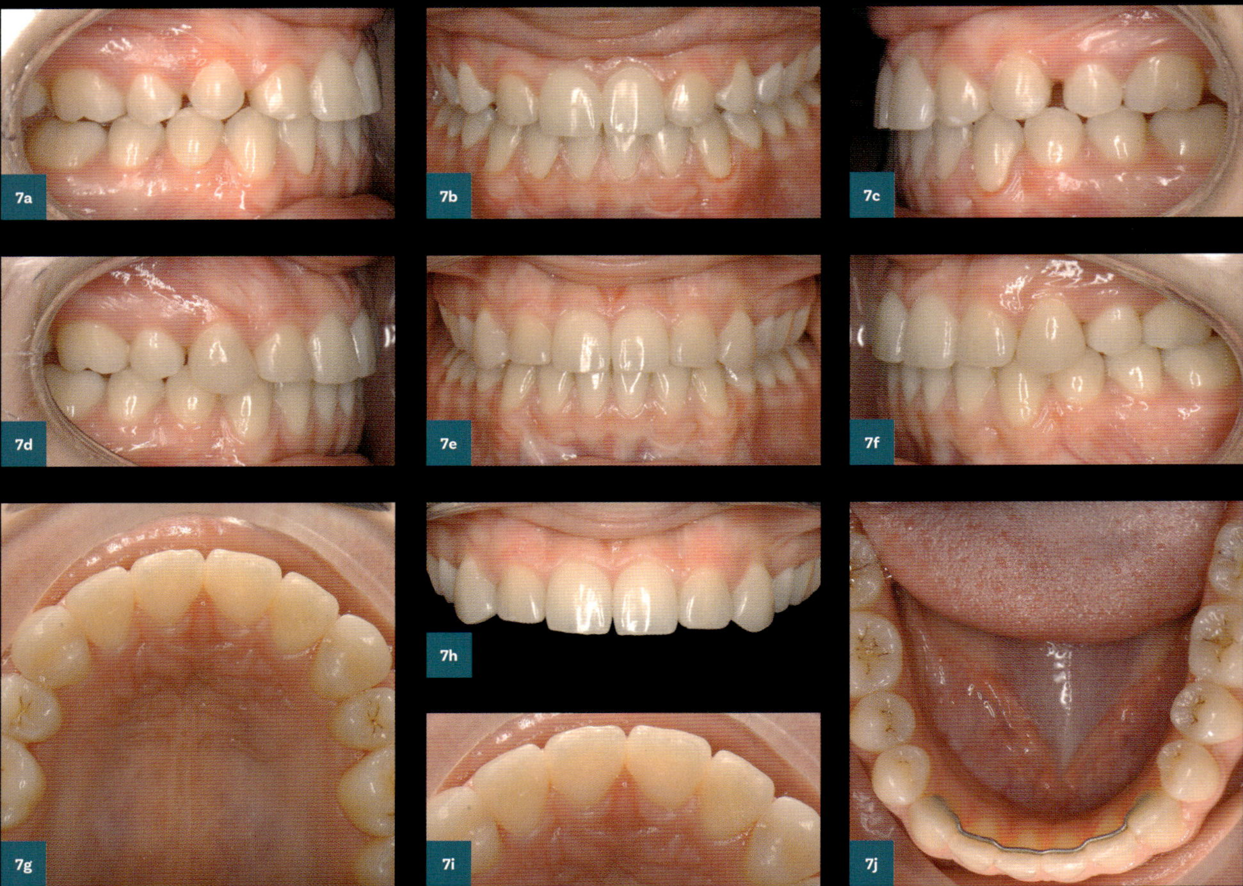

Figs. 7a-j ■ The case has been successfully solved **(a-c)**. In the following images, you can appreciate the aesthetic restoration using composite on the first premolar and the canine.

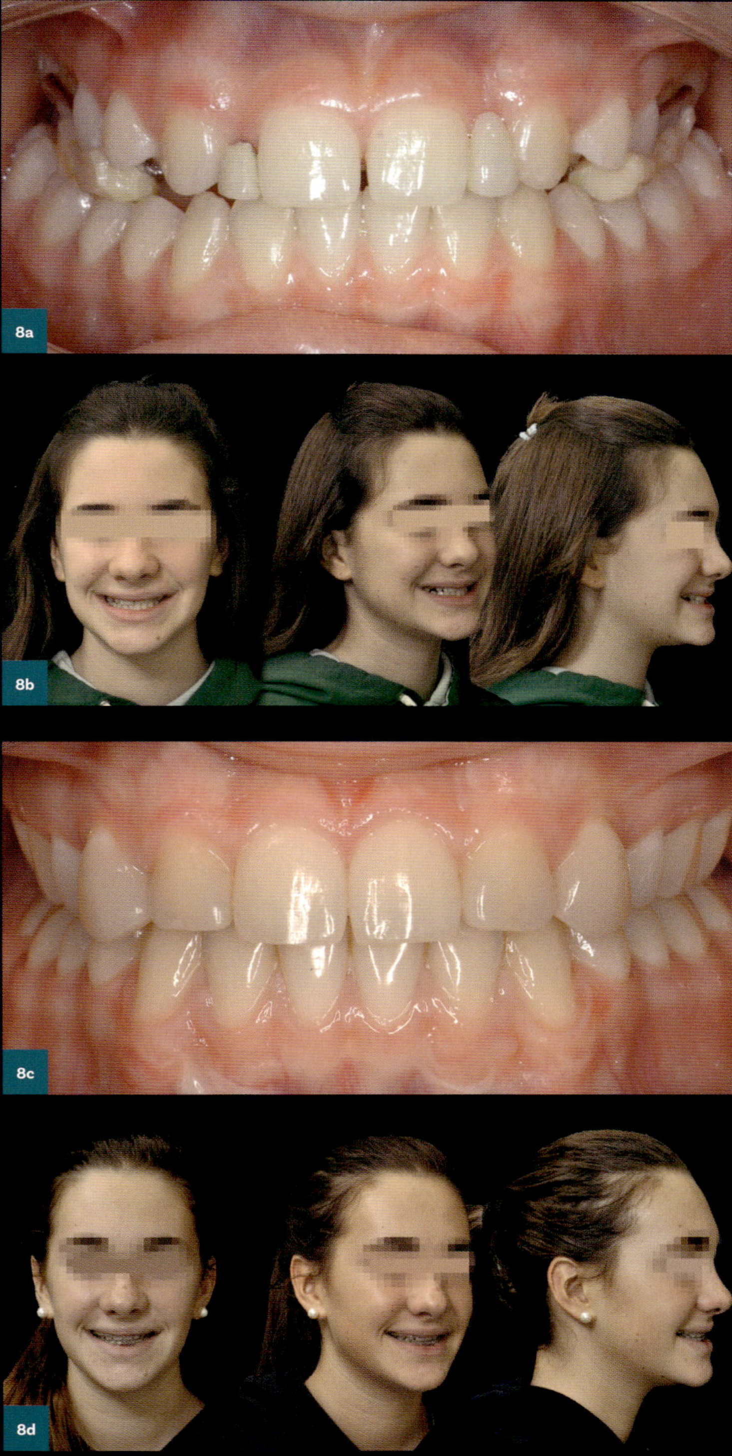

Figs. 8a-d ▪ In a summary of the treatment sequence, the case shows the initial condition both intraorally and through images of the facial profile confirming the case's success.

CONT'D

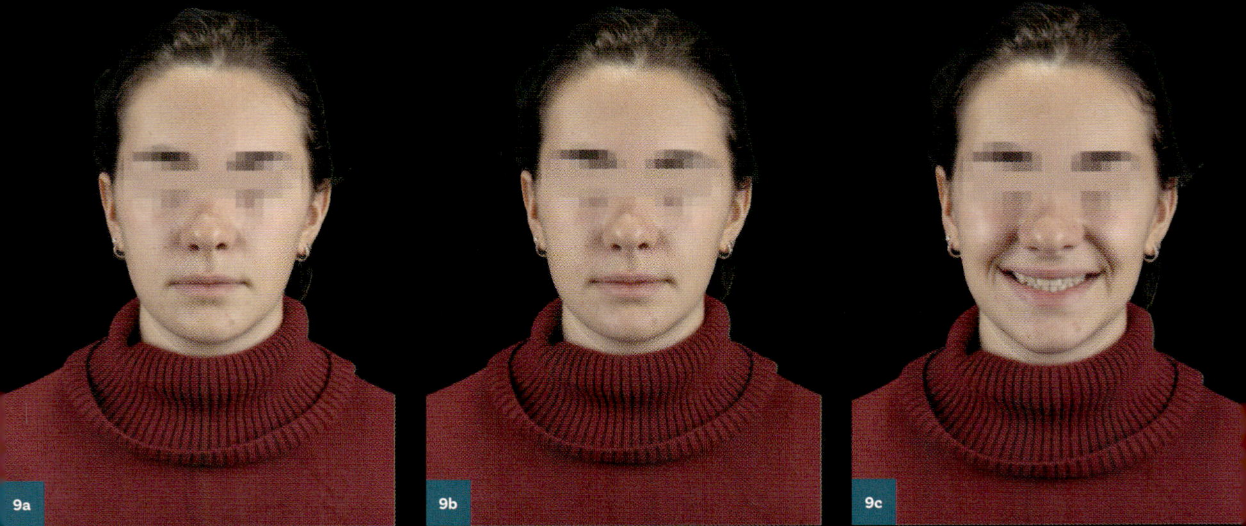

Figs. 9a-c ■ The case after a period of time (18.6 years); note the perfect integration of the patient's smile and the excellent stability of the treatment in terms of the interocclusal relationship and the dental-periodontal transition.

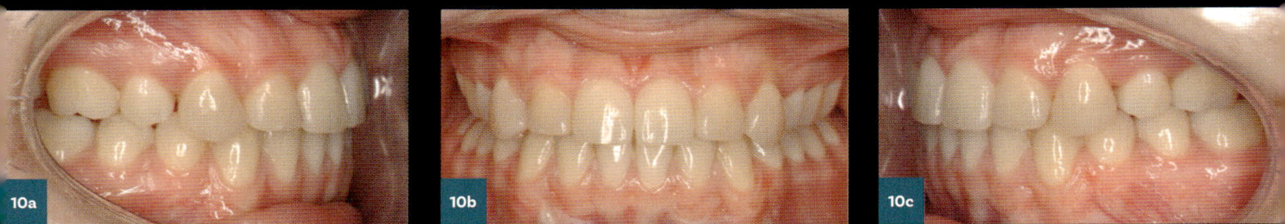

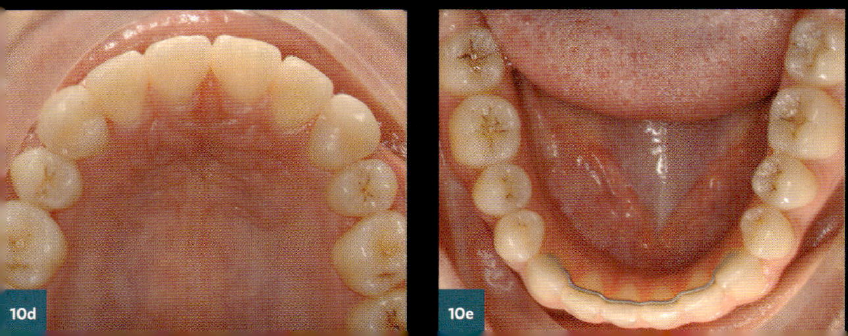

Figs. 10a-e ■ Good occlusal stability. Composite reconstructions (Conservative: Dr Paolo Ferrari, Parma) allow for a favourable transition from adolescence to young adulthood. Subsequently, other minimally invasive restorative options may be pursued without needing a new orthodontic treatment or extensive preparations, given the favourable dental positioning obtained orthodontically.

A rare case of concomitant agenesis of lateral incisors and canines: resolved with adhesive bridges

The concurrent absence of upper canines and lateral incisors is an uncommon condition. Addressing this situation requires therapeutic strategies to preserve spaces and periodontal support. Adhesive techniques are employed on the dependable deciduous canines. Specifically, the premise was created for placing adhesive-type materials . The approach involves using adhesive bridges to substitute the missing teeth. This establishes both aesthetic and structural harmony between the first premolars and deciduous canines. Additionally, it achieves aesthetic balance by incorporating the two upper central incisors.

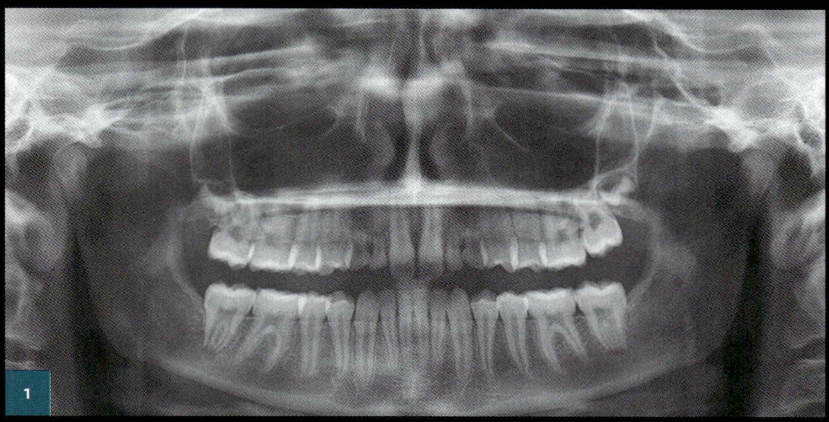

Fig. 1 ■ The radiographic examination testifies to this rare occurrence, i.e., the joint agenesis of the upper lateral incisors and canines.

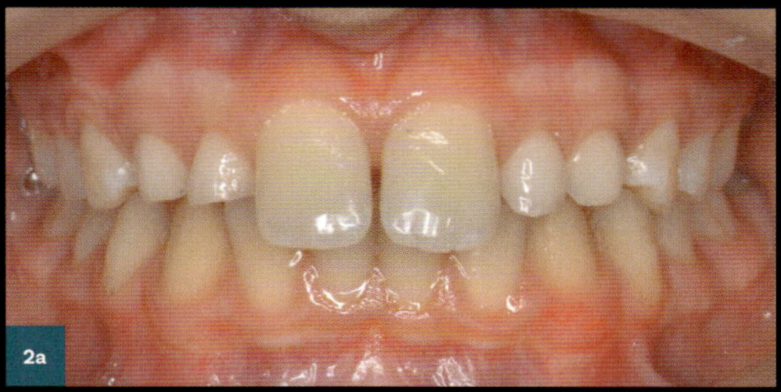

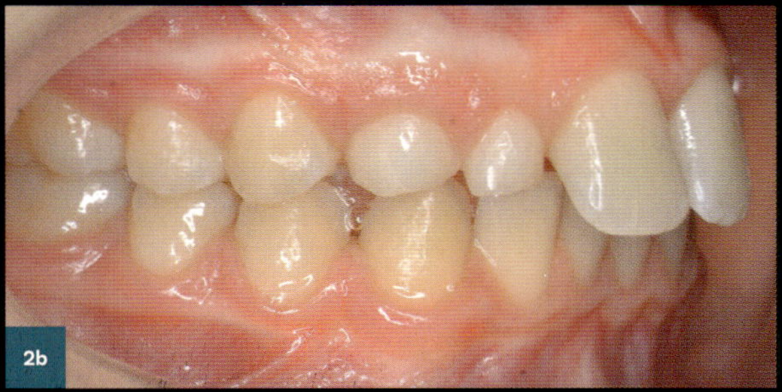

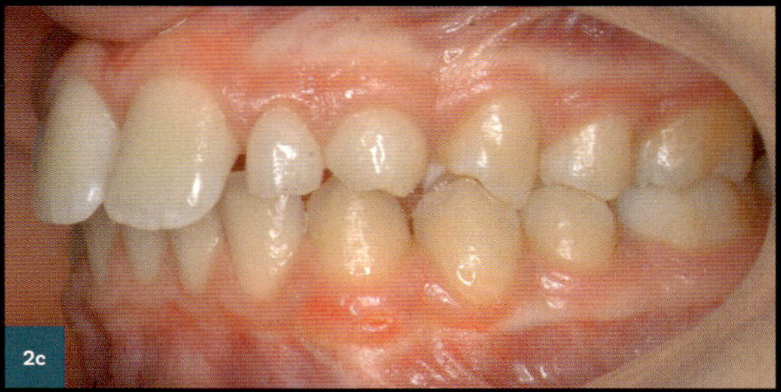

Figs. 2a-c ■ Intraoral photographs show the presence of a dental Class II with increased overjet.

CONT'D >

> CONT'D

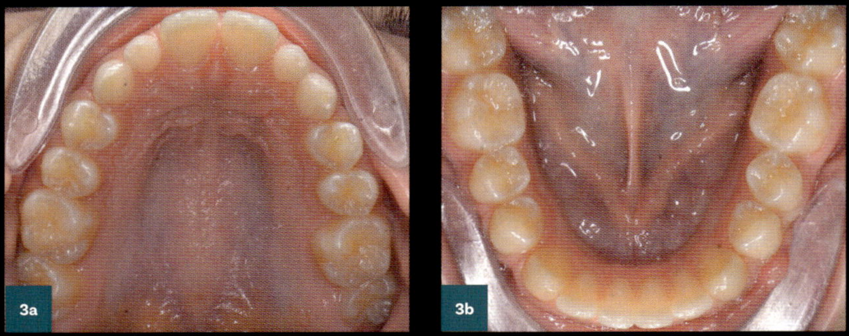

Figs. 3a,b ■ The intraoral occlusal photographs do not reveal noticeable asymmetries.

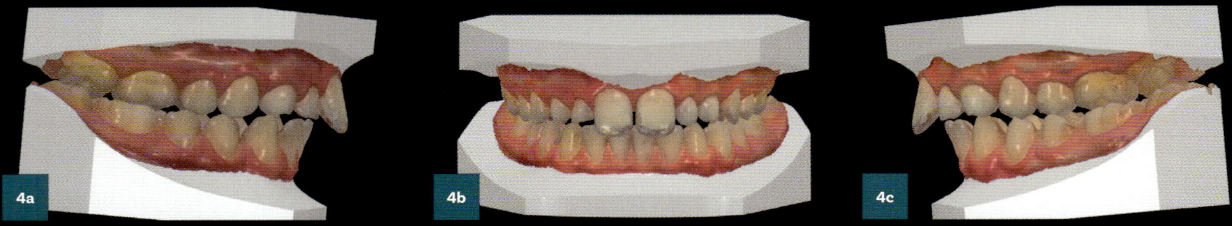

Figs. 4a-c ■ The scan makes the Class II condition more evident and the overjet that needs to be corrected.

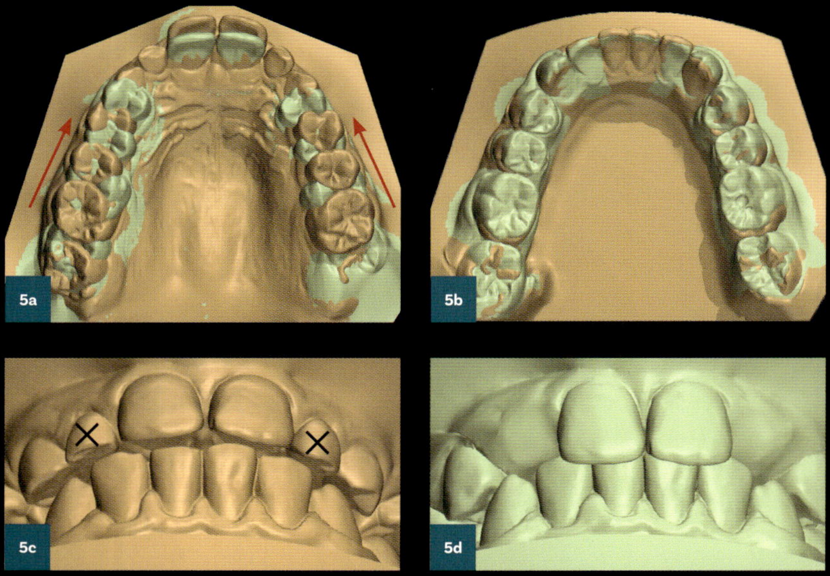

Figs. 5a-d ■ Orthodontic setup to simulate the final position (*in green*) necessary to obtain a correct occlusion and a correction of the overjet after extracting the deciduous laterals.

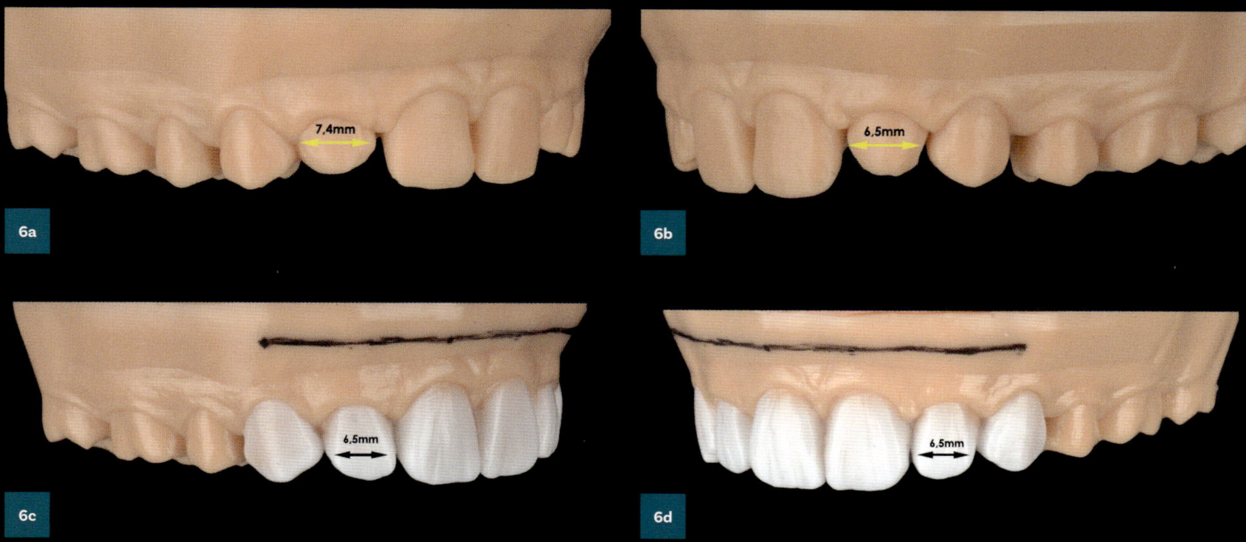

6a 6b 6c 6d

Figs. 6a-d ■ The anterior translation of the deciduous canines would allow adhesive bridges to mask the deciduous canines and stabilize them with permanent premolars.

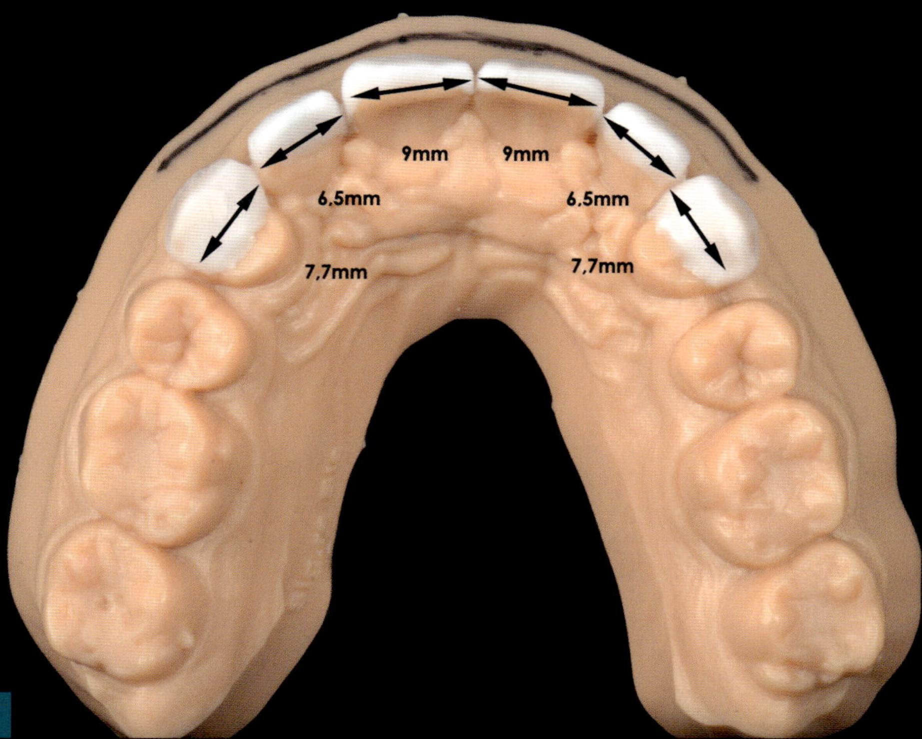

7

Fig. 7 ■ Occlusal view of the duly measured spaces.

CONT'D >

CONT'D

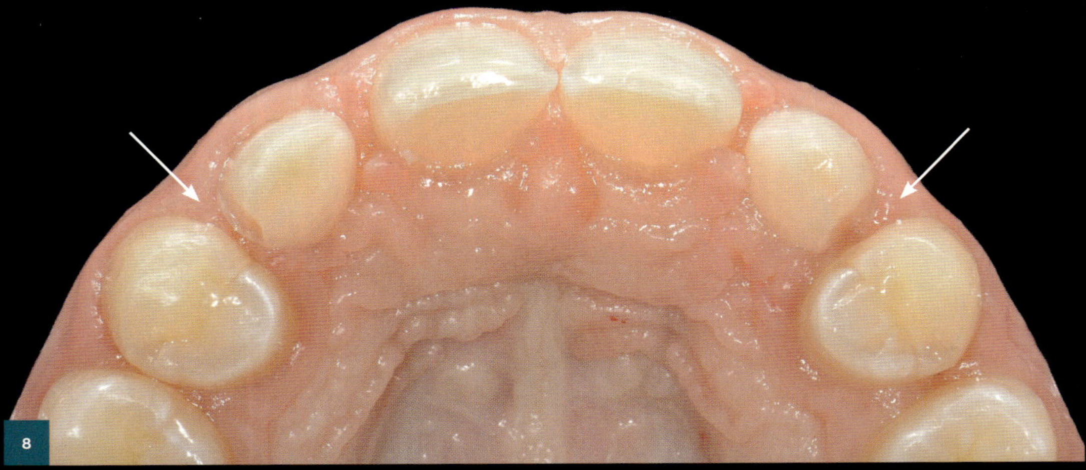

Fig. 8 ■ The clinical picture of minimal preparations performed on the deciduous canines.

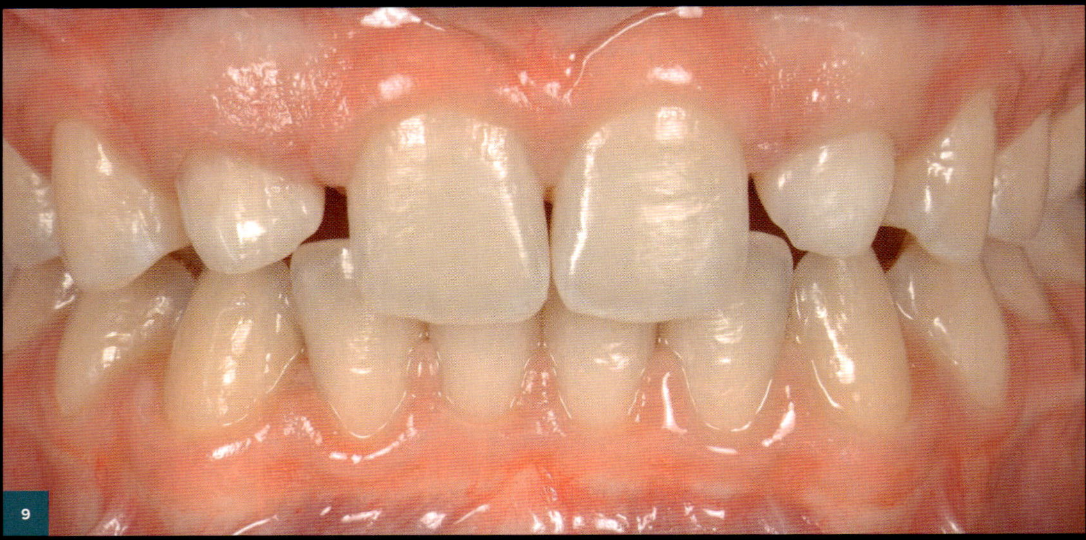

Fig. 9 ■ The provisional restorative solution.

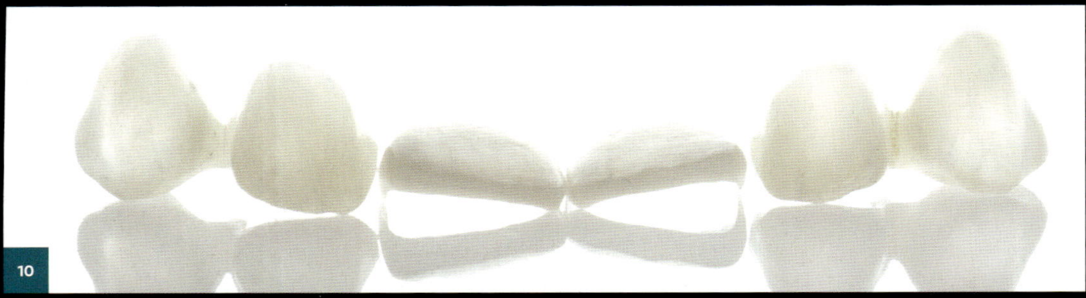

Fig. 10 ■ The lithium disilicate restorations. Single veneers on the centrals and united veneers on the premolars and deciduous canines (Laboratorio Quintavalla, Pozzi, Parma).

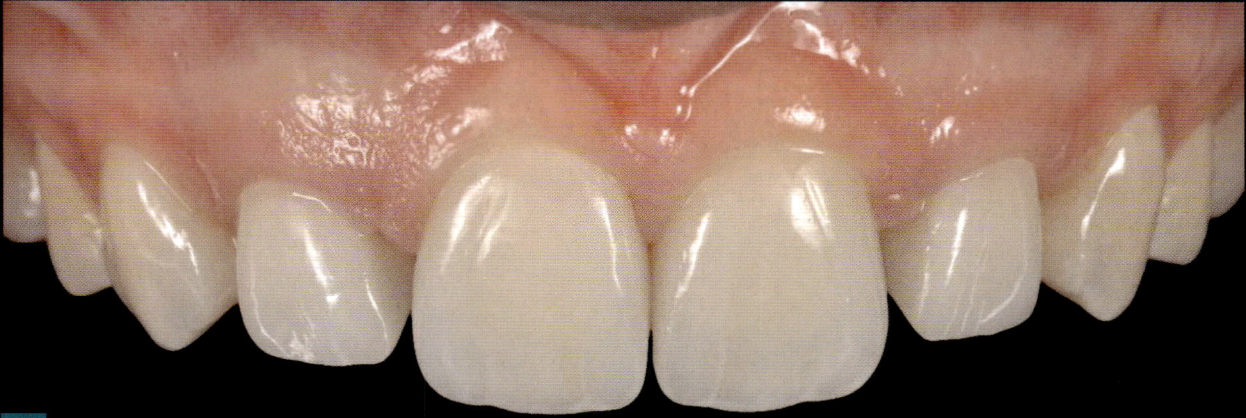

11

Fig. 11 ■ The case once the work was completed (Conservative: Dr. Nikolaos Perakis, Bologna).

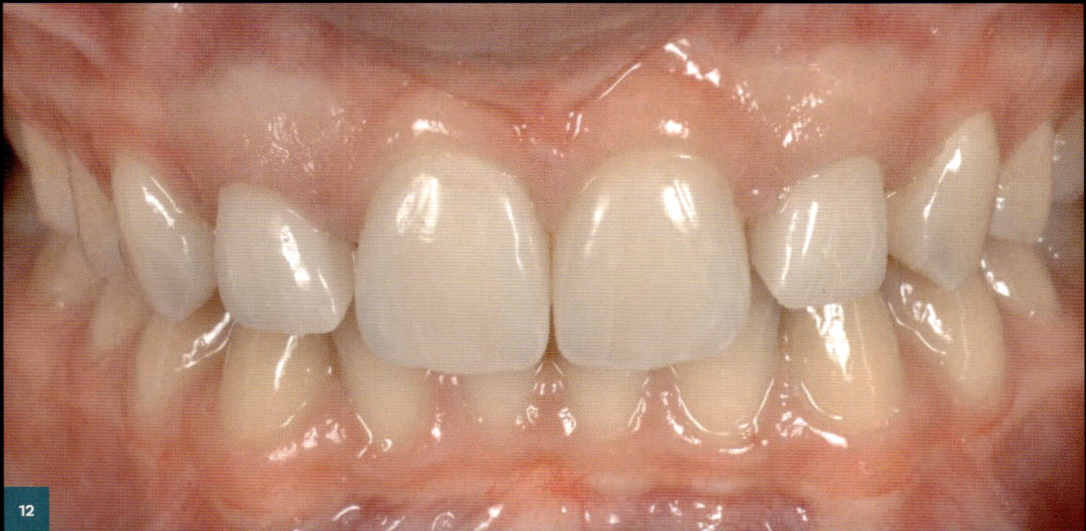

12

Traumatic loss of two upper central incisors in a patient with hyperdivergent Class II malocclusion

The requirement to create a treatment plan for a patient with unfavorable skeletal growth, who lost two upper central incisors due to trauma, prompted the orthodontist to adapt the traditional orthodontic protocol for these specific dysgnathia.

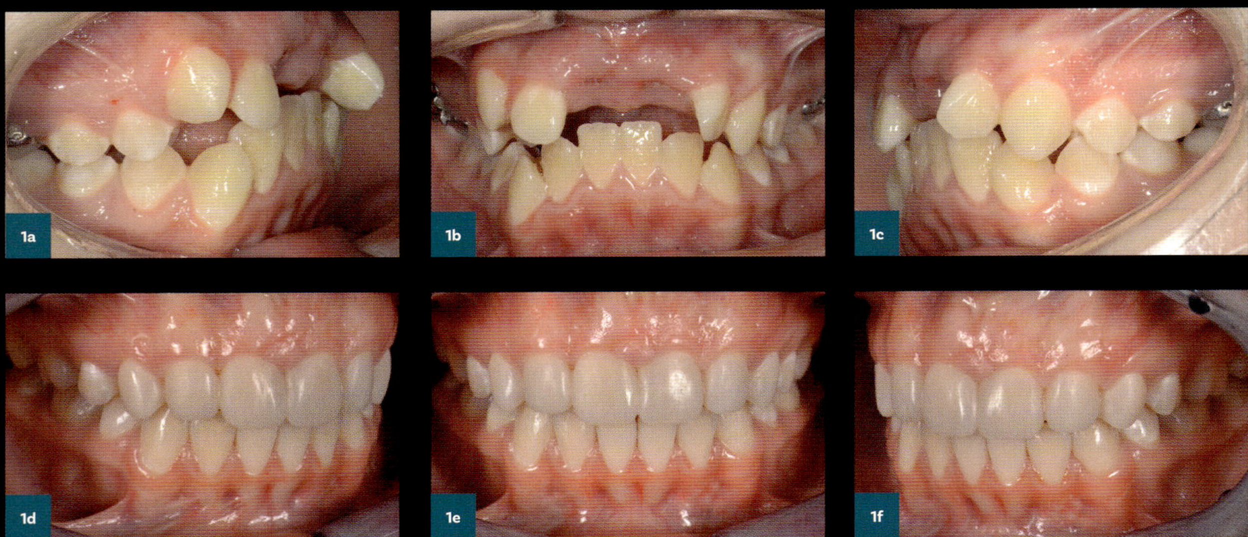

Figs. 1a-f ■ Severe trauma to the upper central incisors caused their avulsion in a 13-year-old girl who needed a restorative solution to enable her to face her adolescence.

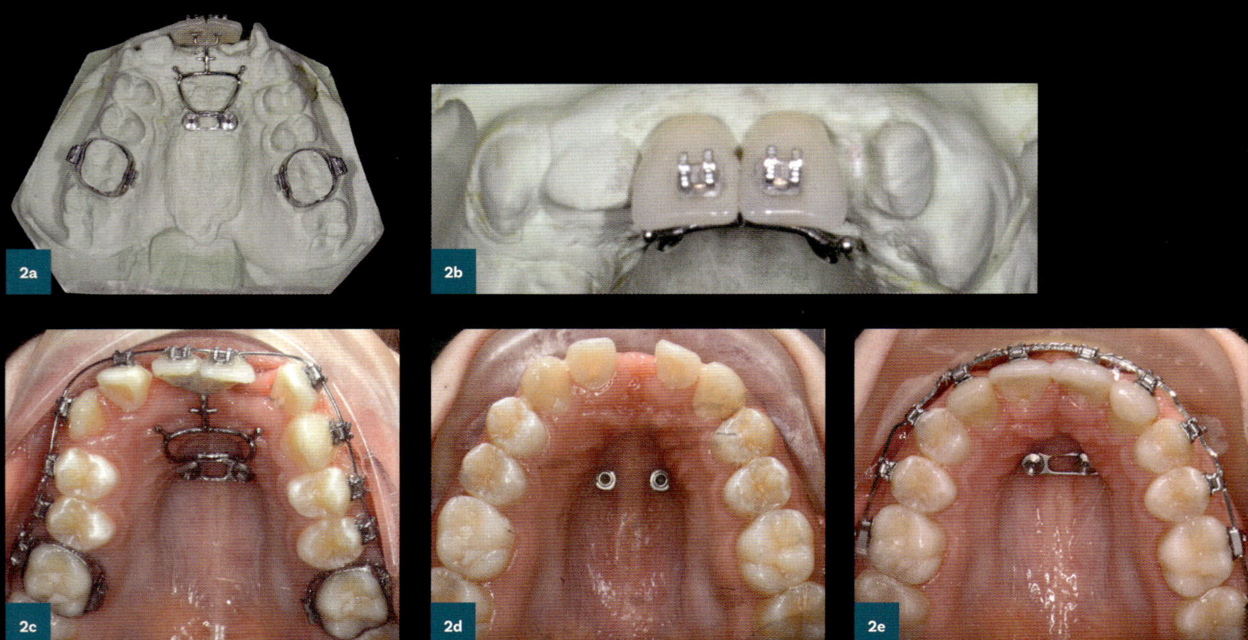

Figs. 2a-e ■ The orthodontic solution necessary to adequately reposition all the dental elements made use of the repositioning of the lateral incisors in a central position through the anchorage provided by two palatal mini-screws (Benefit 2x9 mm); these screws supported the provisional teeth used for mesialization of the lateral incisors.

Instead of the standard approach involving premolar extractions, the traumatic tooth loss prompted the consideration of advancing the upper teeth and extracting only the second lower premolars. This adjustment aimed to achieve symmetry in the case and address the skeletal issue by lowering the posterior fulcrum through mesialization of the lower first molars.
The subsequent aesthetic refinements focused on enlarging the two upper lateral incisors to resemble the lost central incisors due to trauma. This approach facilitated the preservation of all teeth, eliminating the need for osseointegrated implants.

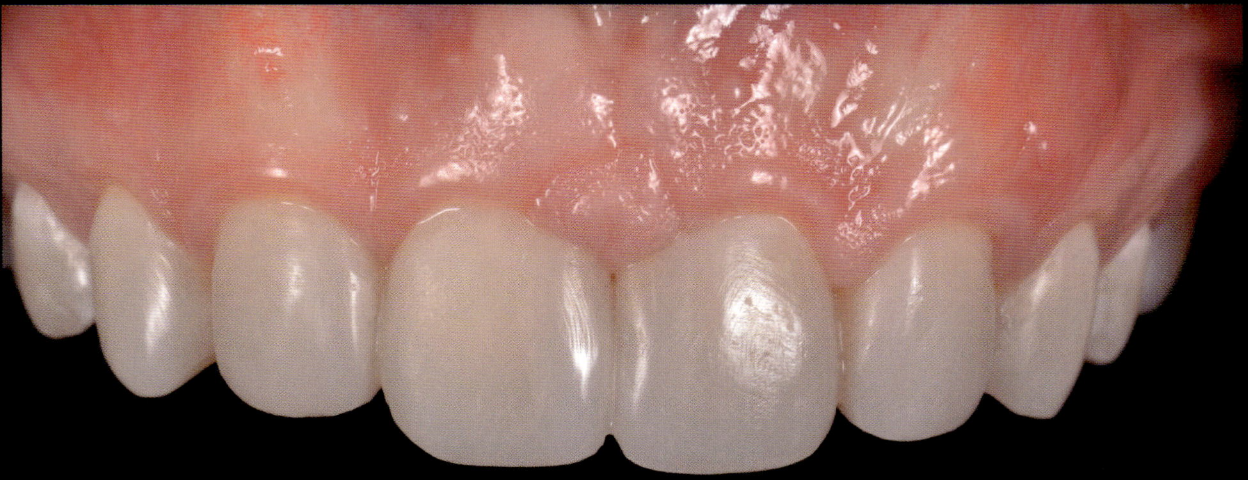

3

Fig. 3 ■ The aesthetic restorative resolution (Conservative: Dr. Nikolaos Perakis, Bologna).

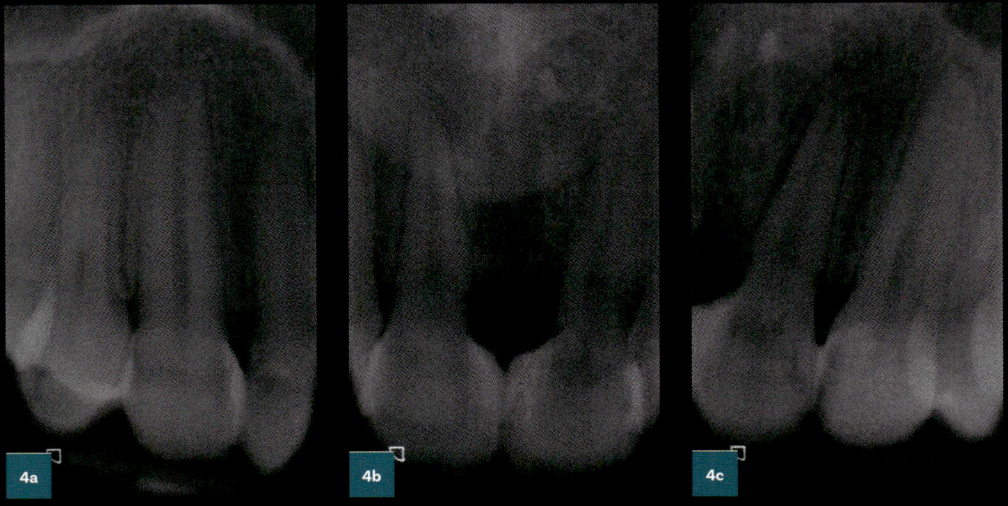

4a 4b 4c

Figs. 4a-c ■ The corresponding radiographic images.

> CONT'D

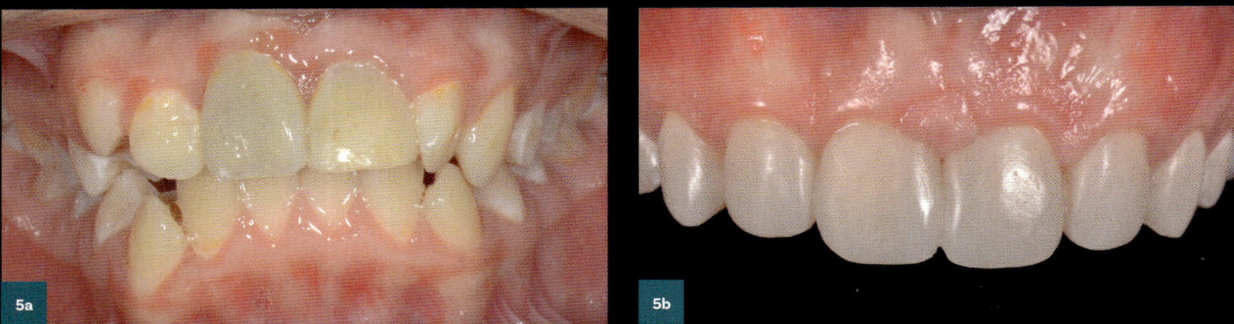

Figs. 5a,b ■ Comparison between the initial therapy phase and the final situation.

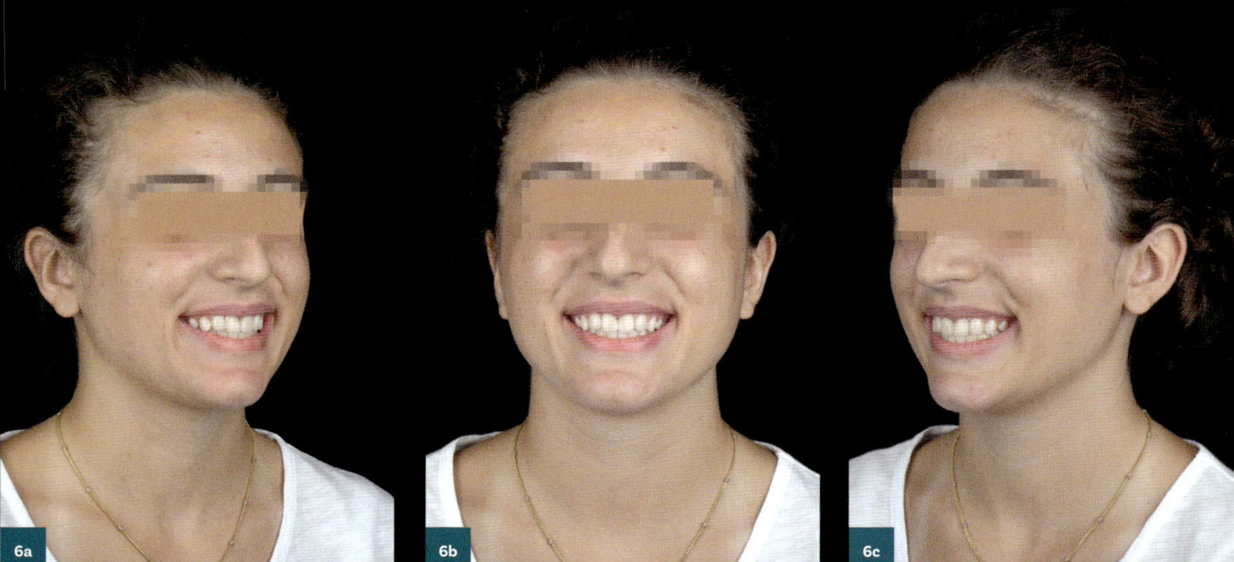

Figs. 6a-c ■ Photograph of the patient once treatment was completed.

Autotransplantion to resolve the traumatic loss of three teeth

The autotransplantation technique, when skillfully applied, has proven to be highly effective in various clinical scenarios. In this instance, it successfully addressed a severe traumatic loss involving three dental elements: the lateral incisor, canine, and upper left premolar. This approach was chosen due to the patient's age—ten years at the time of trauma—and the need to avoid complex orthodontic treatment requiring multiple extractions.

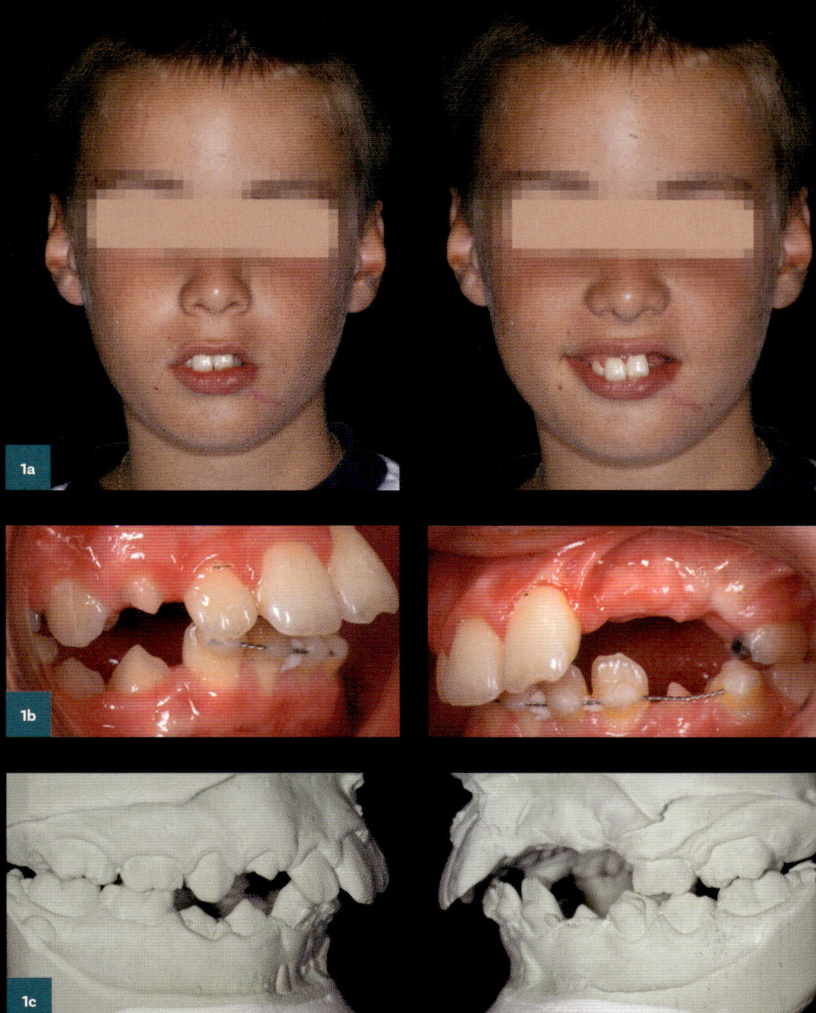

Figs. 1a-c ■ Facial and intraoral images of an 11-year-old boy who had simultaneously lost the premolar, canine and upper lateral on the left side due to a traumatic event. The study of the models allowed a precise evaluation of the case.

> CONT'D

This critical situation facilitated the initial treatment phase, which focused on regenerating bone in the trauma-affected area. After restoring adequate bone volume and considering planned extractions for orthodontic purposes, the lower second premolar was positioned in 23 to mimic the permanent canine. This strategic choice brought the ipsilateral second premolar closer to the first premolar's position, enabling an adhesive bridge to replace the upper lateral incisor.

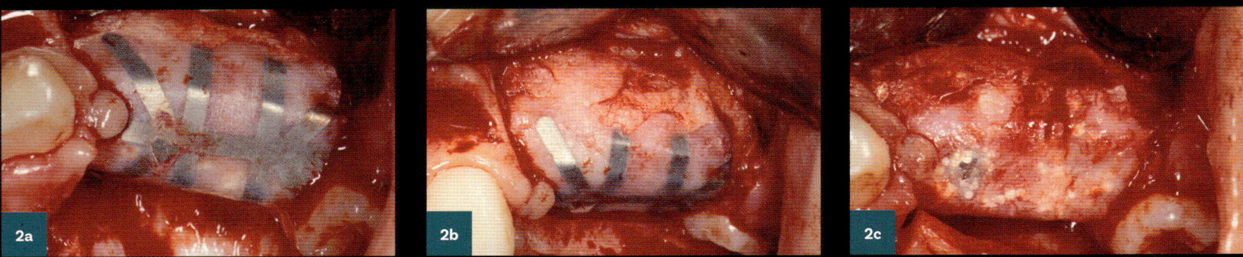

Figs. 2a-c ■ The unconventional therapeutic solution involved (as described in the text) bone regeneration using a membrane (Prof. Massimo Simion). Avulsion of the right upper second premolar for orthodontic purposes and its grafting in the newly formed bone (autologous transplant).

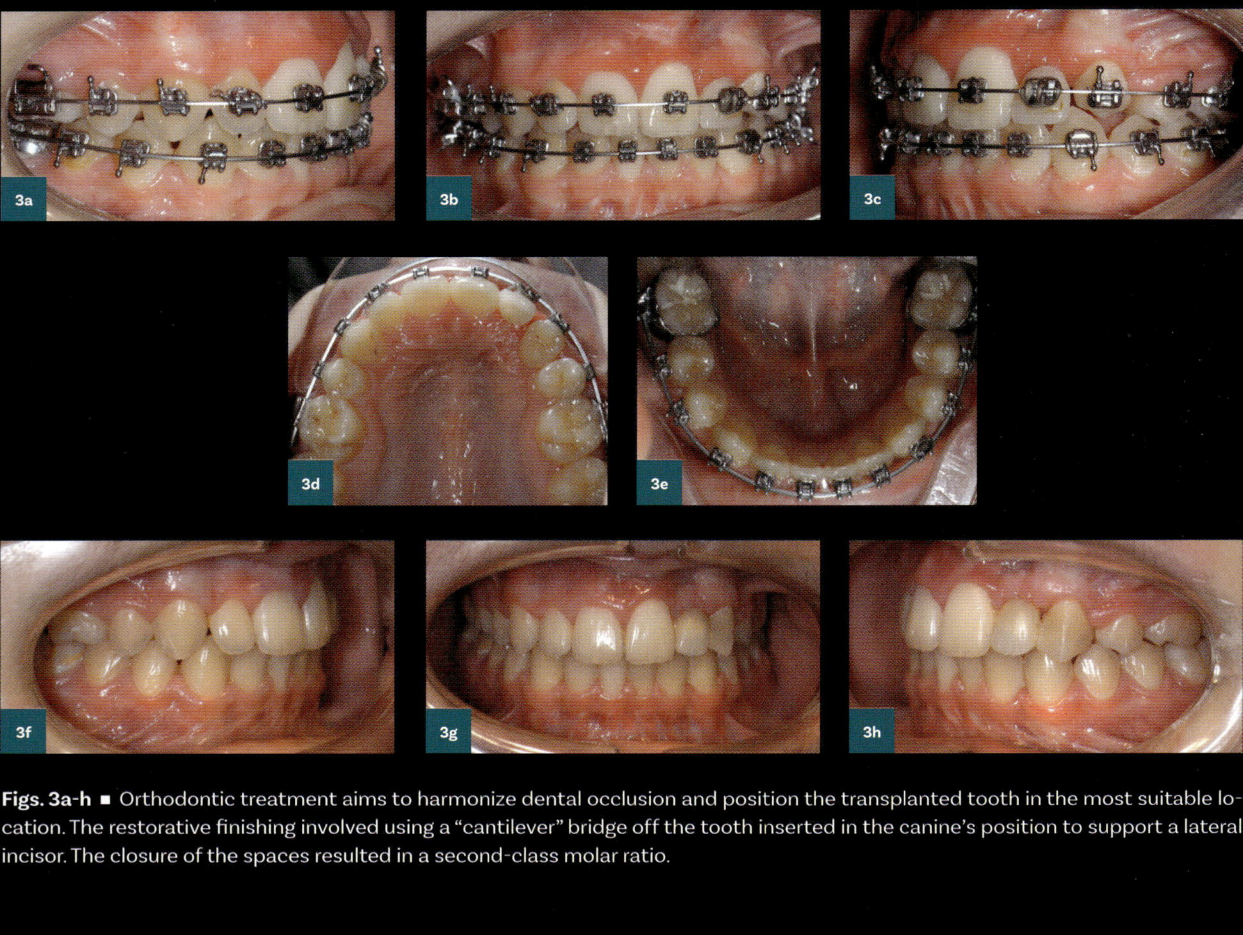

Figs. 3a-h ■ Orthodontic treatment aims to harmonize dental occlusion and position the transplanted tooth in the most suitable location. The restorative finishing involved using a “cantilever” bridge off the tooth inserted in the canine’s position to support a lateral incisor. The closure of the spaces resulted in a second-class molar ratio.

Utilizing a premolar, previously destined for orthodontic removal, as a replacement for the canine, alongside a simple adhesive bridge, enabled the young patient to complete treatment without requiring removable devices or post-growth osseointegrated implants. The successful outcome is supported by the case's impressive 20-year follow-up.

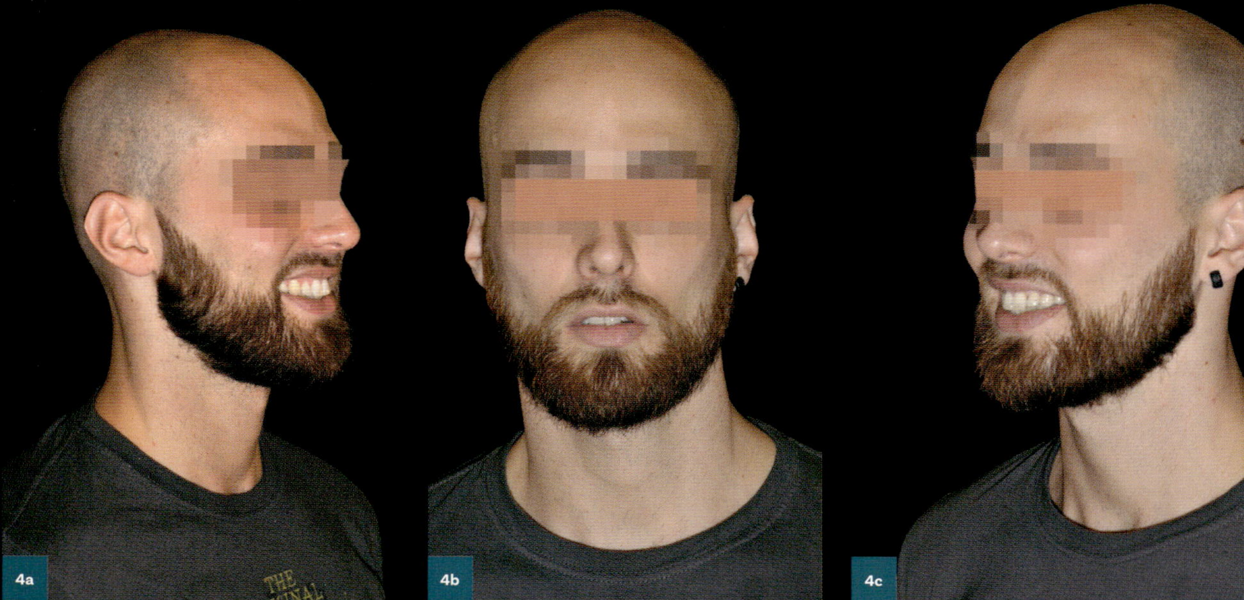

Figs. 4a-c ■ Photo of the patient 22 years later.

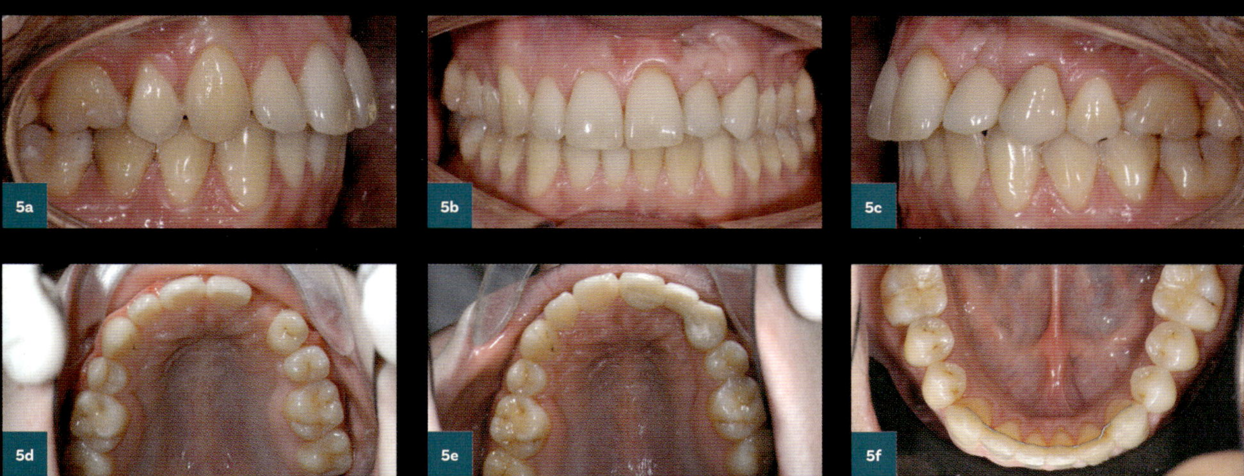

Figs. 5a-f ■ The images show excellent stability of the dental arches and the dental-periodontal relationships, considering the dramatic starting conditions.

Bibliography

1. Cocconi R. Essay II: Space closure vs space preservation as it relates to craniofacial classification. *Int J Esthet Dent.* 2020;15(Suppl 1):S32-S45.
2. Johal A, Katsaros C, Kuijpers-Jagtman AM. Angle Society of Europe membership. State of the science on controversial topics: missing maxillary lateral incisors. A report of the Angle Society of Europe 2012 meeting. *Prog Orthod.* 2013;14:20.
3. Jamilian A, Perillo L, Rosa M. Missing upper incisors: a retrospective study of orthodontic space closure versus implant. *Prog Orthod.* 2015;16:2.
4. Santos Silveira G, de Almeida NV, Pereira DM, Mattos CT, Mucha JN. Prosthetic replacement vs space closure for maxillary lateral incisor agenesis. A systematic review. *Am J Orthod Dentofacial Orthop.* 2016;150(2):228-237.
5. Wright J, Bosio JA, Chou JC, Jiang SS. Maxillary lateral incisor agenesis and its relationship to overall tooth size. *J Prosthet Dent.* 2016;115(2):209-214.
6. Rosa M, Zachrisson BU. Integrating esthetic dentistry and space closure in patients with missing maxillary lateral incisors. *J Clin Orthod.* 2001;35(4):221-234.
7. Rosa M, Zachrisson BU. The space-closure alternative for missing maxillary lateral incisors: an update. *J Clin Orthod.* 2010;44(9):540-561.
8. Rosa M, Lucchi P, Ferrari S, Zachrisson BU, Caprioglio A. Congenitally missing maxillary lateral incisors: Long-term periodontal and functional evaluation after orthodontic space closure with first premolar intrusion and canine extrusion. *Am J Orthod Dentofacial Orthop.* 2016;149(3):339-348.
9. Perakis N, Cocconi R. The decision-making process in interdisciplinary treatment: digital versus conventional approach. A case presentation. *Int J Esthet Dent.* 2019;14(2):212-224.
10. Patroni S, Cocconi R. From orthodontic treatment plan to ultrathin no-prep CAD/CAM temporary veneers. *Int J Esthet Dent.* 2017;12(4):504-522.
11. Zarow M, D'Arcangelo C, D'Amario M, Marzo G. Conservative approach for the management of congenital bilateral agenesis of permanent mandibular incisors: case report and literature review. *Eur J Paediatr Dent.* 2015;16(2):154-158.
12. Saravi B, Vollmer A, Hartmann M, et al. Clinical Performance of CAD/CAM All-Ceramic Tooth-Supported Fixed Dental Prostheses: A Systematic Review and Meta-Analysis. *Materials (Basel).* 2021;14(10):2672.
13. Araujo E, Perdigao J. Anterior Veneer Restorations. An Evidence-based Minimal-Intervention Perspective. *J Adhes Dent.* 2021;23(2):91-110.
14. Spinas E, Aresu M, Canargiu F. Prosthetic rehabilitation interventions in adolescents with fixed bridges: a 5-year observational study. *Eur J Paediatr Dent.* 2013;14(1):59-62.
15. Antonarakis GS, Prevezanos P, Gavric J, Christou P. Agenesis of maxillary lateral incisor and tooth replacement: cost-effectiveness of different treatment alternatives. *Int J Prosthodont.* 2014;27(3):257-263.
16. Dueled E, Gotfredsen K, Trab Damsgaard M, Hede B. Professional and patient-based evaluation of oral rehabilitation in patients with tooth agenesis. *Clin Oral Implants Res.* 2009;20(7):729-736.
17. Nordquist GG, McNeill RW. Orthodontic vs. restorative treatment of the congenitally absent lateral incisor - long term periodontal and occlusal evaluation. *J Periodontol.* 1975;46(3):139-143.
18. Alraheam IA, Ngoc CN, Wiesen CA, Donovan TE. Five-year success rate of resin-bonded fixed partial dentures: A systematic review. *J Esthet Restor Dent.* 2019;31(1):40-50.
19. Tezulas E, Yildiz C, Evren B, Ozkan Y. Clinical procedures, designs, and survival rates of all-ceramic resin-bonded fixed dental prostheses in the anterior region: A systematic review. *J Esthet Restor Dent.* 2018;30(4):307-318.
20. Mourshed B, Samran A, Alfagih A, Samran A, Abdulrab S, Kern M. Anterior Cantilever Resin-Bonded Fixed Dental Prostheses: A Review of the Literature. *J Prosthodont.* 2018;27(3):266-275.
21. Balasubramaniam GR. Predictability of resin bonded bridges - a systematic review. *Br Dent J.* 2017;222(11):849-858.